TROUBLE IN MIND

Trouble in Mind

Stories from a
Neuropsychologist's Casebook

Jenni Ogden

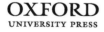
OXFORD
UNIVERSITY PRESS

OXFORD
UNIVERSITY PRESS

Oxford University Press, Inc., publishes works that further
Oxford University's objective of excellence
in research, scholarship, and education.

Oxford   New York
Auckland   Cape Town   Dar es Salaam   Hong Kong   Karachi
Kuala Lumpur   Madrid   Melbourne   Mexico City   Nairobi
New Delhi   Shanghai   Taipei   Toronto

With offices in
Argentina   Austria   Brazil   Chile   Czech Republic   France   Greece
Guatemala   Hungary   Italy   Japan   Poland   Portugal   Singapore
South Korea   Switzerland   Thailand   Turkey   Ukraine   Vietnam

Published by Oxford University Press, Inc.
198 Madison Avenue, New York, New York 10016
www.oup.com

Oxford is a registered trademark of Oxford University Press

Library of Congress Cataloging-in-Publication Data
Ogden, Jennifer A.
Trouble in mind : stories from a
neuropsychologist's casebook / Jenni Ogden.
   p. cm.
Includes bibliographical references and index.
ISBN 978–0–19–982700–8 (pbk. : alk. paper)
1. Clinical neuropsychology—Case studies.
2. Clinical neuropsychology—Popular works.   I. Title.
RC359.O362 2011
616.8—dc23   2011036652

In memory of the most studied single case in history,
HM (1926–2008), who taught us about memory by losing his.

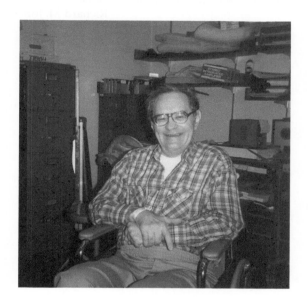

Trouble in mind, I'm blue,
But I won't be blue always,
'Cause the sun's gonna shine in my back door someday.
                                        Richard M. Jones

PREFACE ■

Trouble in Mind is a book that will deepen your understanding of how and why brain disorders change lives. It is written for students studying psychology or medicine, patients who have suffered brain disorders and their families, the health professionals who work with those patients, and the general reader who is intrigued by the brain, mind, and behavior. It is not a neuroscience, neuroanatomy, or neuropathology book, or even a neuropsychology assessment or treatment book. It is perhaps more akin to a neuropsychologist's memoir: a collection of stories about real patients whom I worked with over the years whose behaviors, emotions, or thinking abilities had become disordered, disrupted, or unusual as a result of some type of brain disease or damage.

Patients don't exist in a bubble but are at the center of a complex, interrelated system of family members and health professionals. So although my primary focus is on the patient, every story is enriched by the people in that system as well, caught up in the fallout from what is often a life-changing and sometimes life-threatening brain disorder. Insights into the human psyche come from many sources: the courage demonstrated by a patient who, because of a stroke, has lost the ability to walk and speak but can still comprehend; the denial, anger, grief, and acceptance family members experience as they help the patient struggle with rehabilitation; the empathy and helplessness felt by the neuropsychologist assessing the patient; the exciting discoveries made by the researcher about the workings of the mind because the patient altruistically agrees to participate in an experiment; and the satisfaction therapists gain from watching the patient get a little better and a little stronger every day, until their help is no longer needed.

Ten of the 15 patients who are the stars of this book also featured in the second edition of my textbook, *Fractured Minds: A Case-Study Approach to Clinical Neuropsychology*, published by Oxford University Press in 2005. But in *Trouble in Mind*, the emphasis is on the patients, whose cases—if first introduced in *Fractured Minds*—have been rewritten, with added richness about the interactions between the patients, their families, and the health professionals who dealt with them. I retained 10 of the original cases, either because their disorders were so rare that they were the only patients I ever met who had them or, in the case of patients with more common disorders, because their stories were especially revealing, moving, or uplifting. The five new patients who have made their way into this book allowed me to demonstrate, through their particular stories, a wide range of responses to some of the most common neurological disorders.

Details that could identify patients have been changed, including, in most cases, their given names. Rather ironically, the one exception to this is HM, the famous amnesic. In spite of the thousands of research articles written about him, for 55 years only a small circle of researchers and caregivers knew his identity. On his death in December 2008, his name and image were finally released to the public. As one of the honored few to work with him, I knew his name—Henry Molaison—and face as long ago as 1985, but even today I still think of him as HM. A photo I took of him back then can now see the light of day and is reproduced, along with his real name, in Chapter 7.

To keep the book within reasonable limits, I have not covered the range of disorders included in *Fractured Minds*, but I hope that my selection will satisfy readers who are seeking more information and understanding of some of the very common disorders, such as head injury and Alzheimer's disease, as well as those readers who are simply fascinated by the strange and sometimes bizarre behaviors—such as failing to recognize familiar faces—caused by damage to that squishy gray organ inside our skulls.

In this "sequel" to *Fractured Minds*, only the first chapter discusses clinical neuropsychology and neuroanatomy in any depth. Some readers might want to skip much of that chapter and go straight to following chapters, each of which concentrates on the story of one, or occasionally two, patients with a particular disorder. I have kept detailed research findings and theoretical analyses to a minimum in these case-study chapters, and where especially interesting articles or books are mentioned, I do not cite them formally in the text, to avoid interrupting the story's flow. At the end of each chapter the reader who wants to learn more can find a short section of further reading, including articles, books, biographies of patients, and even novels where one of the fictional characters has the same disorder as the real patients in that chapter and often faces the same struggles and challenges—but in a more literary manner!

So walk alongside me as I enter the hospital wards and rehabilitation units to assess, counsel, and learn from the patients who arrive there daily, shocked and shaken and often changed forever, but harboring strengths they do not yet know they possess, but that will serve them well through the long and challenging months ahead.

ACKNOWLEDGMENTS ■

Thank you to the many patients and their families—those featured in this book and all the others as well—who taught me much of what I know about the importance of having a healthy brain, a strong mind, and a giving spirit. Thank you also to my more formal teachers, mentors, and colleagues, especially Michael Corballis, Suzanne Corkin, the late Dorothy Gronwall, Edward Mee, and Lynette Tippett. Thank you to my many students whose enthusiasm for stories about real patients fed my passion, and to the many great neuroscientists and clinicians whose writings and wise counsel did likewise. I am especially grateful to Ken Heilman, Muriel Lezak, Kevin Walsh, and Barbara Wilson, each of whom has modeled for me what a "good doctor," in all of its meanings, is.

My agent, April Eberhardt, my Oxford University Press editor, Joan Bossert and the wonderful OUP team—especially Tracy O'Hara, Jenni Milton, Arun Prasath, and Jesse Hochstadt—have turned the manuscript into a book and kept me "on task" with patience, good humor, and good judgment. Their faith in this book and their belief that I know something about its subject matter makes all the difference!

Thank you to Michael Leunig, the Australian poet, cartoonist, and cultural commentator, declared an Australian Living Treasure by the National Trust of Australia in 1999, for generously allowing me to reprint in Chapter 11 his heartwarming cartoon "How to Get There," from his book *A Bunch of Poesy* (Angus & Robertson, 1992).

Kind permission to use the title of the great blues song "Trouble in Mind" as the title of this book, and to reprint the first verse of the song's lyrics was granted by Hal Leonard Corporation (**Trouble in Mind**, Words and Music by Richard M. Jones, copyright © 1926, 1937 Universal Music Corp. Copyright Renewed, All Rights Reserved).

The lyrics of the first verse of "Goodnight Irene" are reprinted in Chapter 2. Huddie Ledbetter (1888–1949), better known as Lead Belly, was the first to record the song in 1934 while he was in the Louisiana State Penitentiary, but he had been performing the song since 1908. The lyrics of an earlier version were published in 1886 by Gussie Lord Davis; whether he adapted it from a song he heard or wrote it himself is lost in the mists of time.

Back in the present, various members of my family have contributed with good humor and the occasional insight to discussions on the troubled mind, and have cheerfully ignored my moans about sitting at the computer instead of lying in the sun with a good novel. So here's to all of them, with thanks: John, my husband, and our four children and their families—Caroline and Walter; Jonathan, Sharon, Sophie and Danielle; Josie, Stephen, Belize, Ted and Louie; and Joachim. Almost as many as patients in this book.

CONTENTS ■

TROUBLE IN MIND

1 ∎

Backstory: The Basics of Clinical Neuropsychology

Writers of fiction are warned to put backstory where it belongs, at the back! Backstory is the plethora of peripheral or "historic" background information a writer believes the reader needs to know to fully appreciate why the fictional characters in their novel feel and behave as they do. Fortunately *Trouble in Mind* is not fiction, so I have opted to put the backstory in the front. I believe that students and health professionals in particular will find this chapter a useful introduction to neuropsychology and basic neuroanatomy, and that it will aid their understanding of the theory behind the case studies that follow. I hope it is also of interest to many general readers, providing, up front, answers to some of the questions that are sure to occur to them as they read the case studies. Another advantage of putting the backstory at the front is that it is quickly out of the way, freeing readers to immerse themselves in the world of each patient without being distracted by too much theory.[1]

*****

Brain disorders are among the most common disorders suffered by humans; by the time we are 30, most of us will know someone—a family member or close friend, or even perhaps ourselves—who has had to cope with brain damage of some sort. Perhaps your grandparent was diagnosed with Alzheimer's disease (AD), or your partner suffered a stroke, or you had a friend whose head was bashed in in a car accident and as a consequence struggled at school or work for months, unable to concentrate or function normally in a noisy environment. In my role as a clinical neuropsychologist, I have met many such people over the years, and in the chapters that follow I relate the stories of some of them: people whose lives have been turned upside down when that most mysterious of organs, the brain, is damaged or diseased.

Some patients are able to accept a diagnosis of a terminal brain tumor with apparent calmness, but more often the early reaction is a multilayered one of disbelief, denial, anger, and grief.[2] Families likewise find themselves

---

[1] Throughout the book I use the medical term "patient" rather than "client," as all of the cases I discuss have medical rather than psychological conditions, and usually my first contact with them was when they were medical patients in a hospital. However, "client" is a more appropriate and empowering term for people seen in a psychology clinic, whatever the cause of their problems. I sometimes use the word "participant" when referring to a person (or "subject") who takes part in a research study, even if that person also has a medical disorder.

[2] The suggestions for further reading at the end of this chapter include *A Journey Round My Skull* by Hungarian author Frigyes Karinthy, a fascinating and insightful first-person account of what it is like to have a brain tumor and brain surgery. Other readable biographies and personal accounts of the experience of brain injury and disease include the books by the great Russian neuropsychologist Alexandr Luria and the volume edited by Narinder Kapur.

tipped into an unknown realm—a nightmare that they thought happened to other people and not to them. The doctors, nurses, psychologists, and all the other health professionals who assess, diagnose, treat, and care for these patients have chosen this as their career, and thus do not have these situations thrust upon them. They come to each new patient with experience, knowledge, and professionalism, to do a job to the best of their ability. At the end of the day they can go outside into the sunshine and take up their own lives, thoughts of their patients receding as they engage with their own loved ones. Yet at some point, usually at an early stage of their career, most of the professionals who work with these patients will have a hard time controlling their emotions, and may even have occasions when they have to make a sudden exit from the patient's bedside. It is often a particular patient who sneaks into their hearts—perhaps a small, sad child the same age as their own cheeky daughter, or an old man with the wise eyes of their grandfather who died just last year.

Medical practitioners and psychologists are trained to use science rather than intuition and emotional reactions to diagnose and treat illness, and while an objective and scientific approach is essential, clinicians must also be good communicators and listeners, skills that require more than an ability to express oneself clearly. Many professions that deal with human tragedy have few, if any, training hours devoted to teaching practitioners how to understand and cope with their own emotions, in part because emotions are the most elusive of things to deal with in an academic setting. Psychologists and psychiatrists may be an exception; because an important aspect of their job is to help people express and understand their feelings, learning to understand their own should be considered a prerequisite.

It is a fine balance, caring for people in a professional way without losing empathy. Learning to live with and deal appropriately with their feelings is part of the job of all health professionals (and policemen and firemen and people who work with victims of natural and man-made disasters or who pick up the pieces after a terrorist attack). For health professionals or health care providers, caring is almost as important as knowledge and skills. Of course, if you or someone you loved was faced with having to undergo a delicate neurosurgical operation, and your choice was between an experienced neurosurgeon with an abrupt approach and a novice neurosurgeon with a wonderful bedside manner, I suspect you would choose the experienced surgeon. Let us hope that you would not have to make such a choice. Observe those doctors who are skilled communicators: when they are giving bad or difficult news to a patient they come across as calm, confident and knowledgeable, yet somehow they are gentle and empathetic at the same time. But it takes experience and practice—and humility—to achieve this.[3]

*****

As a discipline, clinical neuropsychology lies midway between *psychology*—the study of human behavior and the nonmedical assessment and treatment of psychological disorders—and *neurology*—the medical discipline concerned with brain and spinal cord diseases and treatments. Thus a clinical neuropsychologist is a psychologist who specializes in the psychological assessment, diagnosis, rehabilitation, and therapy of people with brain disorders. Some neurologists—medically qualified doctors—specialize in clinical neuropsychology; they are often known as *behavioral neurologists*. Clinical neuropsychologists who are

---

[3] In the suggestions for further reading at the end of this chapter I have included references for a number of books—accessible to the general reader—by medical practitioners Pauline Chen, Atul Gawande, Jerome Groopman, Kenneth Heilman, and Danielle Ofri. The practice and writings of these clinicians embody all the characteristics of a "good" doctor.

not medically qualified but have an affiliation with a university psychology department as well as a hospital often carry out research that would best fit into the subdiscipline of psychology called *cognitive neuropsychology*. This is the branch of psychology that focuses on how the mind works, either through experiments on people with undamaged brains (usually psychology students!) or by finding out what patients with brain damage cannot do, leading to hypotheses about the functions of the brain areas prior to damage. Clinical neuropsychologists also carry out applied research with the aim of discovering more about brain diseases, how they affect the mind and behavior, and how the patient can most effectively be helped. The case studies in this book, while all told from a clinical neuropsychology viewpoint, range from those more aligned with cognitive neuropsychology, such as studies of brain-damaged patients that tell us more about memory than about coping with disease, to those more aligned with neurology, such as the cases on head injury and AD.

A practicing clinical neuropsychologist also needs to be an accomplished clinical psychologist—a therapist—as will become evident in many of the case studies that follow. Even clinical neuropsychologists who restrict themselves to research or the administration of neuropsychological tests and do not take an active part in rehabilitation and therapy require some clinical skills. They need to build the rapport necessary to achieve a valid and useful assessment and to discuss in a sensitive manner the often distressing information about a patient's performance. Patients frequently express strong emotions about their illness and their wider situation during their neuropsychological assessment or when involved in a research project, and the clinical neuropsychologist should be able to respond sensitively and constructively.

Every patient in the stories that follow has, in one way or another, triumphed over his or her illness, whether it be by working day after tedious day on rehabilitation exercises, accepting and moving on from an irretrievable loss, or facing up to the certainty of an untimely death. I have often been humbled by the courage and humor of these special people who, while struggling with the extraordinary stress of a brain disorder, have the generosity of spirit to share their thoughts and feelings, draw pictures, put blocks together, and memorize word lists, even when they find these tasks challenging and often embarrassingly childish.

When we see a person with a stethoscope hanging around her neck, we know she's a medical doctor. The neuropsychologist is harder to spot until she sits down beside the patient and opens the case she has been lugging about, pulling out manuals, a stopwatch, paper and pencils, and sometimes colored blocks. Just as the medical doctor uses a stethoscope to listen to and understand the heart, the neuropsychologist uses a battery of tests to look into and understand the mind. But, I hear you say, the mind is surely much more complex than the heart (unless of course you think of the heart in its symbolic sense, as the center of our emotions)? Anatomically the heart is quite simple and how it works is very well understood, but the human brain is the most complex system in the animal kingdom, and probably the most complex system on earth. Although it weighs only about three pounds, it contains more than 10 billion neurons (the nerve cells of the brain). These in turn have trillions of connections with each other. Over the past twenty years neuroscientists have made enormous strides in their understanding of how the brain is put together—neuroanatomy—and how it works. New neurotransmitters—the chemicals that transmit signals from neuron to neuron—are probably being discovered as you read this, and effective techniques for growing new neurons and repairing damaged brain tissue are already well advanced.

But the brain and the mind are not synonymous, although the two are inseparable, at least in the conscious person. Without an active brain there is no mind, and without a mind there seems no point at all in having a brain. This belief is not held by everyone of course; some people think that it is important to keep individuals alive even if, because of an accident or disease that destroys the higher centers of the brain, they are in a permanent vegetative state and their brains are no longer capable of mediating any activity other than perhaps some basic life functions such as breathing. Perhaps one day neuroscientists will discover a way to repair the mind with gene transplants or stem cell magic, or even a brain transplant, but this is a long way off.

There are exciting technologies that allow us to infiltrate the mind and understand a little of how it works. For example, patients or research participants can be given simple thinking tasks to do while their brain activity is measured by an electroencephalogram (EEG), which picks up electrical brain waves. Even more exciting is functional magnetic resonance imaging (fMRI), which shows metabolic changes in specific areas of the thinking brain. As yet EEGs, fMRI, and other similarly sophisticated technologies can only inform us about relatively simple cognitive actions, for example, by highlighting the areas of the brain that are activated when we speak. Often fMRI just confirms what we have known for a very long time from more traditional neuropsychological studies. Even the computer has not made our simple paper-and-pencil tests obsolete, although it plays an increasingly important part in neuropsychological assessments. Computers are especially useful in research when tests need to be given in exactly the same way to every participant, and timing is important, often down to the level of milliseconds. But computers cannot yet assess a patient's fluctuating mood and motivation, two of many factors that are important to evaluate and make

the neuropsychologist will ask the patient about his childhood, education, occupation, hobbies, general health, other physical disorders, personality, relationships, past psychological problems, coping mechanisms, any environmental stressors such as working with toxic substances, and current family and living situation. In short, a neuropsychological assessment includes a more general psychological assessment, because only by knowing who the patient was before the brain damage can we work out how the brain disorder has affected him and how best to approach rehabilitation.

*****

Clinical neuropsychologists need to think like detectives to understand the human mind and how it relates to the brain. The *brain* takes in information conveyed through the five senses, works on that information in the *mind*, and then acts upon it, using *behavior*. The elusive mind can't be directly observed, but must be inferred from the behaviors that result from its workings. For psychologists, the term "behavior" is used to encompass all the actions the mind produces and that we can observe, whether through behaviors that anyone can see by simply looking and listening, or through answers to interview questions or performance on specially designed tests. Behavior includes emotions, motivations, and social interactions as well as more intellectual abilities such as language or the thinking strategies one uses to find one's way around a new city.

One way to conceptualize the mind is to imagine it as a ladder where the first and simplest step is the ability to take in information via our five senses. In humans the visual sense is the most dominant, although audition, touch, smell, and taste can also be important. Clearly if you are blind from birth, either from damage to the eye itself or from damage to the outer layer (cortex) of neural cells at the very back of the occipital lobe of the brain—called the *sensory visual cortex*—any thinking skill that involves vision will be impossible. The next step up the "mind ladder" takes us to *perception*, where we integrate the information received through our senses and make meaning out of them. So for those with intact vision, seeing a chair as lines and surfaces is the visual sensation, but recognizing that those lines and surfaces correspond to a chair involves perception. Chapter 6 tells the story of Michael, who could see but not perceive—and therefore not recognize—objects or familiar faces from sight because of damage to a brain area that mediates visual perception. This area of cortex is also in the occipital lobes and lies adjacent to the visual sensory cortex. An even higher level of perception occurs when sensations from two or more senses are integrated to make a meaningful object or richer concept. For example, as I look out my window and see the trees waving about, I can guess it is windy, but if I can also hear the noise of the wind whistling and moaning, I have a much richer perception of what is happening.

Both sensation and perception are important for the neuropsychologist to understand and assess, but the level of thinking that we are most concerned with is *higher cognition*. This term encompasses everything further up the mind ladder and more complex than perception, such as memory, reading and writing, and understanding. The concept of *attention* is also very important in neuropsychology but is difficult to place on the mind ladder. Sensation, perception, and higher cognition all require some degree of attention, but at the simple sensory level the attention required might be no more than a state of low alertness, such as feeling cold while sleeping, and waking up just enough to pull on another blanket. But attention at the sensation end of the ladder can also be exquisitely focused; for example during meditation you may focus your attention sequentially on the different muscle groups in your body, or on the mantra you are repeating, or on the feel of the sun as it warms your closed eyelids. At the top of the ladder, highly focused attention is often a prerequisite for cognitive functions such as solving a mathematical problem or understanding a difficult passage in a book. Of course it is all too easy to be distracted, even from difficult tasks, and this is especially the case when carrying out complex but well-learned behaviors such as driving a car on a familiar route through busy city traffic. We must maintain at least a low level of general attention to drive, and to allow us to increase and focus our attention quickly if needed.

The higher up we go on the mind ladder the more likely it is that we are dealing with *functional systems* rather than one area of the brain. Functional systems are composed of a number of brain areas working together to produce a behavior. The same group of neurons may be part of many functional systems. As an example, damage to an area of the right parietal lobe may impair the ability to conceptualize how objects are related in space. In turn, this impairment may disrupt many functional systems and result in a wide range of behavioral problems. The patient may no longer be able to do jigsaw puzzles, become easily lost in an unfamiliar environment, have difficulty learning and remembering new tasks that have a spatial component, and even have difficulty performing calculations mentally or on paper that involve carrying figures from one column to another (a spatial task). Janet, the patient I describe in Chapter 3, has these sorts of difficulties along with an even more amazing problem—ignoring half of space!

By carefully observing the behaviors of single individuals or groups of people with damage to specific areas or systems in the brain, and by systematically teasing out finer and finer details of their behaviors and behavioral deficits, we can construct a picture of which brain areas or systems mediate or are essential for which behaviors. With brain imaging techniques like computerized tomography (CT) and MRI, we can map areas of brain damage fairly accurately. Neurologically healthy people—that is, people without brain damage—can also tell us about brain–behavior relationships. By using techniques like EEG and fMRI we can see which areas of the healthy brain are activated when individuals perform simple behaviors. By putting together results of both behavioral and imaging research—using clinical as well as healthy populations—neuropsychologists are mapping the mind onto the brain.

But this is an inexact science, for many reasons. First, the neuropsychological tests that we use are rarely specific enough to pinpoint the simplest and most pure building blocks of whatever behavior or thinking ability—for example, memory—we are interested in. Second, no human brain is exactly alike in its brain–behavior relationships, as each brain has subtle differences depending on genetics and life experience. The final challenge is that we often use damaged brains to assess what the brain can no longer do, so that we can then infer what the damaged part of the brain could have done before it was damaged. Because it is ethically unacceptable to damage human brains for the sake of research, we have to make use of "natural experiments" that provide imprecise lesions and rely on the good will of brain-damaged people agreeing to participate in our studies.

For clinical neuropsychologists, the type of brain damage can also make a difference to their conclusions. At one end of the damage spectrum is *focal damage*: a lesion restricted to a circumscribed area of the brain. If the focal damage is also static, or unchanging (rather than progressive, like a malignant tumor), the symptoms it causes are also likely to be nonprogressive. The most common cause of a static focal lesion is a stroke, caused by a blockage or spasm of a cerebral artery and a resulting loss of blood and oxygen to the part of the brain that artery supplies (see Chapter 2). Focal lesions can also be caused by a different type of "stroke," such as a blood clot that forms within the brain substance (an *intracerebral hematoma*; see Chapter 2). In this situation the area damaged usually shrinks as the blood clot is reabsorbed, often with an accompanying resolution of some or all of the patient's symptoms.

Focal lesions can also be made deliberately by a neurosurgeon—for example. in operations to treat temporal lobe epilepsy. Here the surgeon cuts away the malfunctioning area of the brain—a part of one temporal lobe—that has been causing the seizures. Melody, the young singer profiled in Chapter 8, had her life changed for the better following such an operation. But many years earlier, in 1953, a man who would become famous to neurologists and neuropsychologists as "HM" was the unfortunate recipient of the first such operation to cure epilepsy. HM's neurosurgeon removed the inside part of not one but both of his temporal lobes, resulting in a substantial reduction of his seizures but also causing a dramatic amnesia. For more than half a century after that, HM participated in hundreds of experiments on memory, becoming the world's most studied neurological patient. You can read about HM and his incredible gift to neuroscience in Chapter 7.

In a head injury where the skull is fractured, if a bone fragment, bullet, or perhaps a piece of metal from an automobile accident penetrates the underlying brain, this can also cause a focal injury. The neurosurgeon usually cleans the wound, removing the object and any damaged tissue and debris and leaving a clean focal lesion that does not affect the rest of the brain. Of course sometimes the damage is too extensive and beyond the healing skills of a neurosurgeon. In Chapter 4, you can read about Phillipa, a young teacher and mother who survived a brutal assault by a burglar. Hers is a tragic case illustrating the worst possible outcome of brain damage. The extensive damage to her frontal lobes, the most highly evolved part of the human cortex, took away her ability to teach or parent her children. Perhaps fortunately, it also took away her insight, rendering her unaware of the tragic changes in her personality and life.

Some viruses attack specific areas of the brain, causing focal damage, often on both sides of the brain. For example, the herpes simplex encephalitis virus usually targets the hippocampus, on the inside of the temporal lobes, resulting in severe memory deficits. Brain tumors and brain abscesses are also focal lesions, in the sense that they cause neural death by destroying neurons directly or via pressure effects. However, malignant tumors, while appearing to have a defined boundary on a CT or MRI brain scan, may be widespread with no clear division between diseased and healthy brain (see Chapters 3 and 5). It is therefore important to be cautious when proposing associations between a tumor lesion in a specific area of the brain and the impairments that the patient demonstrates.

At the other end of the damage spectrum is *diffuse brain damage*. This refers to damage that affects many areas of the brain, as in AD and other dementias (see Chapter 14). The damage can often be visualized on a CT or MRI scan or at postmortem examination as *atrophy*, which is shriveled or shrunken brain matter signifying neuronal death and usually affecting large areas of the cortex. Brain atrophy decreases the brain mass and allows the fluid-filled "lakes," or ventricles, in the middle of the brain and the space around the brain to expand. Diffuse brain damage can be progressive as in AD, but this is not always the case. When the damage is caused by a disease that is progressive and will continue to damage the brain over time, like AD, it is much more difficult to study brain–behavior relationships or to predict exactly what sort of problems the individual will face in the coming months. As a result of numerous studies on AD, we can, however, provide some

Many brain diseases cause swelling, or *edema*, in the vicinity of the damage. Edema, which is particularly common in association with malignant tumors, has the effect of increasing the area of nonfunctional brain. As the edema resolves (often when the patient is treated with steroids), the area of nonfunctional brain decreases and often impairments subside dramatically. Massive brain swelling, most common after severe head injury, can compress the brain stem, resulting in the patient's death.

All of the patients whose stories follow started their lives with healthy, normal brains and acquired their brain damage as a result of an accident, disease, or neurosurgery to treat a brain disorder. Thus such cases are said to have *acquired brain damage*. The types of brain damage I have just described—diffuse damage or lesions from disease, accident, and neurosurgery—all fall under the acquired brain damage umbrella. *Developmental* brain disorders encompass the many brain disorders that are apparent from birth. In some cases these may be genetic, as in Down syndrome, and in others they may be a result of some toxin ingested by the mother in the early stages of fetal development, as in fetal alcohol syndrome. Tragically, the perfectly normal brains of some babies are damaged during a difficult birth, for example because of oxygen deprivation. These are also classified as developmental brain disorders. Asperger's syndrome and autism are also developmental disorders, and children who are born with a very low intellectual capacity, often for unknown reasons, also fall into this category. These examples are at the more serious end of the developmental brain disorder spectrum, but there are many less serious conditions that are considered developmental, such as some specific learning disabilities, including developmental dyslexia, where the individual has reading, writing, and spelling difficulties.

Acquired and developmental brain disorders do have a great deal in common, but they differ in many ways as well. Most of the work done in the developmental area is with children, as of course the behaviors and problems that stem from developmental disorders are apparent from an early age. Clinical neuropsychologists are involved in this field along with educational psychologists, but as a very specialized area, and one in which I have had little involvement, I have not included any developmental cases in this book. My patient Kate, described in Chapter 9, is almost an exception to this. She had half her brain removed when she was 18 years old in an attempt to cure her severe epilepsy, a condition she had suffered from since early childhood. Thus although her disorder is acquired, because her brain was compromised very early on, her case has much in common with developmental disorders.

*****

One of the earliest and most important findings about brain–behavior relationships was discovered 150 years ago. Although it was known that the right side, or *hemisphere*, of the brain controlled movement of the left side of the body and vice versa, the discovery that the human brain, while appearing symmetrical, was not symmetrical for language functions was made independently by two neurologists. In 1861 Paul Broca discovered after the death of a patient whose speech was impaired that he had damage in an area in the left anterior (front) part of the brain—now known as *Broca's area*. In 1874 Carl Wernicke discovered that a patient who had lost the ability to understand language had a lesion in a region of the left posterior (rear) part of the brain—now known as *Wernicke's area*. Since that time, numerous studies on brain-damaged patients have proven beyond doubt that in at least 92% of right-handers and 69% of left-handers, the left hemisphere is specialized for the verbal functions of speech, language comprehension, reading, writing, and verbal memory.

In Chapter 2 you will meet two patients, Luke, a gang member who, after a drinking binge, collapsed from an intracerebral hemorrhage that damaged Broca's area, and Irene, a 68-year-old librarian and amateur actress who suffered a stroke in Wernicke's area. These two patients displayed the same language problems as those demonstrated by the two patients described by Broca and Wernicke so long ago. This illustrates the power of the single case study (a careful study of an individual patient as opposed to a group); if we find an association between a specific brain area and a specific behavioral impairment in many single cases, this allows us to hypothesize that the behavior relies to some degree on that brain area. One way of testing this hypothesis is to show that one patient with a particular impairment has damage in brain area A but not in brain area B, and another patient has a different impairment and has brain damage in area B but not in area A. This is termed a *double dissociation*. For example, Luke has damage in Broca's area but not Wernicke's area, and cannot talk in sentences yet can comprehend language. Irene has damage in Wernicke's area but not Broca's area, and can talk in complex—but nonsensical—sentences yet cannot comprehend language. Thus we know that Broca's area is involved in speech and Wernicke's area is involved in language comprehension.

As the technology to analyze the mind becomes more sophisticated—for example, functional MRI and PET scans—the simpler "bedside" neurological and neuropsychological methods of assessment such as double dissociation become less important and in time will no doubt be relegated to the history books. But it will be a long time—if ever—before a machine can completely take over from a careful neuropsychological assessment carried out by an experienced, knowledgeable, wise, and empathetic clinician. It behooves us to remember that just as traditional neuropsychology tools and hypotheses were built on the careful observations and descriptions of neurologists like Broca and Wernicke, so the ever-evolving science of mind with its increasing reliance on sophisticated computers and machines stands on the briefcase of the neuropsychologist—a briefcase filled with blocks, puzzles, and questionnaires, and of course a pad—of real paper—and a sharp pencil!

As neuropsychologists have shown using their simple tests, the left hemisphere is specialized not only for language but for a number of other functions that involve sequential, logical thinking, such as the ability to conceptualize mathematical relationships, to tell left from right, and to carry out skilled acts on verbal command. Julian, the man described in Chapter 5, displays these more unusual left hemispheric problems along with other, even rarer left hemispheric thinking deficits such as being unable to point to specific body parts on the human body.

For many years the left hemisphere was viewed as the dominant hemisphere and very little research was carried out on the functions of the right hemisphere. In fact the right hemisphere was viewed as the minor or nondominant hemisphere, implying that it did not have its own, equally important areas of specialization. More recently it has been established that the right hemisphere is "better" at some tasks than the left, in particular, tasks involving stimuli that cannot be readily described using words, or verbalized. Included are nonverbal memory functions such as remembering patterns and music, interpretation of nonverbal emotional expression, and visual–spatial functions generally. It is now clear that these left–right distinctions are far from absolute. The left hemisphere is capable of quite complex spatial tasks—although many such tasks may be performed better by the right hemisphere—and the right hemisphere has some ability to comprehend simple language and is involved in "extralinguistic" aspects of language, such as voice tone (e.g., pitch, rhythm, the expression of emotion in the tone of voice). Generally, however, the specialization of the left hemisphere for language functions is more pronounced than the specialization of the right hemisphere for visuospatial functions, which have a greater degree of bilateral (both hemispheres) representation.

The concept of cerebral specialization is often exaggerated in the media. The now popular right hemisphere is often touted as the source of creative thinking, the ability to draw, and the "female" traits of sensitivity and gentleness. According to some popular parapsychology books, the right hemisphere is the seat of the subconscious, controlled and subdued by the left hemisphere with its overpowering "male" traits of competitiveness, logical reasoning powers, and poor ability to show emotion. This makes a good story and sells popular psychology books and even cars—"Buy a car for your right creative and passionate hemisphere"—and may be fostered by the political correctness of extolling "female" attributes and criticizing "male" attributes. But there is no evidence for these extreme claims. As an example of the absurdity of such views, the idea that creativity per se is the specialized realm of the right hemisphere appears quite incongruous when one considers the great "left hemispheric" literary writings of humankind. Why these should be considered less creative than great art or architecture is decidedly unclear. Indeed, there is evidence to suggest that musical appreciation, intuitively a nonverbal function, is mediated predominantly by the right hemisphere in nonmusicians but by the left hemisphere or both hemispheres in musicians. It has been suggested that musicians—whose creativity is definitely not in doubt—conceptualize music as a sequential, logical "language," thus explaining its mediation by the left hemisphere.

The current scientific view, backed by considerable evidence, is that whereas each hemisphere has certain specialist abilities (often also represented to a lesser degree in the other hemisphere), in the healthy brain the two hemispheres work as a team, and neither should be considered dominant. When the term "cerebral dominance" is used, it should be qualified by the addition of the specialist functions to which it refers, for example, the (left) hemisphere dominance for language.

The concept of *plasticity of function* is, in one sense, the reverse of specialization. It refers to the ability of some areas of cortex to take on functions not normally attributed to them. The clearest examples of this occur where an entire hemisphere is removed or stripped of its cortex because it is so badly damaged or diseased that it no longer functions normally and often causes uncontrollable seizures and disturbed behaviors, inhibiting the normal functioning of the healthy hemisphere. This drastic but often life-changing neurosurgical procedure is called a *hemispherectomy*. When left hemispherectomies are performed after damage in childhood, the right hemisphere can take over sophisticated language functions, although it appears that some visuospatial abilities are compromised. After the age of about 12 years, language problems are unlikely to recover following extensive damage to the language areas of the left hemisphere. Kate, the hemispherectomy patient whose story is told in Chapter 9, is one of the most amazing people I have ever met. She is the living proof that it is possible to live a normal life with just half a brain.

Plasticity also relates to the concept that there can be a window of opportunity during brain development during which a particular function becomes established. Put in these terms, the hemispherectomy studies suggest that language can become established up to the age of 12 years or so. Ordinarily this takes place primarily in the left hemisphere, but if this hemisphere is damaged before the age of 12, the right hemisphere can take over some of its functions. Children who are isolated completely from language for their first 12 years are never able to establish normal language in either hemisphere.

*****

As with most medical and scientific disciplines, neurology and neuropsychology are well endowed with their own jargon. Whereas jargon should be avoided wherever possible, it is helpful to have a grasp of the most common of these terms. For example, *deficit, dysfunction, symptom, impairment*, and *disorder* are used interchangeably and can refer to any motor, sensory, perceptual, behavioral, psychological, emotional, or intellectual abnormality or loss. A *syndrome* refers to a group of symptoms that characteristically occur together after brain damage.

In many cases, jargon can provide shorthand descriptions for complex disorders. Fortunately, a few simple rules can simplify their interpretation for the beginner; indeed, it can even be fun trying to work out what deficits a patient should have by breaking down the diagnostic label into its component parts. Any label containing *phasia* refers to a speech disorder; *graphia* refers to writing; *lexia* to reading. *Praxia* means to work or perform purposeful actions, and *gnosia* means to know. If the base word is prefixed by an *a-*, strictly speaking it means that that function is completely absent (e.g., *agnosia* means "to not know"); prefixed by *dys-*, it means partial impairment (e.g., *dyslexia* means to have a marked reading difficulty). However, these conventions are often not adhered to, and a patient labeled as having *expressive aphasia* (a problem with expressing one's thoughts with words), may not be totally mute but more accurately may be dysphasic.

Sometimes the main label is preceded by a common English word that signifies the specific type of disorder. Therefore, *visual agnosia* means "to not know what one is seeing" (see Chapter 6), and *tactile agnosia* means "to not know what one is touching." A patient with *dressing apraxia* has difficulty with the actions related to dressing and may try to put his left leg into his right shirtsleeve and his right leg into his left pants leg, thus getting into an impossible tangle! Many of these terms appear in the following case studies and are defined when they first arise.

*****

All of the stories in this book can be read and understood without reading the next section, which provides an introduction to neuroanatomy and the functions of the different lobes of the brain. However, this knowledge will enhance your understanding of how the brain and the mind are related. That said, skipping over this section now, knowing that you can come back to it later if the stories themselves make you more curious about neuroanatomy, is a perfectly sensible strategy. I have included a small number of references to research articles along with suggestions for further reading—novels as well as neuropsychology books—at the end of each chapter.

The brain has three major divisions: the cerebral hemispheres, the cerebellum, and the brain stem. Neuropsychology is most concerned with the cerebral hemispheres. Figure 1.1 depicts lateral (from the side) and medial (split down the middle from front to back) views of the human brain. The *brain stem*, an upward extension of the spinal cord, extends into the *midbrain* in the center of the brain. The brain stem is the life-support part of the brain, as it controls respiration, cardiovascular function, and gastrointestinal function. The *cerebellum* consists of paired structures at the base of the cerebral hemispheres and is concerned mainly with motor coordination, muscle tone, and balance.

The *cerebral hemispheres* are the large paired structures above the midbrain. These are the areas of the brain

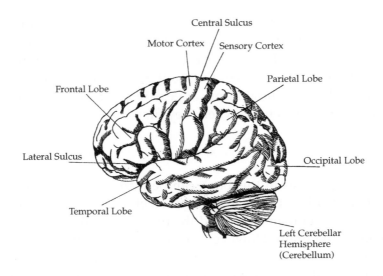

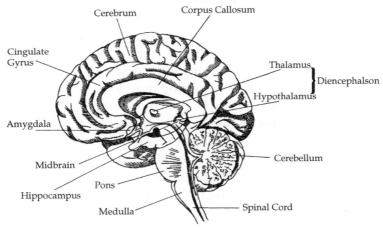

FIGURE 1.1
The human brain. The upper figure is a lateral, or side, view of the left hemisphere, and the lower figure a medial view of the right hemisphere, drawn as if the brain had been split lengthways down the center. (Reprinted from Ogden, J. A. 2005. *Fractured Minds: A Case-Study Approach to Clinical Neuropsychology, 2nd Ed.*, p. 7, with kind permission from Oxford University Press, New York.)

concerned with thinking and higher forms of human behavior. They are covered by a highly convoluted layer of nerve cells called the *cerebral cortex*, or *gray matter*. I will describe the divisions or lobes of the gray matter in more detail a little later. The clusters of axons, or fiber tracts, that connect the nerve cells in a given area of the cortex to other parts of the brain form a layer directly below the cortex called the *white matter*. Deep within the hemispheres are further paired structures of gray matter called the *basal ganglia*. Diseases of the basal ganglia include Parkinson's disease (Chapter 12) and Huntington's disease (Chapter 13). The two hemispheres are separated by the *longitudinal fissure*, a deep groove that runs from the front of the brain—the *frontal lobes*—to the back of the brain—the *occipital lobes*. The other main fissures are the *central sulcus* (sulcus is another word for fissure or gully) separating the frontal from the *parietal lobe*, and the *lateral sulcus*, separating the *temporal lobe* from the frontal and parietal lobes. A tough band of fibers called the *corpus callosum* lies under the longitudinal fissure and allows information to be transmitted between the two hemispheres. Within each hemisphere, smaller fiber tracts connect different parts of the hemisphere.

A system called the ascending *reticular formation* (RF) controls the overall arousal level of the cortex. The RF is a diffuse system of neuron chains traveling up through the brain stem. All the major sensory pathways send impulses to the RF, which relays them to the *thalamus*, consisting of paired gray matter structures deep in the brain at the upper end of the brain stem. The thalamus serves as a relay center for motor pathways, many sensory pathways, and the RF. On reaching the thalamus, the impulses are relayed to the cerebral cortex, where they influence the level of mental alertness or sleep. The RF is often damaged when a person suffers a closed head injury in an accident (see Chapters 10 and 11) or when a small baby is shaken aggressively.

Within the brain lies the *limbic system*, which is involved in emotion, motivation, and memory. Two of the areas included in the limbic system are the *hippocampus*, an essential area for the laying down of new memories (see Chapters 7 and 8), and the *amygdala*, which is involved in aggression.

The brain has three coverings, called the *meninges*. The outermost thick, tough covering is called the *dura mater* (Latin for "tough mother"), which adheres to the inner surface of the skull. The delicate, filamentous middle membrane, called the *arachnoid mater* ("spider mother") is attached by cobweb-like strands of tissue to the fine *pia mater* ("little mother"), which adheres closely to the cortex. The *subarachnoid space* lies between the arachnoid mater and the pia mater and is filled with *cerebrospinal fluid* (CSF). Blood vessels also lie within the subarachnoid space. An inflammation of the meninges is called *meningitis*; one symptom of meningitis is a stiff neck, caused by the muscles of the neck contracting strongly (called "guarding") to prevent bending of the neck and the consequent painful stretching of the inflamed meninges.

The *ventricles* are lakes of CSF located deep within the hemispheres. The lateral ventricles, large paired structures in the center of each hemisphere, connect in the middle to form the third ventricle and, below that, the fourth ventricle. The CSF is continuously formed within the ventricles and circulates through them and around the outside of the brain and spinal cord within the subarachnoid space. Excess CSF drains into the venous system from the subarachnoid space. If one of the small apertures between the ventricles becomes blocked, the CSF cannot flow out and the ventricles increase in size, causing increased pressure within the skull (*intracranial pressure*). This condition, known as *hydrocephalus*, can be corrected by a neurosurgeon placing a valve, or shunt, into the blocked ventricle to allow the CSF to flow out continuously through a tube into a body cavity.

The blood supply to the brain, or *cerebrovascular system*, is too complex to describe here, but in simple terms it involves two pairs of cerebral arteries that carry the oxygenated blood from the heart around the brain. The *internal carotid arteries* supply the anterior parts of the brain, and the *vertebral arteries* supply the posterior parts of the brain. The internal carotid and vertebral arterial systems are linked at the base of the brain by a ring of vessels lying in the subarachnoid space, a clever design feature called the *Circle of Willis*. If one of the main arteries becomes blocked, the blood can pass around the circle to reach the deprived area. The Circle of Willis is a frequent site of weakenings on the artery wall, called *aneurysms*. If an aneurysm bursts, it expels blood around the brain in the subarachnoid space, causing a *subarachnoid hemorrhage*. A blockage in an artery away from the Circle of Willis can result in the blood and oxygen supply being cut off to the part of the brain that artery supplies, resulting in an area of brain death, called a *stroke* (see Chapter 2). The venous system carrying away the used, deoxygenated blood includes *superficial veins*, which drain the lateral and lower surfaces of the hemispheres, and *deep veins*, which drain the internal area of the brain. The cerebral veins empty into channels called *venous sinuses* within the coverings of the brain, and these in turn empty into the large internal jugular vein.

The cortex, or gray matter, of each hemisphere can be divided up in a number of ways, but the simplest is to conceptualize it as four lobes. In clinical neuropsychology the lobes are often viewed as separate areas and are frequently linked to specific abilities or functions, but they are in fact divisions of convenience rather than true anatomic divisions. Nevertheless, these divisions serve a useful purpose in discussions of brain–behavior relations. The four cortical lobes of the left hemisphere are labeled in the upper drawing of the brain, and the right hemisphere is divided up in the same way. The large frontal lobes form the anterior part of the brain, and the parietal, temporal, and occipital lobes make up the portion posterior to the central sulcus.

All three posterior lobes (in each hemisphere) are involved in the awareness, perception, and integration of information from the outside world delivered via our five senses, although the connections of the posterior lobes with the limbic system ensure that the way we experience the world is influenced by our mood, motivation, and past experiences. Generally, the parietal lobes are involved in functions involving tactile sensations, sense of position, and spatial relations. The strip immediately behind the central sulcus in the parietal lobe is called the *sensory strip*. It contains in its neurons a "map" of a person in which different regions correspond to different areas of the body, more or less in the same spatial order as they occur in the body itself but with body parts that are very sensitive, such as the lips and fingers, being represented by larger clusters of neurons. The nerve fibers from the body map in the left hemisphere cross over such that they activate sensations on the right side of the body, and the body map in the right hemisphere connects to the left side of the body. Thus, damage to neurons in the foot area of the body map in the left hemisphere will cause a loss of feeling in the right foot, and damage to the tongue area in the right hemisphere will cause an area of numbness on the left side of the tongue. The remainder of the parietal lobe has less specific functions. The left parietal lobe has a bias toward sequential and logical spatial abilities, such as perceiving the details within a spatial pattern (see Chapter 5), whereas the right parietal lobe is more involved with the holistic appreciation of spatial information, such as appreciating an entire scene. The left parietal lobe also appears to mediate the ability to calculate, which involves both logical and spatial concepts. The right parietal lobe is especially good at conceptualizing complex spatial relations, and people with right parietal lesions often have extreme difficulty copying complex patterns or working out how to put jigsaw puzzles together (see Chapter 3).

The temporal lobes are concerned primarily with hearing and smell, but they are also involved in integrating visual perceptions with other sensory information. The hippocampus, a part of the limbic system lying inside the temporal lobes, plays an essential role in memory (see Chapters 7 and 8) and also allows the integration of emotion and motivation with the sensory information relayed from the outside world to the posterior lobes of the hemispheres. The left temporal lobe is concerned more with verbal and sequential functions; it includes the language comprehension area (see Chapter 2) and is involved in new verbal learning and memory. The right temporal lobe tends to be more concerned with nonverbal functions, such as the interpretation of emotional voice tone and emotional facial expression and the appreciation of music and nonlanguage sounds. It also appears to play a part in nonverbal learning and memory (see Chapter 8), although this role is not so clear as the left temporal lobe's role in verbal memory.

The occipital lobes are the visual lobes; they mediate sight, visual perception, and visual knowledge. A patient with a large lesion of the right occipital lobe may have a complete defect (loss of vision) in the left visual fields of both eyes (and vice versa for a left occipital lobe lesion), and a patient with lesions of the primary visual cortex, at the very posterior end (called the pole) of both occipital lobes, will be unable to see, even though the eyes function normally. This condition is termed *cortical blindness*. Very specific visual field defects can also occur if the visual pathways are damaged at other points. For example, a lesion in the right temporal lobe that damages the optic fibers that travel through the brain from the eye to the occipital cortex will result in a visual field defect in the upper left quadrant of both eyes. Lesions of the cortex of the occipital lobe can result in a number of strange disorders, particularly when the lesions are on both sides of the brain. For example, Michael, the man described in Chapter 6, can see and describe the form of objects, but is unable to recognize what it is he is seeing. This condition is called *visual agnosia*.

The large frontal lobes lie anterior to the central sulcus and are concerned mainly with acting on knowledge relayed to the posterior part of the cerebral cortex from the outside world. They can be divided into three zones. The *primary zone*, or *motor strip*, is immediately in front of the central sulcus and is mapped like the sensory strip in the parietal lobe. But the motor strip is concerned with movement of the parts of the opposite side of the body rather than with touch. The *secondary zone* lies in front of the motor strip and puts actions together, so that we can perform motor patterns like riding a bicycle. In the left frontal lobe these regions also include a major motor area (Broca's area, discussed earlier) involved in talking, or speech, but not in comprehension of language (see Chapter 2). The large area at the very front of the frontal lobes is called the *prefrontal cortex*. This is an extremely high-level part of the brain and much more developed in humans than in any other animal. These lobes are often called the executive lobes, as they are concerned with *executive functions* such as forming abstract concepts and planning and executing actions based on the information received from the posterior cortex. They also enable us to have insight into our own behaviors and inhibit us from doing things we know we shouldn't do—but perhaps would like to do! Alcohol intoxication affects the prefrontal lobes, which explains why people who are drunk often behave in ways they are ashamed of when they sober up. The inside, or medial, parts of the two frontal lobes are part of the emotional limbic system, and this allows executive functions to be modulated by the individual's emotional and motivational states. Thus we find that people who suffer serious damage to the prefrontal lobes have emotional problems and also problems with thinking abstractly and making good decisions (see Chapter 4). The prefrontal lobes are also concerned with alertness—via their association with the reticular formation—and the ability to attend in a general sense or to focus attention on a particular task. As any teacher knows, this is a prerequisite for learning. Attention is really a process, and is mediated by many areas and systems in the brain, including the parietal lobe.

As you read the chapters that follow, you will understand at a deeper level how the brain works and what happens to the mind when different parts of the brain are damaged. Reading about Phillipa and what happened to her when her frontal lobes were severely damaged after a brutal assault by a burglar gives a whole new meaning to the soft, worm-like, gray convolutions that lie inside our skull just above our eyes.

■ Further Reading

Broks, P. 2003. *Into the Silent Land*. London: Atlantic Books.
Chen, P. W. 2007. *Final Exam: A Surgeon's Reflections on Mortality*. New York: Knopf.
Gawande, A. 2002. *Complications: A Surgeon's Notes on an Imperfect Science*. New York: Picador.
Gawande, A. 2007. *Better: A Surgeon's Notes on Performance*. New York: Picador.
Gawande, A. 2009. *The Checklist Manifesto: How to Get Things Right*. New York: Metropolitan Books.
Groopman, J. E. 2003. *The Anatomy of Hope: How People Prevail in the Face of Illness*. New York: Random House.
Groopman, J. E. 2007. *How Doctors Think*. New York: Houghton Mifflin.
Heilman, K. M. 2002. *Matter Of Mind: A Neurologist's View of Brain–Behaviour Relationships*. New York: Oxford University Press.

Heilman, K. M. 2009. *Postgraduate Year One: Lessons in Caring.* New York: Oxford University Press.

Kapur, N. (Ed.). 1997. *Injured Brains of Medical Minds: Views From Within.* New York: Oxford University Press.

Karinthy, F. 2008. *A Journey Round My Skull.* Translated by V. D. Barker. Reissued with a new foreword by O. Sacks. New York: New York Review of Books.

Lezak, M. D., Howieson, D. B., and Loring, D. W. 2004. Part I. Theory and Practice of Neuropsychological Assessment. In: *Neuropsychological Assessment, 4th Ed.* New York: Oxford University Press.

Luria, A. R. 1987. *The Man with a Shattered World.* Reissued with a new foreword by O. Sacks. Cambridge, MA: Harvard University Press.

Luria, A. R. 1987. *The Mind of a Mnemonist.* Reissued with a new foreword by J. S. Bruner. Cambridge, MA: Harvard University Press.

Ofri, D. 2003. *Singular Intimacies: Becoming a Doctor at Bellevue.* New York: Beacon Press.

Ofri, D. 2005. *Incidental Findings: Lessons from My Patients in the Art of Medicine.* New York: Beacon Press.

Ofri, D. 2011. *Medicine in Translation: Journeys with My Patients.* New York: Beacon Press.

Ogden, J. A. 2005. Introduction to Clinical Neuropsychology. In: *Fractured Minds: A Case-Study Approach to Clinical Neuropsychology, 2nd Ed.* (pp. 3–27). New York: Oxford University Press.

Ogden, J. A. 2005. The Neuropsychological Assessment. In: *Fractured Minds: A Case-Study Approach to Clinical Neuropsychology, 2nd Ed.* (pp. 28–45). New York: Oxford University Press.

Sacks, O. 1970. *The Man Who Mistook His Wife for a Hat.* New York: Summit Books.

2 ■

Lost for Words: Two Tales of Aphasia

Luke was one of those people whose very presence fills up a room. In this case the room was a six-bed ward in the neurosurgery ward at Auckland Hospital, and I had no trouble finding a 28-year-old Maori man among the pale-faced, pajama-clad older men who lay sleeping or reading in the other beds. This late in the afternoon, visitors had been shooed away until after dinner, so the small crowd around Luke made him even more noticeable. Powerfully built, with a mane of tangled black hair and tattoos on both arms and his bare chest, he was sitting bolt upright in his bed, a low shaft of sunlight catching the large greenstone pendant suspended from a piece of leather around his neck. His left hand was hovering over a board covered with letters and numbers, and as I approached his bed he looked up at me, his strong face shadowed with fear. Around him sat three young Maori, a woman and two men, all, like Luke, with arms generously tattooed. I noticed a leather jacket thrown on the end of his bed, the gang patch clearly visible. Luke's visitors looked and smelled hot in their leather pants and tight-fitting black T-shirts. The silence was palpable.

I walked up to the bed and smiled at them, introducing myself as a psychologist. Luke peered at me through dark, bloodshot eyes and tried to speak, but when an unintelligible noise came out of his mouth, he looked down at the communication board and slowly, with much hesitation, pointed in turn to various letters, glancing up at me between each "word."

"V-O-C-E G-O-M-N H-E-P M-E."

"What's he trying to say?" the young woman whispered.

I turned to Luke, who was now gazing at me. "Voice gone, help me?" I asked, and he nodded vigorously. He winced, and I saw the blood drain from his brown face as his left hand shot up and clasped his head.

"And your head is giving you hell," I added. He nodded almost imperceptibly this time, his forehead still covered by his huge hand, the skull and crossbones on a large silver ring on his little finger winking in the sunlight. The young woman, who appeared about 18, was crying now as she stroked his right hand, which lay motionless on the white sheet.

Luke's doctor had asked me to attempt an informal assessment of Luke's understanding of what had happened to him, and to find out how he was coping with his situation. I had read his hospital file and spoken to the charge nurse, who suggested I also talk to his visitors. They had been the ones who had brought Luke into the hospital, and one or more of them had been at his side ever since. According to them, they and the other members of their gang were Luke's *whanau*—family—and the young woman holding his hand had been noted as his next-of-kin in his hospital admission form.

I knew from his file that Luke had collapsed at a party the evening before. At first his friends thought he was drunk, but when he awoke from his semicomatose state the next day, unable to speak and weak down his right side, they realized this was more than a hangover, and took him to the emergency department at Auckland Hospital. A CT brain scan revealed that Luke had suffered a *cerebrovascular accident* (CVA)—a general term that refers to a stroke or brain hemorrhage due to a blockage or rupture of an artery or vein. In Luke's case the CVA was a collection of blood within the brain substance of the lower posterior region of the left frontal lobe. He was transferred to the neurosurgery ward, and now, a few hours later, was fully alert but very frightened as he desperately tried to spell the words that his lips refused to form, using a communication board of letters and numbers given to him by the speech pathologist.

Luke was now lying flat, his eyes closed but the color in his face a little better. "Is it OK if I talk about what is happening to you with your friends here?" I asked him. Luke held his left hand up, the thumb and forefinger clasped in an "O," then reached over his body to clasp the woman's hand.

"Sharon's his girl," said one of the men. "I'm Jimmy and he's Hawke." He nodded toward the man sitting next to him. "We're whanau."

"You brought Luke in, and have been with him ever since? You must be pretty tired."

"Yeah, but no bugger's told us nothin' yet. What's goin' on?"

"Luke had a small bleed into the left side of his brain; the part that's important for speaking and also controls movement of his right arm and hand. It's a sort of stroke."

"But he's not an old bastard, he's only 28. I thought you had to be old to have a stroke?"

"You're right, but that's a different sort of stroke when a blood vessel gets blocked up and blood and oxygen can't get to a part of the brain. The type of stroke Luke has had—when a blood vessel bursts and you get a blood clot in the brain—can happen to younger people, although it's pretty uncommon."

"He'd been on a bloody drinking binge, stupid bugger. P'raps he fell over and hit his head?" said Hawke. "I seen this happen to Charlie—he was one of the bros—he came off his motorcycle and bashed his head in and that was the end of his loud mouth; couldn't walk either for bloody months."

"Sounds as if Charlie had a severe head injury," I replied. "It doesn't look as if Luke's problem is a result of falling and hitting his head, which is good. A small bleed like this into the brain might have been precipitated by the drinking binge, but that is pretty unlikely. He was probably just unlucky. An intracerebral hematoma—that's what it's called, it just means a blood clot inside the brain—it can happen to someone with high blood pressure, and heavy smoking isn't good either. But sometimes it just happens for no apparent reason in perfectly healthy people."

Luke was gazing at me now and he appeared to be listening. His girlfriend blew her nose loudly and then asked in a whisper, "Will he get better?"

"It's too early to know, but he's doing pretty well given he had the bleed only last night. Most people who are young and healthy like Luke recover really well. The blood is usually reabsorbed in time, and with rehabilitation Luke will gradually learn to speak again and the weakness on the right side of his body will get better. But I'm afraid it will take time and probably a lot of hard work."

"Shit." The word exploded from Luke's mouth and we all looked startled, Luke as well. He tried to say something else but nothing comprehensible emerged.

"There you go, you're already beginning to get better," I grinned, looking down at his still-startled expression. I decided not to explain just yet that single swear words are often the first words spoken after damage to the speech area of the brain. It has been suggested that these emotionally motivated expletives can be produced by the normally mute right hemisphere and thus are the first words to find expression when the left hemisphere is silenced.

*****

After the age of about four, most of us take for granted our effortless ability to produce and understand complex and structured strings of words to communicate with others who speak the same language. When this ability is taken from us without warning, it is hardly surprising that our overriding emotion is often fear. For Luke and his friends, the fear did not spring from knowledge about the relationship between language deficits and left brain damage, but was fear of the unknown. In their experience, only very old people suffered strokes that led to speech problems. Although they were aware that motorcycle and car crashes could result in head injuries, causing speech problems and limb weaknesses, they had never before experienced a drinking binge that had such a devastating result.

A careful assessment confirmed that Luke was suffering from *expressive,* or *Broca's, aphasia.* His most severe difficulties were in speech and spontaneous writing—ways of expressing language—in contrast with his reasonably intact ability to comprehend language. This syndrome is named for neurologist Paul Broca, who first described it in 1861.[1] His patient, commonly referred to as "Tan" because that was the only utterance he could make, was found at postmortem to have a lesion of the *third frontal gyrus,* now

[1] Broca, P. 1861. Remarques sur le siège de la faculté du langage articulé suivie d'une observation d'aphémie (perte de la parole). *Bulletin de la Société Anatomique,* 6, 330–357 (Translated in R. Herrnstein and E. G. Boring. 1965. *A Source Book in the History of Psychology.* Cambridge, MA: Harvard University Press.)

known as *Broca's area*. This remains the area most frequently associated with expressive aphasia. The other most important area lies immediately adjacent to Broca's area and contains the motor neurons for the tongue and lips. Lesions deep to Broca's area (i.e., lesions beneath the cortical surface of the area) have also been shown to produce expressive aphasia.

Luke's hematoma was in Broca's area, and his symptoms were a classic illustration of Broca's aphasia: a severe nonfluency of speech, which may be so extreme as to render the patient mute. More often, speech is limited to a few stereotyped expressions or expletives. Less severely affected patients may be able to provide sensible one-word answers to questions and even produce short "sentences" with many hesitations, but these are often *agrammatical*: the patient is more likely to produce nouns and verbs than grammatical modifiers and prepositions, resulting in unmelodic speech. Names of familiar concrete objects are easier to articulate than common grammatical terms such as "or," "if," "but," and "where." For example, a Broca's aphasic may answer the question "What is wrong with you?" by saying in an effortful and staccato manner, "Peech gone, can't palk, talk." Nearly every sound requires a fresh start, and many words are incorrectly pronounced. Words beginning with letters like "p," "b," or "m," which are formed at the front of the mouth, are easier to say than letters like "s" and "t"; so "speech" may sound like "peech," and "talk" may be articulated as "palk." Verbs usually appear in their simplest form, so the patient says, "Me go" rather than "I am going."

The right hand is often weak or paralyzed, because the left brain lesion that causes Broca's aphasia may encroach on the adjacent hand area of the motor strip. Writing done with the nonparalyzed left hand is nonfluent, like the patient's speech. Copying may be better than writing spontaneously or to dictation. Words are misspelled, correct letters are poorly formed, grammatical words are left out entirely, and perseveration of letters—writing the same letter repeatedly—may occur.

Some patients have difficulty swallowing food and saliva, although this usually fully recovers over days to weeks. Many patients with Broca's aphasia also suffer from *oral apraxia*. Apraxia refers to a difficulty miming or performing learned motor skills on command. Thus patients severely affected with oral apraxia may be unable to poke out their tongues or whistle on verbal command or in imitation of the examiner. Language comprehension is usually impaired to some degree. Simple requests are often understood, but patients with severe Broca's aphasia are unlikely to understand a three-step command, even if each step is simple. Even when only a "yes" or "no" response is required, some patients may have difficulty comprehending more complex language input. Often the comprehension of numbers and symbols is also impaired.

Generally, Broca's aphasics are alert and appear to interact with their caregivers and family in an intelligent, unconfused manner. Their nonverbal memory—memory for pictures, faces, patterns, and melodies—is good; they have no difficulty recognizing doctors and other caregivers, and they can follow a simple daily schedule. They are often emotionally fragile and easily angered or reduced to tears.

*****

I made a time to see Sharon alone the following day, and she told me what she knew about Luke's past. He grew up the eldest of 10 children in a poor area of Auckland. He was miserable at school and left when he was 15, having failed in many of his academic examinations. Since then, apart from a few laboring jobs from time to time, he had been financially dependent on the unemployment benefit.

He was initiated into a Maori gang soon after leaving school and passed his time riding motorcycles with his mates, committing petty thievery, playing billiards, smoking marijuana, consuming large quantities of alcohol, and playing the guitar and singing the blues. He had been a heavy smoker since the age of about 13, and drank large quantities of alcohol, mainly beer, at least four nights—or days—a week. When I asked about head injuries, Sharon, after talking with Jimmy and Hawke, told me that they could remember his suffering at least three minor injuries over the past few years from fights and minor motorcycle accidents. More by good luck than sensible living, he appeared to have avoided a serious head injury. For the past five years Luke had been living with his mates in a rundown "gang" house, although he went through periods of visiting his family. Sharon had been living with him for about a year.

Luke's parents were finally contacted—they had no phone—and arrived at the hospital with five of Luke's nine siblings, ranging from the one closest to him in age, a 26 -year-old brother who still lived at home, to the youngest, who was only five years old. His father had been unemployed for most of his adult life, and Luke's mother looked exhausted and very worried. Getting to the hospital by two buses from their house in a poor area of Auckland was time-consuming and difficult, and even the bus fare was too expensive to allow visits very often during the time Luke remained in the neurosurgery ward. He had sporadic visits from some of the other gang members, but after the first two days Sharon was his only regular visitor.

During the first week after his stroke, Luke was unable to utter more than single words, but he was able to use his communication board to spell out ungrammatical and misspelled sentences of three or four words. He would quickly become frustrated and angry when he was unable to make himself understood, and the words exploding from his mouth were often swear words. On one occasion, he became so angry that he threw the communication board at the speech pathologist and then swept his water jug and glass off his bedside table with his left arm. He appeared to comprehend the lecture he subsequently received from the speech pathologist and the doctor, and their threat to have his arm tied to the bed did not have to be carried out.

Assessment of Luke's language functions demonstrated reasonable comprehension of spoken and simple written English, although he had difficulty comprehending grammatical function words (the "little words" used to connect phrases in sentences) such as "above" and "below." For example, when asked to point to the picture that best illustrated the sentence "The cat is under the chair," he was just as likely to point to a picture of a cat on a chair as a cat under a chair. According to Luke's mother, his reading had been poor before his hemorrhage, so it was difficult to assess whether his comprehension of more complex written passages was impaired.

Luke also had apraxia of the left arm. When asked, "Show me how you brush your teeth," he made large circling movements in the air. He understood the command and could nod in confirmation when I performed the correct movement, but he could not copy my movement accurately. In contrast, he could use a real toothbrush correctly. He also had oral apraxia and was unable to pretend to whistle, blow a kiss, or sip through a straw.

A second CT scan performed two days before Luke's discharge from the hospital showed that the area of hemorrhage had reduced considerably as the blood was reabsorbed, and he was fortunate in that the cortex and underlying white matter did not appear to have been extensively damaged. By the 10th day following his hemorrhage his right arm and hand had gained some strength, and he could articulate short sentences with few function words such as "Phone Mum. Clothes, umm... [*patting his arm*] coat,...black, umm...." At this point, the psychologist suggested the word "leather." "Yes, yes, leather coat, jacket, jeans pease, please." His speech sounded strained and had impaired prosody; that is, it sometimes lacked the normal intonations and melody. Luke's ability to repeat simple sentences had improved, although he became muddled if the sentences were more than about five words long, were grammatically complex, or were ungrammatical. For example, Luke could repeat "Auckland is in New Zealand," but he had difficulty with "Wellington is north of Christchurch and south of Auckland" and "The boy eat the food." At this point there was nothing more that could be done for him in the acute neurosurgery service, and Luke was transferred to a live-in rehabilitation unit.

I visited him there a few days later. In response to my greeting and query about how he was doing, he pointed to his head and said with a grin, "Trouble...mind."

Sharon, who was also visiting him, laughed and said, "You mean 'Trouble In Mind,' silly." She turned to me. "That's one of his favorite blues numbers!" Then out of Luke's mouth came:

Trouble in mind, I'm blue,
But I won't be blue always,
'Cause the sun's gonna shine in
my back door someday.

Sharon and I looked at Luke in amazement. He was singing—with every word clearly enunciated in his mellow voice!

"Wow, I think we'd better get you started on melodic intonation therapy," I told him. "It uses music to help you produce words more easily."

Melodic intonation (MI) therapy was first developed in the 1970s, based on the observation that some patients with Broca's aphasia are able to produce words while singing, in contrast to the severe impairment of their normal speech. This led to the idea that combining slower speech with intoned patterns with a precise rhythm and distinct stresses on words would assist the patient in expressing longer, more complex sentences. And sure enough, the speech pathologist found that Luke's ability to repeat sentences improved if she sang a sentence with a strong intonation pattern, and she began to incorporate MI therapy into her twice-daily sessions with Luke. At first she asked Luke to copy her after she sang, using only two or three pitches, simple two- and three-syllable words ("wat-er," "hos-pit-al"); then she expanded to two- and three-word phrases ("Show me," "I am hun-gry"), with the syllables or words normally accented in speech being sung in the higher pitch. At the same time, Luke was asked to emphasize the rhythm of the "melody" by tapping his left hand on the table in time with each syllable—a strategy demonstrated to facilitate improved speech. Luke quite quickly graduated to longer sentences, such as "I would like some orange juice," and he began to use melody and rhythm to express himself to Sharon and his friends when he couldn't find the spoken words. Usually he would do this by first humming a well-known simple melody—more often than not, "Mary had a little lamb"—and then singing the same melody with the sentence he wanted to express inserted. He became particularly good at singing, to the tune of "Mary had a little lamb," the sentence "Sharon I love you I do." This invariably gave Sharon a boost, which she sorely needed at times during the long rehabilitation process. One of the first sentences he spoke in a normal, "nonsinging" voice was "Sharon, I love you," followed by "Get me outta here!"

Not all people with Broca's aphasia are helped by MI therapy. The best candidates seem to be those with good auditory comprehension skills relative to their ability to produce and repeat speech, and those who are able to track how they are improving or failing to improve. As a singer,

Luke really enjoyed MI therapy, and there was no doubt that it helped his speech recovery, although the speech pathologist used other forms of speech therapy with him as well. In addition, spontaneous recovery as the hematoma was reabsorbed was probably also occurring, and thus his improvement was probably due to a combination of factors.

This difficulty highlights one of the common problems in assessing the usefulness of rehabilitation methods for aphasia and other cognitive and motor problems following brain damage. To assess the effect of a particular therapy strategy, it is necessary to adhere strictly to a carefully designed program that allows the influence of the therapy to be discriminated from various other recovery mechanisms. One way to do this is to design an experiment using the patient as his own control: take baseline measures of various aspects of language and other deficits, such as apraxia, before commencing a therapy strategy aimed at improving one aspect of the patient's disorder. If the therapy is effective, all elements of the targeted aspect of the disorder will improve more quickly than will other aspects. If the therapy is stopped after a short time, the patient's improvement in the targeted aspect should stop or slide backward but improve again when the therapy recommences.

This single-subject study design is often more practical and ethical than assessing whether a therapy strategy works by comparing two groups of aphasia patients, one with therapy and the other without. Even so, in a busy rehabilitation unit, it is difficult to use single-case designs stringently, particularly given the attraction of approaching the patient's numerous problems from as many therapeutic angles as possible over the same period. There are ways to assess multiple therapies within the same single-case study design, but the practicalities of carrying out such complex experimentation with every patient unfortunately work against its regular implementation. It is understandable that from the patient's point of view trying every therapy that might be of use is a more attractive proposition than becoming a participant in a carefully designed rehabilitation program where different therapies are introduced according to a strict and drawn-out time frame.

Luke's therapy program was multidimensional, and the efficacies of individual interventions were not assessed. He received not only speech and physical therapy, but also individual and family psychological counseling, which appeared especially helpful in enabling him to cope with the cessation of his alcohol consumption, forced on him by his confinement in the rehabilitation unit. In the first two weeks there, he escaped three times and was found in a nearby hotel bar. No doubt the other drinkers thought that his strained and staccato speech was a result of intoxication. It was made clear to Luke that his escapades would not be tolerated, and if they continued he would be discharged from the unit. Hospital staff kept a close watch on him for the next month, and during this period he became quite depressed and apathetic and would participate in speech and physical therapy sessions only if he was continually encouraged. Counseling sessions that included his family and friends seemed to help Luke, and his mood and motivation gradually improved. He found that keeping active helped him fight his need for alcohol, and as he gained control over his desire to drink, he began to feel justifiably proud of this achievement.

Another helpful intervention was suggested by Sharon. She, Jimmy, and Hawke took turns spending the day at the rehabilitation unit, going to every therapy session with Luke. Their participation in speech and physical therapy not only encouraged Luke but often added a much-needed humorous touch to the sessions as they would often crack up at Luke's attempts to talk in sensible sentences or to perform some physical exercise. This interaction seemed to alleviate Luke's frustration with his slow progress and cause him in turn to laugh at his friends' attempts to copy him! He would then gamely try again. The presence of cheerful friends at therapy sessions may well have a negative effect on progress for some people, and the details of a rehabilitation program must be tailored to fit the individual. Luke's mates were there for him between therapy sessions when he wanted to relax; they were sensitive to his moods and knew when to leave him, when to cheer him up, and when to listen to him express his feelings. They became skilled at understanding Luke's body language, and at times were able to relieve him of the weary task of using words to try to communicate important ideas to staff.

Sharon brought in his guitar, and he would spend thirty minutes or more playing and singing with his friends or by himself before he became tired. Sometimes the words of songs came spontaneously and sometimes he just hummed, and he had no trouble forming chords with his good left hand. While at first he could only strum with his right hand, he slowly began to pick out blues breaks as his fingers strengthened and his fine finger movements became more coordinated.

Billiards also became a regular feature of Luke's day. At first a friend would help him push the billiard cue, but gradually he gained the strength and coordination to manipulate the cue himself. His friends even agreed to cut down on their smoking habits to encourage Luke to do likewise. The knowledge that Luke's hemorrhage may have been in part a result of his heavy smoking had been salutary for them.

Luke was discharged to live with his parents three months after his hemorrhage, and continued to attend speech and physical therapy twice a week for a further three months as an outpatient at a hospital closer to his home. It was a day for celebration when an assessment of his language functions six months after his hemorrhage demonstrated that his ability to speak spontaneously and with normal intonation was almost back to normal levels. He still occasionally missed function words and at times had trouble finding the right word, although when cued by the first letter he could normally produce it. His repetition was now good and he had no difficulty understanding complex language. He had completely recovered from his apraxia and had regained reasonable strength in his right arm.

At this point I gave Luke a full neuropsychological assessment. I found that his performance was average on tests that required him to learn lists of words and short stories, as well as on tests that required visuospatial skills, like making patterns with colored blocks and finding his way about the neighborhood. His performance was in the low average range on verbal tests including providing the meaning of words, reading, and understanding abstract verbal concepts such as those conveyed by proverbs like "A rolling stone gathers no moss." His level of verbal ability may have been in part a result of his left frontal damage and aphasia, but was also a reflection of poorer verbal skills before his hemorrhage. He had always been a poor reader and as a Maori had struggled with the European-style schooling system. In addition, many of the neuropsychological tests available to assess him in the 1990s were culturally inappropriate, although the visuospatial tests—such as copying a complex geometrical pattern—were less so than the verbal tests.

This problem highlights the importance of developing appropriate tests for different cultural groups, both in terms of the test items and in the scores that we consider "average." I'm reminded of another Maori gang member I assessed many years ago. Jake had crashed his motorcycle and ended up with a severe head injury. I didn't see him until some months later, when I was called in by the physical therapist, who was ready to expel him from her sessions because of his refusal to cooperate with the exercises she was giving him for his weak left arm, the result of damage to the right motor strip of his brain. I soon discovered that Jake thought his arm was weak because it had been broken. I used simple drawings to show him how the brain controlled his body and explained that the physical exercises the therapist was asking him to do over and over again were to stimulate his brain and help it—and therefore his arm—recover. His amazed expression when he realized his brain was connected to his arm was almost funny, but poignant as well.

I had been asked to assess his intelligence and looked into my arsenal of tests to see if I could find anything that might be "culturally appropriate." He did reasonably well on a few of these, but then I tried a test that assesses abstract thinking. It involved questions such as "How are a cat and an elephant alike?" The correct answer is to say that they are both animals (or mammals). This is one of the easiest sorts of questions and Jake had no problem here. But when I got to the harder questions he began to look frustrated. I came to the question "How are a poem and a statue alike?" (The "correct" answer is that they are both art forms, or creative works.)

Jake was stumped, and he shrugged. "Dunno."

I thought for a moment and then asked, "How are a legend and carving alike?" He grinned triumphantly, and banging his chest with his left fist said: "Well, they both come from here. They both have soul." Jake's abstract thinking was fine; it was the test content that needed fixing. Later in this chapter I will devote some space to the complex and often controversial issues around providing assessments and therapy that are culturally fair, especially for indigenous peoples.

Following his six-month assessment, Luke and his therapists had a meeting and decided that his recovery had plateaued at near-normal levels. Any further improvement would occur slowly and Luke's best strategy now was to get on with as normal a life as possible. Luke shifted from his parents' house into a house with Sharon and two of her friends. He didn't return to the gang house he had lived in before his accident, as he had given up his gang membership. I was never clear as to whether this was on his own initiative or because he was booted out, perhaps because of his new close association with "whities." With the help of the rehabilitation unit, he was able to obtain a part-time job doing light work weeding and planting in a plant nursery. A year later he was working at the nursery full time and had a steady partner—not Sharon, who had moved to another town where she was able to get a job. Luke no longer rode motorcycles and had traded his in for an old car. He reported that he drank alcohol no more than once a week, and even then he kept his alcohol consumption to moderate levels. How true this was I don't know, but I do know that he had given up smoking cigarettes, although he admitted to a joint once in a while. He said he felt that his speech had improved even further and gave him trouble only when he was tired or had had a couple of drinks. He grinned when he said this was one of the reasons he had cut down on his alcohol consumption; everyone thought he was drunk long before he really was.

Luke declined the offer of a final follow-up assessment, but his comments provided a much more appropriate outcome measure. "I reckon that the important thing is me getting on okay, and it doesn't matter too much what all them tests show. Seems to me I might do better not to know how you fellas think I'm doin' and just get on with my life. Don't take it personal, I've got you lot to thank for my job, and giving up all those bad habits like drinking and smoking and others I won't mention in your presence! The only thing I'm really sorry about is giving up the motorcycle. I just might get another one now I know I'm okay again. I think that hemorrhage put some sense into my nut, so I'll be the guy in the slow lane from now on!"

*****

Luke came from a minority culture, and this was an important consideration in both his assessment and rehabilitation. Superficially, it might seem that the findings of clinical neuropsychology should be applicable to all ethnic and cultural groups. This is probably the case when we consider the overall picture. It seems likely, for example, that damage to Broca's area will potentially give rise to problems with speech regardless of the patient's ethnicity. It is at the level of detail that we must question our assumptions about cross-cultural brain–behavior similarities. For example, many Australian aborigines demonstrate an uncanny ability—from the point of view of white cultures—to navigate, without a compass, their way across vast deserts and to track animals by recognizing footprints. Most white Australians have no idea how the aboriginal people achieve this, let alone being able to do it themselves. There have been a small number of culturally specific neuropsychological tests designed, such as a test that requires the recognition of different footprints for Australian aborigines and a horse recognition test for Pueblo Indians. On these tests, members of cultures other than the group the tests were designed for do very poorly. As neuropsychologists, we must ask whether the Australian aborigines and Pueblo Indians have evolved highly sophisticated and specialized topographical orientation and visuospatial abilities or whether they learn these skills as children. Either way, findings like these are intriguing and have implications for how the mind has evolved and how it works.

In the case of specialized evolution, we might expect to find in aborigines a cortical area or neural system specialized for topographical and visuospatial abilities that is absent in ethnic groups not possessing such impressive skills in these areas. Perhaps these skills are associated with a greater development of systems in the parietal lobe—the brain's "spatial" lobe—or are mediated in part by the same system that enables a city dweller to find his way around a new city. If, on the other hand, each individual must learn the skill anew, questions arise about the way development organizes the functional systems of the brain and whether given the same learning environment, the brains of members of other groups have the same potential for developing these skills as the brains of aborigines.

In practical terms, the different abilities of different ethnic groups, whether innate (present at birth) or learned, should influence how we interpret impairments after brain damage. To interpret test results correctly, we require normative data—appropriate comparison scores—for that particular group of people. Normative test data are usually grouped according to age and sometimes by gender, level of formal education, and socioeconomic group. Ideally, we should also have normative data on the performance of different ethnic, cultural, and even subcultural groups such as "gang members," and in recent years there has been a greater focus on this area of neuropsychology. Normative test data alone will not solve the problem of cross-cultural assessment, as the manner in which tests are given, the cultural similarity of the neuropsychologist or other health professional to the patient or client, the content and format of the tests themselves, and the way both the test scores and the patient's test "behaviors" are interpreted also contribute to a true, repeatable, and helpful assessment.

The form an assessment should take to optimize its usefulness for a particular person is an important but difficult issue in countries that include many ethnic groups in various stages of assimilation by the dominant culture. Often all we have available to assess a client of an ethnic minority are tests developed for Europeans or white

Americans to be given by a white neuropsychologist. The validity of giving a person from another cultural group such an assessment will increase with the client's level of acculturation into the dominant culture. For example, a part Native American man who has been raised in a large American city by a white American mother, who has succeeded in the Western education system, and who identifies primarily with white Americans will probably be reasonably well served by the same test battery and conditions as his white American peers.

But many Native Americans who require a neuropsychological assessment following, for example, a stroke or a head injury are unlikely to have succeeded in a Western school system based on white American values, skills, learning conditions, and test measures. In addition, many Native Americans forced into close social contact with white Americans may not feel truly comfortable in a white American world and may have long since given up hope that their white American friends and acquaintances could understand that their worldview is fundamentally different from that of the Native American. The danger here lies in the white American neuropsychologist's interpretation of the Native American patient's test performance and information about the patient's life that is gathered from an interview. These cautionary remarks are not restricted to the situation in the United States but are equally appropriate for many westernized countries—including Canada, South Africa, Australia, and New Zealand—where the indigenous people and minority ethnic groups have been, and often still are, oppressed and dominated by the white culture. Similar issues surround the cross-cultural assessment and treatment of people from immigrant groups.

A separate question that rightly concerns many neuropsychologists pertains to the morality of giving a client of another culture, however acculturated, no choice regarding the "ethnicity" of an assessment. Often, faced with a client from a different culture, our choices are limited to not performing an assessment at all or to performing one as sensitively as we can while consulting with people of the client's culture. Cultural consultants may be able to advise us about how best to put the client at ease during the assessment as well as suggest culturally appropriate interpretations of some of the data.

*****

Irene, the second aphasic patient I want to tell you about, also lost her language following a stroke, but that was about the only thing she had in common with Luke. She was a fit, healthy, well-educated, and comfortably well-off 68-year-old white woman when, in a matter of seconds, her life changed forever. Irene had worked for 35 years as a librarian, was a lover of books and the stories they held, and was an amateur actress who performed the stories of others, but at the end the ability to tell her own story was taken from her. Thus my version of how the stroke affected her has been cobbled together without the benefit of Irene's thoughts and insights.

It was a sunny Saturday afternoon in early December, and Irene's daughter Daisy and Daisy's husband, Peter, were sitting near the front of a small theater watching "Cinderella," that year's Christmas production put on for the children of the town by the local amateur drama company. Daisy had watched Irene acting in plays from Shakespeare to comedy ever since she could remember, but this was the first time she had watched her mother and Renie, her own 16-year-old daughter—playing the part of Cinderella—on the same stage. Daisy and Peter were laughing as much as the rowdy kids that surrounded them as the wicked stepmother—Irene herself—stormed around the stage, yelling at poor Cinderella sitting in her rags at the hearth, then turning to the children in the audience, trying—without success—to get their support.

"Sweep up the cinders, you useless wretch," she shouted as she shook a broom at Cinderella. The ugly stepsisters crowded around her, and she stroked their hair and cried, "My beautiful daughters, tonight you will be the belles of the ball!" Turning back to the audience, her dress hitched up to expose bright orange and purple bloomers, she asked, "Which of my beautiful daughters do you think the prince will take for his wife?"

"Cinderella! Not your ugly daughters!" shouted the children.

The wicked stepmother glared and waved her finger at her excited audience. "Never, never...." She seemed to hesitate but then went on, "Dreadful rubbish isn't here." She stumbled and would have fallen if the ugly stepsisters hadn't caught her. Finding her balance, she said something else that was unintelligible, but Daisy was already on her feet and Cinderella had left the hearth and was running toward her grandmother. The curtain came down as the actors on the stage gathered around Irene, and at last a hush fell over the youthful audience as they realized something was wrong.

Four long hours later, Daisy, Peter, and Renie, still dressed in her Cinderella rags, listened to the neurologist as he explained what had happened to Irene, who lay asleep in a bed in the neurology ward, exhausted by the ambulance ride and the drawn-out examinations and MRI brain scans.

"Your mother has suffered a significant stroke affecting the left side of her brain," he told them. "We've done an angiogram of the arteries that supply her brain, and it shows a complete blockage of a division of the left middle cerebral artery, which supplies the parietal and temporal lobes. When the blood supply is cut off, part of the brain is deprived of oxygen, and can die. I'm afraid it doesn't look good. We've started her on medication that hopefully will limit any further damage, but we'll just have to wait and see."

"Why would she have a stroke?" said Daisy. "She keeps fit, and she's never smoked. She's really careful with her diet and eats really healthily. She's not even a little bit over-weight. I know she gets her cholesterol and blood pressure checked every year and she's never had any problems." Daisy's voice faltered as her tears got the better of her, and Renie put her arms around her mother, her own tears fall-ing freely.

"It's the common stroke of old age, I'm afraid. But you're right, your mother is very unlucky. As you say, she has none of the usual risk factors. Have others in her fam-ily had strokes?"

"Yes, Mum's father died of a stroke when he was in his late fifties. And Mum had breast cancer when she was 55; could that have anything to do with her having this stroke now? She's been doing so well since then." Daisy's tears started afresh.

"No, I don't think her breast cancer would have any-thing to do with it, but her father's stroke suggests that there may have been a genetic factor."

"What's the matter with her speech?" Renie asked, her voice shaking. "She seemed very muddled and I don't think she could understand anything we said to her."

"She probably has a receptive aphasia—that means she has lost the ability to comprehend speech—which makes sense given that her stroke has affected the left temporal lobe of her brain; that's where the part that comprehends speech is. But she won't be in any pain and probably has very little insight into what has happened to her. Later she may be puzzled by being in the hospital."

"What about other problems. Will she be paralyzed?" Peter asked.

"No. The stroke doesn't appear to have extended to the motor areas nearer the front of the brain. I think she has a loss of feeling in her right side, but hopefully that will resolve. She is also likely to have lost a section of her vision in the upper right quadrant of both her eyes. That's a result of damage to the optic tract that carries the signals from her eyes to the visual cortex at the back of her brain."

"She'll hate that," Renie said. "She loves reading and it will be dreadful if she can't see to read."

"She'll quickly adapt to the visual field defect, and not even notice it. That won't affect her reading, I don't think. But I'm afraid that she mightn't be able to read for a different reason. Just as she can't understand what you say, she won't be able to understand what she reads either."

"Can't you do anything, give her something to help?" Renie sobbed.

"It will be a day or two before the speech pathologist can test her speech and reading properly, and hopefully the medications we're giving her might shrink the area damaged by the stroke. What she needs now is rest, and you could probably do with some as well."

I met with Daisy two days later and found out more about Irene's life. Her husband had died eight years earlier, and Irene had retired from her librarian position when she was 65. She was an educated woman with a postgraduate university degree in English and further qualifications in library studies. But her passion was drama, and over the past 40 years Irene had been involved not only in acting roles but as a playwright, director, and stage manager. She had even turned her hand to designing and making costumes and backdrops. When her only grandchild—named for her but called Renie to avoid confusion—had begun to show an interest and talent in acting through her school, Irene had been delighted, and their already close relationship became even closer. Renie was devastated by her grandmother's collapse, especially as "Cinderella" had been the first production they had been in together.

Although at this early stage I was unable to assess Irene's cognitive or memory abilities because of her communication difficulties, with the use of specially designed aphasia tests the speech pathologist was able to assess the many different aspects of language. The neurologist's first impression was right; Irene had *receptive*, or *Wernicke's*, *aphasia*. This type of aphasia—sometimes called *jargon aphasia* for obvious reasons—is named for neurologist Carl Wernicke, who in 1874 described 10 aphasic patients whose main difficulty was an inability to comprehend speech.[2] He had autopsy data on four patients, and each had a lesion that damaged the left posterior superior temporal lobe, now known as *Wernicke's area*. Patients with Wernicke's aphasia experience two main difficulties: a severe deficit in comprehending both spoken and written language, and fluent, grammatically correct but nonsensical speech and writing. Because patients are unable to understand what is said, they can't repeat things accurately. Their fluent speech and writing is full of *phonemic paraphasias* (substitutions based on pronunciation) and *semantic paraphasias* (substitutions based on meaning). For example, "bell" might be substituted with "dell" or with "ring, ring." Nonexistent words (*neologisms*) may also occur. The way in which words are put together (*syntax*) is largely preserved, giving the speech a normal, melodic sound. With close attention and knowledge of the patient, it is often possible for the listener to gain some meaning from a conversation. The patient may seem unconcerned about or even unaware of these problems, and often evinces confusion and an apparent loss of intelligent behavior, although these are difficult to assess given the patient's comprehension deficit. Although usually impossible to test, verbal memory (memory for words, conversations and stories) is often impaired as well,

[2]Wernicke, C. 1874. *Der Aphasische Symptomenkomplex*. Breslau: Cohn & Weigert (Translated in *Boston Studies in Philosophy of Science, 4*, 34–97).

especially if the temporal lobe damage is as extensive as it was in Irene's case.

Irene was almost a textbook case of Wernicke's aphasia. For the first week, most of the time she did not seem particularly upset or frustrated by her difficulties, and she happily chatted to visitors or medical staff whenever there was a gap in their conversation. Understandably, Daisy and Renie were very upset by the difficulty in communicating with her, and spent hours at her bedside struggling to make sense of what she was saying. They brought in her favorite books and were dismayed to find she could no longer read sensibly. Just like her spontaneous conversation, when she was shown a page of writing she attempted to read it aloud, but her words often came out as paraphasias, although occasionally she read single words correctly. She couldn't write sensibly either, and even when Renie asked her to write her own name, she only managed the "Ir" before hesitating and finally writing "eee." One day Renie brought in a child's picture book of "Cinderella" and Irene appeared delighted with it, pointing to the wicked stepmother and saying, "Bad girl, no mum, mother," then laughing and pointing at herself. Renie pointed to the word "Cinderella," and Irene looked puzzled until Renie pointed to a picture of Cinderella. Then she looked pleased and said "Severella, no not that one, call her Reen," pointing to her granddaughter.

The following transcript from a taped conversation I had with Irene about two weeks following her stroke provides a good illustration of her fluent but confused oral language and impaired comprehension, typical of Wernicke's aphasia.

Jenni: Do you remember acting in a play just before you had your stroke?
Irene: That is a good one, I know.
Jenni: Do you know what the play was called?

Irene: Oh yes, it's a girl but not the others.

Jenni: What others?

Irene: The mean ones and the matter, matter, the bigger one.

Jenni: Do you mean the sisters and the ugly stepmother?

Irene: Oh yes, I don't know that all right!

Jenni: What part did you play?

Irene: That one I could do.

Jenni: What about Renie? What part did she play?

Irene: That's not one of them—gracious, where is it all going?

Jenni: Do you know where you live?

Irene: By the tea over there [*pointing out the window to the harbor*].

Jenni: By the sea do you mean?

Irene: Something over there.

Jenni: Somewhere over there?

Irene: Can you make up that one? [*laughs*]

Jenni: I can't understand everything that you say. Do your words make sense to you?

Irene: No, not too much.

Jenni: It must be frustrating. Do you know in your head what you want to say?

Irene: No, yes, upside down. It works out then gets mus, musted, before it's there. And then the other one is not there.

Jenni: I think you're saying that on the way out the words get muddled and then you can't think of the next word.

Irene: Yes, something to do with that.

Over the next two weeks the nursing and occupational therapy staff tried to occupy her, taking her for walks and settling her in the patients' common room, where at first she chatted away to the other patients, although they couldn't understand much of what she was saying. She would look at magazines and picture books but could not read them, apart from picking out individual words here and there. By the third week she began to refuse to get out of bed, pushing the nurses away and even shouting unintelligibly at them. On one occasion she swept her full dinner plate and cup of tea off the table to spill across her bed, shouting at the nurse, "Go back from here, leave it, leave me." Pushing the table violently away, she lay down in her bed, tears streaming down her face.

Daisy was very concerned by this change in her mother's mood; before her stroke, even when all the chips were down she had managed to stay positive. When she had been diagnosed with breast cancer in her early fifties, she had not only courageously faced her own illness, surgery, and chemotherapy, but had initiated a fund-raising and support group for breast cancer victims. One of her initiatives had been to write a script for a humorous play about breast cancer. She gathered together a small group of breast cancer survivors and turned them into amateur actors. Every weekend for a number of weeks they entertained, educated, and gave hope to many women as they hammed it up for various local women's groups. Irene not only directed the play but was also one of the actors. Then two years after her final chemotherapy treatment, without warning, her husband died from a heart attack. Within three months, after a time of grieving, she was fully engaged in life again, enjoying her work as a librarian, working with the drama group, and spending quality time with her family and friends. Her retirement from the library on her 65th birthday had, for Irene, marked the next exciting phase in her life, allowing her to devote much more time to her beloved drama, a passion she now shared with her granddaughter.

And now Renie was the only person who could sometimes calm Irene when she withdrew and refused to eat or talk. It is impossible to know what Irene's thoughts and feelings were over this period. Had she lost her "inner speech" along with the ability to construct and understand coherent verbal language? If we cannot think and reason verbally, can we experience emotions fully? Depression often follows left hemispheric damage, and one hypothesis is that in nonbrain-damaged individuals the right hemisphere is "depressed" and the left hemisphere "happy" and the two balance each other. However, when the left hemisphere is damaged, the depressed mood of right hemisphere becomes dominant.[3] But perhaps a more likely explanation is that the language problems that often accompany left hemispheric damage cause such dreadful frustration that despair is almost sure to follow. For Irene, a woman who had gained so much fulfillment from reading and drama, the loss of her language must have been intolerable. Perhaps she didn't know "consciously" what had befallen her, but her depression indicates that she had some level of awareness.

Irene's many friends—especially those from the drama group she had given so much to over the years—visited daily, and the nurses had to keep a close watch to ensure she wasn't overwhelmed, especially given her struggle to understand them or to be understood. She became increasingly frustrated and upset by the conversations of the other patients and by staff as they went about their duties, so she was moved to a single room in the neurology ward. As Christmas drew near, many patients were discharged, and the nurses decorated the ward with tinsel and Christmas lights. A Christmas tree twinkled merrily in the patient's common room. Irene, who had always loved Christmas, remained locked in her sadness. After discussions with the family, her neurologist decided that she could be

[3] Janet, the patient described in Chapter 3, has hemineglect resulting from a right parietal lobe malignant tumor. Her inappropriate cheerfulness is a possible example of the reverse condition, where her mood is dominated by the intact "happy" left hemisphere.

discharged from Neurology on Christmas Day and stay with her daughter until early in the New Year. She would then be transferred to the rehabilitation unit, where she would continue to have speech therapy as well as physical and occupational therapy. But the family were prepared for the possibility that her language comprehension might not improve, since the stroke had damaged Wernicke's area irreversibly. After six weeks in the rehabilitation unit her case would be reviewed. At that point, if no further recovery seemed likely, the family would need to find a nursing home for her long-term care.

*****

Broca's aphasia and Wernicke's aphasia are perhaps the best-described acquired language disorders, but there are a number of other aphasia types. At the least impaired end of the aphasia "spectrum" are disorders of word finding. Ask anyone older than 60 and they will complain about their increasing difficulty in remembering people's names and even the names of common objects. They know they know the name, it's on the "tip of their tongue," but they can't quite capture it. Following localized brain damage to many areas of the left, "language" hemisphere, adult patients of any age can experience this same phenomenon, but often in a more extreme fashion. This mild type of aphasia is called *anomia*. At the other extreme is *global aphasia*, usually following a very extensive left hemisphere stroke that damages both Broca's and Wernicke's areas and the connections between them. Globally aphasic patients can neither speak fluently—not even using jargon like Irene—nor comprehend language. They can't repeat words nor read or write. Most have numbness and a weakness or paralysis of the right side of their body, because the massive lesion encroaches on both the motor and sensory strips.

Between these two extremes lies every possible variety of language disorder. Some language disorders—the *dyslexic* disorders—affect only writing, reading, or both, but not speech or comprehension of speech. The range of language impairments is hardly surprising given that the brain areas lesioned are rarely identical across patients. In addition, there are individual differences in the brain areas that mediate different language skills. Most notably, the area that mediates fluent speech extends beyond Broca's area in some people. This individual variation has been demonstrated during neurosurgery for epilepsy where the epileptic brain tissue is excised while the patient is awake. The brain itself has no pain sensors, so after a local anesthetic to numb the scalp and skull while the skull is opened, the neurosurgeon can stimulate different areas of the cortex to see if language or comprehension is interrupted in the awake patient; if it is, the corresponding area is not excised.

Although some patients, like Luke and Irene, have language disorders that fit one of the "classic" aphasia types rather well, in general the complexity of language disorders is not well served by labeling specific types of aphasia. In practical terms, it is often more useful simply to describe all the patient's impairments and to plan a rehabilitation program that addresses each impaired aspect of language in a way that is appropriate for that person. Concurrently, as with all rehabilitation programs that focus on neuropsychological impairments, it is important to address the psychosocial problems that result from the patient's changed status and to work actively toward preventing long-term psychosocial problems from developing in the future.

The ability to communicate with others is clearly one of the most valued functions we possess. Verbal language is generally considered the most important communication medium for humans, although there are cases of people who are unable to communicate verbally but can do so successfully in other ways. Often, however, even these nonverbal means of communicating are essentially a language. Sign languages of the deaf, for example, use the fingers, hands, and arms to produce letters and words and the visual or tactile system to receive the language, rather than using the tongue and mouth to produce language and the auditory system to receive it. If Irene had been skilled at sign language before her stroke, it is likely that she would have lost the ability to communicate in this medium as well as the ability to communicate using speech.

True nonverbal communication involves the expression and comprehension of gestures that have the same meaning for the communicator and the receiver and that cannot easily be expressed in words or with symbols. When Irene became angry and withdrawn, her daughter felt distressed because Irene was nonverbally communicating her frustration and sadness. The expression and understanding of emotions add richness to our relationships and communications, but our ability to use emotional, nonverbal communications to succeed and sometimes simply to survive in our complex human world is severely limited.

Presumably, the evolution of verbal language went hand in hand with the increasing ability of the human species to reason and think abstractly. Humans were thus able to increase the complexity of their mental, social and physical worlds. Modern humans could not survive in the world they have constructed without the ability to think and communicate with symbols and words. Emotional and other forms of nonverbal expression, although often communicating subtleties of meaning that words could never fully communicate, are nevertheless not specific enough to allow us to go about our daily activities easily and successfully.

The breakdown of language is devastating for the patient and distressing for everyone with whom the patient tries to communicate. Losing the ability to comprehend language appears, for a number of reasons, to be more disabling than losing the ability to express language while retaining the ability to comprehend it. When patients have severely impaired comprehension, their own expressed language becomes incomprehensible. When comprehension is reasonably intact, most individuals who are unable to speak or write fluently can find other, nonverbal ways to express themselves. In addition, if they can comprehend, it is likely that they have "inner speech" and can think and reason in words. Thus their inability to express themselves in words, although extremely frustrating and debilitating, is less likely to impinge on their sense of self, their intellect, and their personality.

Luke and Irene differed not only in the aphasias they had, but also in the types of lesion and the probable courses of recovery from that lesion. Luke's brain damage was caused by a hemorrhage into the brain tissue—a *hemorrhagic stroke*. As the blood was reabsorbed, many of the neurons that had been "stifled" by the blood began functioning again, although others were probably permanently damaged. Luke's youth may well have contributed to his ability to recover, both because of the relative plasticity of his brain—that is, other neurons were probably able to take on the functions of the damaged neurons—and because his health was generally good. Also, his energy levels and motivation to recover were high.

In contrast, Irene's stroke was caused by the blockage of an artery, preventing oxygen from reaching the neurons in a large area of cortex and resulting in their death—an *ischemic stroke*. Some patients with Wernicke's aphasia, especially if they are younger than Irene and manage to remain motivated during the long and tedious rehabilitation period, can show some improvement over time.

Substantial improvement would suggest either that some pockets of neurons were only transiently damaged rather than destroyed by the stroke or that, over time, other cortical areas were able to take over some functions. The form the aphasia or other cognitive impairment takes is related to the location of the damage, not the type of damage. The pattern of recovery or the rate at which the impairments worsen is, however, related to the type of damage. If Luke's lesion had resulted from an ischemic stroke that killed the neurons in Broca's area, he probably would not have recovered his speech to the same extent, and if Irene's aphasia had been caused by a hemorrhagic stroke into Wernicke's area, she might have recovered some of her language ability.

Although Luke's and Irene's loss of language—the cognitive ability that separates humans most clearly from all other animals—was the primary focus of this chapter, their very different stories illuminate a number of important issues. Brain damage does not respect race, culture, gender, or socioeconomic group. A massive stroke that affects the left side of the brain will render a physicist with private health insurance and a homeless drug addict paralyzed and aphasic in the same way, although of course the physicist will probably receive better medical care and rehabilitation. But if the brain damage is severe, no amount of rehabilitation will be able to repair the damage and return the sufferer to his or her former self. Fixing a broken mind requires a cooperative effort and a holistic approach, sometimes with rich rewards and sometimes with only tragedy at the end.

*****

On Christmas Eve, I arrived in Neurology and joined the small group of nurses, interns, night porters, and therapists gathered at the nursing station. At 9 p.m. all but the dim floor lights along the corridors were turned off, and as patients and their visitors sat in their darkened rooms, a long procession of nurses, each holding a candle, wound their way through the softly lit hospital corridors, their voices harmonizing as they sang their way through everyone's favorite Christmas carols. When they had gone, taking their Christmas blessings on to the next ward, I remained behind, chatting to the nurses and helping them eat a large Christmas cake brought in by a grateful family member. Then Daisy appeared, hurrying along the corridor.

"Have the carol singers been?" she asked when she reached us.

"Yes, they were lovely, as always," the nurse replied. "Have you come in to pick up Renie? She's in with her grandmother."

"I'm sorry I missed them; I felt I had to spend a little bit of time at my office party. All my workmates have been so understanding, and I've hardly seen them over the past three weeks," Daisy explained. "Did my mother enjoy the carols, do you think?" she added, her voice sounding a little sad.

The nurse smiled at her. "I'm sure she did. And tomorrow you'll have her home with you. I think she'll be much happier when she's back in a familiar place."

I was ready to leave as well, so I walked with Daisy down the corridor. I wanted to say my own goodbyes to Irene and Renie. We reached the open door of Irene's room and stopped. The room was dim, with the only light coming through the window from the streetlights far below. Renie was sitting by Irene's bed, a red hat with a bell perched on her head, her long blonde hair loose down her back. She was holding her grandmother's hand as Irene lay quietly, her eyes closed. At first I thought the singing was coming from the CD player, but then I realized it was Renie's sweet voice. Daisy looked at me, her eyes overflowing. I heard her whisper: "Irene used to sing that song to

Renie to send her to sleep when she was a little girl. Did you know that Irene means 'peace'?" She took my hand and squeezed it as we stood there listening.

> Irene, goodnight, goodnight,
> Irene goodnight,
> Goodnight Irene, goodnight Irene,
> I'll see you in my dreams.

Daisy moved quietly into the room to join her mother and daughter and I tiptoed away, home to my own family. During the night, while sleeping, Irene had a second massive stroke. She did not wake again.[4] For Daisy and Renie, it also brought a kind of peace. They knew the vivacious woman that had been Irene could never have been content living in a prison of meaningless words.

■ Further Reading

Fox Garrison, J. 2005. *Don't Leave Me This Way: Or When I Get Back on My Feet You'll Be Sorry.* New York: Harper Collins.

Ogden, J. A. 2005. The breakdown of language. Case studies of aphasia. In: *Fractured Minds: A Case-Study Approach to Clinical Neuropsychology, 2nd Ed.* (pp. 83–98). New York: Oxford University Press.

Pinker, S. 1994. *The Language Instinct: How the Mind Creates Language.* New York: William Morrow.

Sacks, O. 1970. The President's speech. In: *The Man Who Mistook His Wife for a Hat* (pp. 76–80). New York: Summit Books.

Sacks, O. 2010. Recalled to life. In: *The Mind's Eye* (pp. 32–52). New York: Knopf.

[4]Irene died more than 25 years ago and, because of the importance to her story of "her" song, I have retained her real given name. To protect her identity I have taken minor poetic license with other facets of her life, taking care to preserve the essence of her personality.

3 ■
Left Out, Right In! The Artist with Hemineglect

Late afternoon on a sunny Friday, Janet McKenzie ran her car into the left side of her garage doorway. She had spent the day at work, where she was the personal secretary for the boss of a small art supply company. As an amateur artist herself, she loved her job, and had become friendly with a number of local artists who bought their supplies from the company. But today had been especially pleasant because it was her birthday—she had achieved the half-century mark—and her work colleagues had not allowed such a milestone to go past unnoticed. They had decorated her office and even hung a "Happy Birthday" banner over the main entrance, and to her surprise, some of their artist customers had appeared at midday to join the small, close-knit group of employees in a celebratory birthday lunch.

So when she found herself jolting to a sudden stop at her garage door, she put it down to a lapse of attention because she was dreaming, not only of her lovely day but also about the birthday celebrations her family were planning in her honor that night. When George, her husband, suggested that perhaps she had overindulged at lunch, she laughed, saying she didn't think fruit juice could impair her judgment to that extent!

But that evening at her birthday party, something much stranger happened. When the time came to blow out the 50 candles on her large birthday cake, Janet blew out all the candles on the right side, leaving those on the left still burning. She seemed unaware of her bizarre behavior, and when George pointed to the still-burning candles, she remarked that they looked so pretty it seemed a shame to blow them out. Only after he told her that she wouldn't be able to cut the cake did she finally extinguish the candles on the left.

Two days later George heard thumping sounds in the bathroom and found Janet lying on the floor, dazed, disoriented, and incontinent. She was unable to describe what had happened, but it seemed likely that she had suffered a generalized seizure. He called an ambulance and she was admitted to the neurosurgery and neurology ward of Auckland Hospital, where a neurological examination revealed a sensory loss in her left arm, a mild left *hemiplegia* (weakness on one side of the body), a left visual field defect (a blind area at the left side of her visual field), and a tendency to ignore her left side. A computed tomography (CT) scan showed a large mass in the right parietal lobe of her brain. The following day the mass was biopsied. The histology results took a few days to come back, but confirmed the presence of a grade 2 astrocytoma, a malignant tumor of moderate aggressiveness. Janet was given steroids to reduce the swelling surrounding the tumor, and as a result her condition rapidly improved, so that by the time I first saw her she was no longer confused or disoriented.

*****

"Bed rounds" on neurosurgical wards can be depressing affairs, and this one was no exception: a young man with a serious spinal tumor, a woman with a subarachnoid hemorrhage lying motionless with a cold towel over her eyes, a gang member with a severe head injury and total unawareness of where he was or what had happened to him, and a mother of three school-age children who had to face the news that the results of the biopsy carried out a few days previously showed that her brain tumor was not the benign type she had been praying for.

But then we reached Janet's bed. She looked like a bright-eyed bird sitting propped against a pile of pillows, her short, dark hair sticking up haphazardly around a dressing on the right side of her head. One leg—her left—protruded from the white covers, looking rather uncomfortable hanging awkwardly over the side of the bed. She was wearing a pink nightgown and matching bed jacket, but her left arm was outside the bed jacket sleeve, and we could see that the strap of her nightgown had slipped down, revealing her left shoulder and in danger of slipping further to expose her left breast.

The nurse smiled and touched her bare shoulder. "Janet, how about putting your arm into the sleeve."

"No, thank you," replied Janet, her dark eyes twinkling up at the nurse. "I'd rather leave it like it is if you don't mind."

"It looks rather uncomfortable," the nurse commented, "and whatever will your visitors think?"

"Well," Janet said, her arm lying slack by her side, "I'm starting a new off-the-shoulder fashion. I would think it might cheer the visitors up."

"Let me help you; it's difficult to manage by yourself," cajoled the nurse, trying to keep a straight face.

Janet was laughing now but said in a firm tone, "Perhaps I'll do it later, but I think I'll leave it like this for now, if it's all the same to you doctors and nurses!"

As the nurse leaned over and rearranged Janet's attire so that it was somewhat more modest, the neurosurgeon looked across at me, standing in the huddle of people that accompanied him on his teaching rounds. "Jenni, would you like to give Janet some of your bedside tests, so we can get a better idea what's going on?"

I was about a year into collecting my data for my doctoral research on the bizarre neuropsychological disorder called *hemineglect*, and already it was clear that it was surprisingly common on this neurosurgery and neurology ward. So far I had discovered that almost half of the acute patients admitted with damage to one side—or hemisphere—of their brain ignored or neglected visual stimuli in the side of space opposite to their brain damage. Because hemineglect was more likely to be a problem for patients who had suffered a large stroke in the right hemisphere of the brain or, as in Janet's case, had a malignant tumor there, the neglected side was usually the left. But in most cases the neglect lasted only a few days, and as I already knew from having tested her the day before, patients with signs as dramatic as Janet's were relatively rare.

So here was an excellent teaching opportunity, and I was confident that the new intern and the nervous medical student would find Janet's performance on my simple paper-and-pencil hemineglect tests a fascinating introduction into the bizarre world of the disordered mind. It was only too common to find junior doctors so overwhelmed by the enormity of having to learn about the brain that they completely dismissed the importance of also learning about the mind. Their knowledge about the complex thinking functions at risk following brain damage seemed to stop at the smorgasbord of problems associated with dementia, a disorder that they conceptualized in a vague sort of way as a loss of memory and gradual dropping off of the intellect. Their understanding of more specific and, especially, less common cognitive (thinking) disorders was usually limited to a few facts about Broca's and Wernicke's aphasia, language disorders with odd names that they found interesting to observe but would leave to the speech pathologist to assess and treat.

I positioned Janet's table across her bed and, standing on her right, placed a simple screening test for visual hemineglect on it. I could almost feel the intern's impatience as he looked down at the horizontally positioned sheet of paper covered in randomly scattered short lines. A long way from the sophisticated tools of neurosurgery! I placed a pencil in Janet's right hand and asked her to cross out each line, holding the page steady for her as her left arm lay, apparently useless, at her side. She crossed the sixteen lines on the right of the page and then put her pencil down, leaving 22 lines on the left untouched.

"Have you crossed them all out?" I asked.

"Yes, I've got them all," she replied. "Can't you give me something harder than that? I'm not a five-year-old!" She chortled and winked at the medical student standing next to me.

The intern on her left offered his opinion. "She's got a left visual field defect, so she can't see the lines on the left. Look, she doesn't even seem to realize I'm standing over here." He was correct; Janet didn't turn toward his voice when he spoke but continued to look at me.

I slid the page horizontally across her table toward me so that it was on Janet's far right; that way her left visual field defect would be less likely to restrict her view of the paper. I tapped the page to attract her attention. "Janet, I want you to look at the page again and see if there are any lines you missed. If there are, draw a line through them."

Janet responded by crossing the same lines again, remarking, "I think I've crossed out some of these before."

Next I asked Janet to copy line drawings of a three-dimensional cube and a five-pointed star. In both cases she copied only the right sides of the models, and even these were muddled. (Figure 3.1 shows drawings by Janet and other hemineglect patients.) I then asked her to draw the numbers on a clock face, with the "12" already in place to ensure that her attention was directed to the correct starting point. She placed the "1" correctly, and then proceeded to put in the numbers "2" to "12" around the perimeter, but only on the right side and more closely spaced than on a clock, such that by "six o'clock" she had reached "10." She drew "11" and "12" falling off the bottom of the clock, leaving the entire left side empty (see Figure 3.1).

Finally I asked Janet to copy a simple line drawing of a scene consisting of, from right to left, a tree, a house, a fence, and another tree. She dutifully copied—albeit roughly—the tree on the right and then the house before putting her pencil down, saying she had finished (see Figure 3.2). I pointed to each of the items in the model drawing of the scene and asked her to name them. She did so correctly. I then asked her if she would draw in the fence.

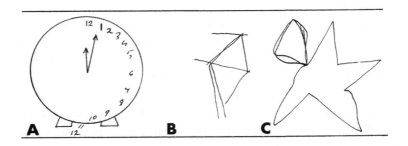

FIGURE 3.1
Drawing tests of hemineglect. *A:* Janet's attempt to place the numbers on a clock face. *B, C:* Copies of a cube and five-pointed star by other patients with left hemineglect.

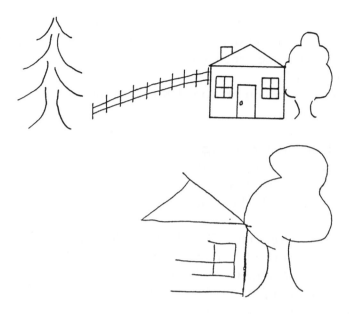

FIGURE 3.2
Asked to copy a simple scene (upper drawing), Janet drew only the right
side (lower drawing) and said she had copied it all.

"Well, I will if you really want me to, but it will probably blow down in the next wind!" she replied, drawing a
rough version of the fence.

"Now copy the rest of the scene," I requested.

"That really is all I can draw," she insisted.

I pointed to the tree on the left.

"That tree? I can't draw trees," she informed me, and I
could not induce her to draw it.

The neurosurgeon then took over and tested the strength
and sensation in Janet's arms and legs. To a casual observer,
it appeared that Janet was hemiplegic—that is, that her
entire left side was paralyzed. But the neurosurgeon was
not fooled. "At worst she's got a mild weakness and significant sensory loss in her left arm, but her left leg is probably
not weak. It's difficult to be certain given her neglect."

"How do you know it's neglect?" asked the intern. "Look, she doesn't use her left arm at all, and she couldn't raise her left leg when you asked her to. Surely that's a hemiplegia?"

"Janet, can you lift your left arm in the air?" asked the neurosurgeon.

Janet did so, although she raised it slowly, and it quickly fell to her side again.

"Good," praised the doctor. "Now lift both your arms high in the air." Janet's right arm rose but her left arm remained slack by her side. "Put your left arm up as well," he reminded her.

"No, it won't move," said Janet, "Bloody hunk of meat. When I get home I will give it a piece of my mind."

The neurosurgeon lent over and pinched Janet sharply on her right upper arm. "Stop that," she said. She lifted her left arm, somewhat sluggishly, and tried to smack his hand away.

The neurosurgeon looked over at the intern and grinned. "Doesn't seem too hemiplegic to me," he remarked. He turned back to Janet. "Let's get you out of bed and see what your walking is like."

With support, Janet managed to walk reasonably well using both legs, but then, chuckling loudly, she began to hop, holding her left leg off the ground. "It's a good job I used to be an acrobat in a circus, because it helps me put my knickers on when I'm standing on one leg!" she remarked.

"Why are you hopping?" I asked.

"Well, how else am I to get around?" she replied, looking pleased with herself.

As we left Janet's room and formed a group in the corridor, the medical student turned to me, her voice excited.

"That's amazing! Is that hemineglect? We were told about that in a psychology lecture, but I thought it was one of those rare disorders that we'd never see."

*****

Hemineglect, also known as *unilateral spatial neglect, unilateral inattention,* or simply *neglect,* has as its main symptom an apparent unawareness or unresponsiveness to stimuli in the side of space opposite the brain damage. In behavioral terms, when we see left hemineglect as a consequence of a right hemisphere lesion ("lesion" is a term used to indicate any type of localized brain damage), what we observe is a patient who misses the words on the left side of a page when reading, writes only down the right side of the page, ignores or is uncharacteristically rude to people standing on the left, collides with the left wall when walking down a corridor, turns only to the right when walking or using a wheelchair, puts on makeup or shaves only on the right half of the face, and in severe cases, eats only the dinner on the right side of the plate and then complains of being hungry! Usually "side of space," or *hemispace,* is defined as the side to the left (or right) of the patient's body midline, but sometimes when an object is neglected, it appears that the patient mentally divides the object itself in half, even if the entire object is on the patient's "good" side, and then neglects the side opposite her brain lesion. Thus when Janet was asked to copy a cube, she copied the right side only, and as I discovered later on more detailed testing, she did this even when the model was displayed in her right hemispace. Although neglect can occur following both left and right hemispheric damage, the more severe and lasting cases usually follow right hemispheric lesions, very often large lesions involving the parietal lobe in the posterior half of the brain and encroaching on the subcortical basal ganglion structures lying deep within the brain.

Cats and monkeys can also demonstrate neglect of the side of space opposite a brain lesion, but their neglect occurs just as often on the right as on the left, because in nonhuman animals the two brain hemispheres are very similar in the functions they mediate. This contrasts with the human brain, where in the majority of people the left hemisphere is dominant for verbal functions and the right hemisphere for spatial, nonverbal functions.

In humans, neglect of visual stimuli seems to be the most common form of the disorder, probably because vision is our dominant sense. But neglect of sounds (*auditory neglect*) and of touch (*tactile neglect*) can also occur. Neglect of the limbs opposite the brain-damaged side is also quite common (*body* or *motor neglect*), which can interfere with rehabilitation when teaching patients to walk on the neglected leg or use the neglected arm, even if their limbs are not physically weak. Whatever function or modality is neglected, it is clear that the neglect is not the result of physical problems caused by the brain damage, although physical difficulties often also occur, making the diagnosis of neglect difficult. For example, many patients who have a large lesion in the posterior part of either side of their brain often have some damage to the optic tract, resulting in their field of view being blocked out on the opposite side. Thus when they look straight ahead they will have a blind section, or visual field defect—sometimes a complete semicircle called a *hemianopia*—on one side. But if they move their eyes or their whole head toward the blind section, the intact part of their visual field will move as well. Thus people with a visual field defect often learn to compensate by moving their head and eyes. In contrast, a patient with left hemineglect may continue to ignore objects on the left or the left side of objects even if the head and eyes are moved toward the object or if the whole object is placed in the intact right visual field.

Similarly, the motor strip in the cortex (the outer layer of neurons of the brain), controls movement of different parts of the body, and if the arm "area" of the motor strip on the right is damaged by the lesion, the left arm will be weak or paralyzed. But patients who *neglect* their own limbs will seem reluctant to use them, so that the limbs appear physically weak, even if there is no damage to the motor strip and they are not, in fact, physically weak. Thus Janet's left leg hung out of the bed, and her left arm lay unmoving by her side. But sometimes she moved a limb without thinking, for example, when she tried to stop the doctor from pinching her arm. Janet probably did have a small degree of physical weakness of her left arm, but not enough to explain her apparent severe hemiplegia.

However, although her refusal to raise her arm appeared to be a conscious and almost defiant action, it was not one she had unambiguous voluntary control over. Neglect is a neuropsychological disorder known as a "higher cognitive disorder" because it involves a disruption of higher-order thinking. A lower cognitive order would be, for example, visually perceiving the form of an object without "thinking" about what it does or how it is related to other objects. Janet's inattention to sensations and limbs on her left was not a consequence of her deciding to be difficult. It was even more intriguing and hard to understand when we heard her making excuses—often ridiculous ones—for not using her limbs, such as "It's a good job I used to be an acrobat in a circus" or "I'm starting a new fashion." Perhaps when patients find themselves suddenly bereft of some ability that they have previously taken for granted, and can see no obvious cause for it—for example, they don't have a broken arm—they try to rationalize it for their own peace of mind. But this is not the whole story, since even neuropsychologists who know all about neglect can display it, just like Janet, if they sustain the appropriate brain lesion. Indeed, some days later, after her neglect had been explained to Janet, I heard her telling a friend all about the disorder while continuing to neglect her own left arm, and complaining that the nurses had forgotten to bring her a cup of tea although it was in clear view on the bedside table to her left.

Curiously, patients like Janet, with left-sided neglect from a right hemispheric lesion, not uncommonly joke about their problems, and in cases where this is extreme or clearly inappropriate, it suggests a lack of awareness about the seriousness of their condition that itself seems to be the result of the right hemispheric lesion. Some researchers have even hypothesized that the right hemisphere is the "depressive" hemisphere and the left hemisphere the "happy" one. They suggest that when the left hemisphere is damaged, the healthy right hemisphere may dominate emotional expression, resulting in the "catastrophic" depressive reaction sometimes seen following left hemispheric damage. When the right hemisphere is damaged, as in Janet's case, the patient may appear indifferent or even amused by the resulting disorder, perhaps because the damaged "depressed" hemisphere cannot appropriately moderate emotional responses. Whatever the cause, patients with neglect often seem amused by their own comments.

*****

I had met Janet for the first time the day before the teaching round, four days after she had been admitted to hospital. To judge how any sort of brain damage has affected a person's mind and personality, it is important to determine, as carefully as possible, what that person was like and what his or her cognitive strengths and weaknesses were prior to the brain damage. Often family and friends are the best source of this information, supplemented with knowledge about formal qualifications, vocation, and hobbies, all viewed within the appropriate cultural context. Thus when I arrived at Janet's bedside and introduced myself, I was pleased to find her husband with her, which gave me the opportunity to gather information about what Janet was like when she was well—information that Janet herself might not have been be able to provide very reliably, given her neurological status.

George described her as an energetic, intelligent woman with a great sense of humor. Janet told me she had left school when she was 17 and had worked as a typist before marriage. They had two children, and during their school years Janet was an active member of various community groups and enjoyed amateur landscape painting and pottery. When she was 45 she enrolled in a part-time course in business management at the local polytechnic institution and completed the course with excellent grades two years later. Since then she had been working full-time in the art supply company.

So from this information I knew that before her tumor grew large enough to affect her in such a dramatic way, she was of above-average intelligence, socially capable, and judging from her artistic hobbies, she very likely had well-developed visuospatial abilities (e.g., conceptualizing and drawing objects in space). This last might be especially important given the site of her tumor in the right parietal lobe, as this area of cortex is important in the mediation of general visuospatial abilities. Thus if she now performed poorly on drawing tasks I could be reasonably confident this was a result of her brain damage and not because she had always been poor at drawing—a common excuse given by hemineglect patients!

Two days earlier, Janet had undergone a burr-hole biopsy—a procedure where a small hole is made in the skull to allow the surgeon to remove a sample of the tumor tissue for pathological analysis. Janet had recovered well and was keen to do a few standard neuropsychological tests. Indeed, she told me that she didn't think there was much the matter with her and seemed unconcerned about the mass in her head that she had been told was probably a malignant tumor. This lack of concern was clearly not a result of confusion, because on a series of tests designed to give an estimate of verbal intelligence she scored in the "Superior" range, and her scores on tests of verbal abstraction were particularly impressive. These results demonstrated that her frontal lobes, the areas that are most important in mediating these abilities, had not been affected by her tumor.

Patients with large frontal lesions can display an indifference to or denial of their illness, but so can patients with parietal lesions, especially those who also have neglect. This disorder is called *anosognosia*, a word that like many neuropsychological terms is more easily remembered if broken into its parts. The root of the word, *gnosia*, means "knowledge," prefixing it with an *a-* turns it into *agnosia*, or "no knowledge," and prefixing it with *anoso-* turns it into anosognosia, or "denial of knowledge." Anosognosia can refer to a denial of illness shown by behaviors such as a wheelchair-bound stroke patient with no movement in his left limbs saying that he will be back at work as a builder within a week and appearing to believe this, or a patient's denying that a body part—usually a limb that has a loss of sensation or is paralyzed or neglected—belongs to her.

For example, at one point, Janet pointed to her left arm, which had a loss of sensation and usually lay motionless by her side. "Remove that arm from my bed!" she demanded.

"But it's your arm," I explained.

Janet laughed and agreed, "Well, you could be right I suppose, but it doesn't seem to belong to me!"

Another variant of the same disorder is termed *misoplegia*, or "dislike of the hemiplegic limb." Janet displayed this when she called her arm a "bloody hunk of meat."

Because the logical, sequential type of thinking required for mathematics and for verbal abilities is mediated more by the left than the right hemisphere, I was intrigued to discover that Janet scored poorly on mental arithmetic problems. But when I explored her difficulties further by asking her to do some simple additions on paper that required carrying figures from one column to the next, it became evident that her problem was a result of her left spatial neglect. For example, in solving 128 + 394, she added 8 to 4 correctly and correctly placed the "2" of the "12" under the right-hand column, but she placed the "1" below the "2" rather than carrying it over to the middle column. She then added 2 and 9 together and wrote "11" in front of the "2." She neglected the "1" and "3" on the left of the numbers entirely, giving a final answer of 112! Whether she was doing sums in her head or on paper, her errors arose because she was unable to carry numbers over to the left and also neglected numbers on the left. In contrast, an *acalculia* ("not able to calculate"), resulting from a left hemispheric lesion, is an inability to understand how to perform calculations by using logical thinking, for example, a difficulty understanding the concepts of "subtract" and "divide."[1]

I gave Janet a book to read aloud, and she proceeded to read fluently but missed two or three words on the left of every line. When the passage clearly did not make sense, she would occasionally insert a word that was not on the page. A year later, her daughter said she would receive letters from her mother written down the right side of the page. Her writing was also difficult to read because of her tendency to repeat some letters. For example, when writing "Janet" she would reiterate the curves of the "n" three or four times, and when writing "hospital" she would repeat the "l" a number of times. Although this could be viewed as *perseveration* (i.e., repeating the same behavior), which is commonly associated with frontal lobe pathology, the reiteration of letters in cursive writing is also found following right parietal lesions. In these patients, it is categorized as a type of *spatial agraphia*, a problem with the spatial aspects of writing.

---

[1] Julian, the man described in Chapter 5, has a true acalculia.

On visual tests that clearly involved spatial functions, such as completing jigsaw puzzles of objects where the object was not known and putting colored blocks together to form the same pattern as in a model, Janet's performance was abysmal—not that this worried her in the least, although her husband looked very concerned! Indeed, her attempts were so bad that they demonstrated not only neglect of the left side, but also a more generalized inability with spatial concepts, which is common following parietal lesions of either hemisphere but more pronounced after right parietal lesions.

Another task I gave Janet showed that her neglect was not just for scenes, objects, and pictures in the real world, but also affected her imaginary world. I asked Janet to imagine walking through the door of her bedroom and describing the furniture in front of her and on each side of the room. According to her husband, she correctly named all the furniture in the room but said everything was on the right side. When asked what was on her left, she replied, "Nothing much, except I think a window." I then asked her to draw in the furniture on a plan (top down) view of her bedroom, with the doorway placed at the top so that the side of the room she had previously imagined was to her right was now on the left of the page and vice versa. She drew the bed, the chest of drawers, a couch, and the shower and toilet cubicles all in the opposite side of the room, now on the right side of the page.

On verbal memory tests where Janet was asked to remember lists of words and short stories, her performance was excellent, but on nonverbal tests where she was asked to look at designs and then draw them from memory, she scored poorly. As verbal memory is primarily a function of the left temporal lobe and nonverbal spatial memory a function of the right temporal lobe, this made sense. Although her tumor did not appear to encroach directly on her temporal lobe, which lies directly below the parietal lobe, it may well have affected it given the size of the tumor and the swelling around it, as well as the connections and interactions between the different lobes of the hemisphere. In addition, Janet's left neglect meant that she would not attend to the left of the designs and thus not remember them. However, she had no difficulty with some nonverbal visual tasks such as remembering faces; she recognized me each time she saw me. As research has shown, perception and recall of human faces is a very specialized sort of nonverbal memory, and thus her intact ability here was not a surprise.[2]

I wondered if, when she looked at faces, she saw only half of them. So one morning I asked her if I could draw something on her face using a black eyeliner brush. She looked slightly surprised, but agreed, perhaps thinking I had finally taken complete leave of my senses. I drew a large black circle on her right cheek and a large black cross on her left cheek, and then pushed her wheelchair into the bathroom, where there was a large mirror.

"What do you think?" I asked her.

"Funny-looking makeup is what I think! Why did you draw that on my cheek?"

"Draw what?" I asked.

"That bloody circle. It looks ridiculous."

"Yes, I suppose it does rather. Is there anything else that looks ridiculous?"

"No. Isn't that enough?" she replied, making a face at her reflection.

"What about your other cheek, the other side of your face. Is there anything wrong with that?"

"Not that I can see. Are you trying to trick me again?"

"No. But I did draw a big cross on your left cheek, here," I said, placing my finger on the cross. "Can you see it now?"

---

[2]Michael, the man described in Chapter 6, has prosopagnosia, an inability to recognize familiar faces.

"Perhaps I can, I don't know. But I'd like to get rid of that silly circle if you don't mind."

"OK. Here's a tissue with makeup remover on it. You wipe the black marks off your face," I told her. She took the tissue and scrubbed vigorously at the black circle.

"And what about the black cross?" I reminded her. At that, she made one casual wipe across her left cheek, leaving most of the cross still visible.

"That will have to do," she said. So I cleaned off the cross and wheeled her back to her bed.

On a later occasion when I tested her, Janet demonstrated another bizarre aspect of hemineglect. When I showed her a picture of a symmetrical object such as a desk, she identified it correctly, but of course she could do this from the details on the right only. More surprisingly, when shown a picture of a toothbrush with the handle on the right side of the picture, she also identified it correctly, demonstrating that she must have attended to the brush on the left side of the picture. However, when she was shown a picture of a car colliding with a tree that was on the left side of the picture, she identified it only as a car, and neglected to comment on the fact that it had crashed into a tree. So it seemed that she could be motivated to attend to the left side of drawings of objects only if she could not identify an object from the information on the right side of the drawing.

Janet did not always ignore people standing to the left of her bed, as do some patients with neglect. One man I assessed would either completely ignore his visitors if they stood on his left side or swear at them. As soon as they came around to his right side, he would greet them warmly. On one occasion, I made the mistake of sitting down on his left side to test him. I managed to get his attention, but when I asked if he would cross out lines on a page (he had done this before), he snarled, "I'm not doing any more of your stupid tests, so shove off." I asked him if he would like me to sit on his other side, and he replied, "Well, that would certainly be better for me, wouldn't it!" I moved around to his right side, and he smiled at me and happily began the crossing-out-lines test. He still neglected the lines on the left of the page, but his attitude toward me remained pleasant. According to his family, his "normal" personality was mild and kind, and he never swore.

When Janet's biopsy results came back, she was scheduled to have the tumor "debulked"—as much of it removed as possible—before starting radiotherapy treatment. A follow-up CT scan five days postoperation showed that the tumor was considerably smaller and the swelling much reduced as a result of her ongoing medication with steroids. At this point and again three months later, I repeated some of the visuospatial and neglect tests. She demonstrated a marked reduction of neglect and a small improvement on tests of visuospatial construction, such as copying patterns using blocks. Her copies of drawings remained muddled, but five days postoperation she copied the fence on the scene test spontaneously, although she still neglected the left tree. After considerable encouragement, on the crossing-out-lines test, she crossed all but three of the lines on the extreme left side. She was still inclined to ignore her left limbs, but she would raise her left arm and walk using both legs if asked to do so. She still frequently collided with the left wall or left side of a doorway, and throughout her illness was never able to compensate for her left visual field defect.

*****

When Janet began rehabilitation, soon after the operation to debulk her tumor, two bracelets with bells were put on her left arm to see if the noise they made would draw her attention to that arm. She was taught to talk herself through tasks; for example, when walking, she was to say to herself, "right leg forward, right heel and toe down, left leg forward, left heel and toe down." When writing or reading, she was encouraged to tie a bright red ribbon around her left wrist and to move her left arm on the table at the side of the paper or book. She was to tell herself to look toward the red ribbon whenever she reached the right side of a line. Janet's family were all instructed in these techniques and told to interact with her from her left side as much as possible.

Janet's neglect declined significantly over the three-month period of her initial rehabilitation, and her awareness of her left limbs improved markedly. As is often the case, it is impossible to say how much of her recovery was due to spontaneous recovery (and the debulking and shrinking of her tumor and its surrounding swelling by surgery, radiotherapy, and steroids) and how much was due to active rehabilitation. There is a view that rehabilitation should begin early if neglect persists for a month or more, to ensure that the patient receives training that will stimulate appropriate synaptic reconnections (i.e., connections between neurons) and lessen the possibility of the patient's developing behaviors and movements that foster faulty connections.

Five months after her operation, Janet returned to her job on a part-time basis, but she was unable to function at her previous level. She could not find her own way to work, and indeed was unable to go anywhere outside her own backyard without someone to guide her. When her husband decided to test her by asking her to direct him while he was driving from their home to her workplace, she got them hopelessly lost, although she had driven the route herself hundreds of times both as driver and, since her illness, as passenger. Maps didn't help, and even traveling on a bus was a problem, because she quickly became disoriented and didn't know where to alight. Even if the bus driver told her where to get off, she would then be left standing on the sidewalk with no idea which way to turn. Of course, if she had to make a decision, she would turn right, and not left! Even at work she frequently lost her way when taking messages from one floor to another in her office building. Although some of this difficulty, especially in the early and late stages of her illness, was related to her ignoring turns to the left, her spatial disorientation problems were more general than that.

Once she got to work, she was faced with other conundrums. For example, she was no longer able to use the word processor to type memos because her left hand was too clumsy to touch-type, and when she tried to type with two fingers or her right hand only, she was very slow to find letters on the left side of the keyboard. Although she generally remained optimistic—or as her husband commented to me, unrealistic—she did at times become upset by what she perceived as the charity her employers were extending in allowing her to continue in her position. By the time Janet was finally forced to resign from her job, her visual and motor neglect had increased again to a severity that equaled that when she was first admitted to the hospital. This time it did not spontaneously recover, and rehabilitation was to no avail.

*****

Following Janet's initial admission to the hospital, Janet and George's lives were dominated by the health system. Janet's surgery was followed by daily trips to the hospital as an outpatient for radiotherapy treatment that made her nauseated and constantly tired, then by time-consuming and exhausting visits to the physical therapist and occupational therapist three times a week for three months of rehabilitation, along with her regular checkups with the neurosurgeon. George dreaded these visits to the surgeon, fearing each time that they would be told that Janet's tumor had increased in size again.

But when, two years after her surgery, they were given the news that a CT brain scan confirmed extensive regrowth of the tumor, Janet remained calm. She refused further medical treatment other than steroids to help reduce the swelling around the tumor, but agreed to return to physical therapy for two months. However, it soon became apparent to the therapist that Janet's hemiplegia and neglect were too severe for rehabilitation. Accepting her invalid status with limited awareness, and with George taking early retirement to look after her, Janet spent her time watching television and talking to family and friends who visited her. Most days George would set her up at the kitchen table with large sheets of paper stapled to a board, and with a palette of paints and brushes on her right. She would work happily for an hour or so painting vague scenes, and sometimes the right sides of faces, all squashed into the right side of the paper. George called it her "Picasso phase," as Janet could no longer conceptualize how a tree or a face should be put together, even on its right side.

A year after she left her job she stopped taking steroids, which had caused her face to swell, and her behavior became increasingly inappropriate as the months wore on, possibly as a result of the tumor and swelling encroaching on the frontal lobe. Her speech became *dysarthric* (slurred) as a result of a left-sided facial weakness, but she retained her conversational ability, and her unabated sense of humor, while often bizarre, proved a blessing for her family and friends in her final months.

When Janet died, four long and difficult years following her diagnosis, George became quite seriously depressed, partly as a grief reaction to Janet's tragic illness and death, and partly because he suddenly found himself with nothing worthwhile to do with his life. He no longer had Janet to care for day and night, and he had given up his job. After seeing a clinical psychologist for several months, he gradually began socializing again and took up some new hobbies. His life took on new meaning when his daughter asked if he would look after her two preschool children four days a week while she worked. After caring for Janet, he found two healthy and active kids fun to care for, and his helper role at the local play school soon banished any hint of depression.

Janet's neglect and other visuospatial problems were caused by a malignant tumor, which although impeded in its growth by surgery and radiotherapy, ultimately caused her death. Certainly Janet initially benefited from surgical and steroid treatment, followed by rehabilitation, but because her brain damage was not static (as in a stroke), any rehabilitation gains were only short-term. In cases like this, surely only the patients and those who care for them can decide what level of treatment and rehabilitation, if any, is worthwhile. If in the final months or weeks the patient would prefer to watch television soap operas, listen to music, or even just sleep, rather than repeating "research-driven" and clever—but tedious— tests or "therapeutic" exercises three times a week, then their own choices are surely the best "rehabilitation" they can have. But it never fails to move me when a patient with so little time left willingly agrees to participate in research, knowing that it can never help them, simply because they want to help others. Getting to know these courageous and generous people is surely the most humbling and rewarding aspect of the work of any clinician or clinical researcher.

■ Further Reading

Genova, L. 2011. *Left Neglected*. New York: Gallery.
Heilman, K. M., R. T. Watson, and E. Valenstein. 2003. Neglect and Related Disorders. In: K. M. Heilman and E. Valenstein,

eds. *Clinical Neuropsychology, 4th Ed.* (pp. 296–346). New York: Oxford University Press.

Ogden, J. A. 2005. Out of mind, out of sight: A case of hemineglect. In: *Fractured Minds: A Case-Study Approach to Clinical Neuropsychology, 2nd Ed.* (pp. 113–136). New York: Oxford University Press.

4 ■
The CEO Has Left the Building: Control and the Frontal Lobes

Phillipa batted her eyes at the doctor who was standing with me at her bedside. "You're pretty cute. When I get out of this place—wherever I am—we could have a good time together."

"So where do you think you are?" asked the recipient of her attentions. He, along with everyone else on the ward, was well accustomed to Phillipa's inappropriate behaviors.

"It's no bloody hotel, that's for sure—too many bloody beds in the room. So you tell me, smarty-pants!"

"You're in Auckland Hospital, in the neurosurgery ward. You came in nearly two months ago now; don't you remember?" the doctor replied, grinning at her.

"Of course I remember. What do you think I am, a bloody idiot?" Phillipa looked annoyed for a moment but then chuckled. Her face was marked by deep scars, and her inch or so of brownish hair was not yet long enough to conceal the surgical scars on the left side of her scalp.

"No, we know you're brighter than most of us in here." The doctor nodded his head toward me. "This is Jenni Ogden; she's a psychologist. Tell her what you used to do."

Phillipa scowled at me. "Who are you? Another one of these school inspectors all over the place? You know what I am. I'm a teacher, and I don't need you coming to check up on me."

"Hullo, Phillipa," I said. "I'm not an inspector. I'm just a student. I'm doing some research in psychology for my PhD and wanted to talk to you about possibly being involved in my study."

"PhD, huh. That's pretty bright. You and me could run rings around this bloke here. Fancies himself as a doctor. But he's cute; gotta give him that."

*****

I was in the early stages of my doctorate, and Phillipa was the first patient I assessed who displayed many of the bizarre behaviors that commonly follow severe damage to the frontal lobes. I had read her file, and in fact had already seen her in action when assessing other women in the same room. She would greet anyone who passed by her bed by calling out loudly: "Hullo, you there. Come over here and talk to me." It did not seem to matter to Phillipa whom she greeted in this manner: another patient's visitor, a doctor she did not know, or the woman who cleaned the floor. Most people looked embarrassed, replied with a brief "Hullo," and moved rapidly away. Their exits would be punctuated by loud swearing from Phillipa or comments such as "You snaky bastard, run for your life!" On one occasion I had seen the nurse quickly pulling the curtain around her bed after Phillipa began to undress, gaily unconcerned about exposing her naked self to the other patients and their visitors.

But this was the first time I had met her formally, as I hoped she would now have recovered sufficiently from her dreadful head injuries and subsequent surgery—almost two months previously—to cope with my neuropsychological tests. She had been brutally beaten over the head with an iron bar when she surprised a burglar who had broken into the primary school where she taught. It was a Saturday afternoon and she had gone to the deserted school to catch up on some work preparation. By chance, the headmaster also decided to do some weekend work and, coming in shortly after the assault and finding clear signs of a break-in, discovered Phillipa lying in a pool of blood and deeply unconscious. Without doubt, she would have died if she had lain there much longer. The frontal bone of her skull had been shattered, and the underlying brain was badly damaged on the left. To save her life the neurosurgeon had to do what amounted to a partial left frontal lobectomy—cutting away the anterior part of her left frontal lobe, the *prefrontal lobe*. Fortunately, the more posterior cortex of the frontal lobe wasn't damaged, preserving Phillipa's ability to speak. She had sustained some moderately severe damage to the right prefrontal lobe as well, so it was not surprising that she was left with a severe "frontal lobe syndrome."

Her assaulter was caught and jailed for many years, but Phillipa's term was for life. She was only 35 when the assault happened, an intelligent woman with a university degree in English literature who worked as a primary school teacher in a small town north of Auckland. She and Larry, her husband, had led a busy life with their two children, just eight and 10 years old. Physically, Phillipa recovered very quickly from her head injury and neurosurgery. Within a month, although weak down her right side, she was able to sit up in bed or in a wheelchair. Her physical

disability paled into insignificance compared with her cognitive and psychological problems. I met with Larry to find
out about the Phillipa he had known before her brain
damage.

"She was a practical, positive person who didn't suffer
fools gladly. She could do three things at once and hardly
ever seemed to get tired or uptight, even when the kids
were acting up and she had another two hours' marking to
do," Larry told me, his eyes sad. "And although she had a
great sense of fun, and the kids in her class loved her, she
was really pretty conventional. I think that's what is hardest about these changes in her personality. She's so—well,
immodest—now sometimes." He blushed, and then stumbled on. "She would never have sworn in public like she
does now, and before, she would never get undressed in
front of people, not even in front of our own children. I
know it's just her brain damage talking, but if she continues like this I can't see how we could cope with her at
home."

*****

The prefrontal lobes include the area of frontal cortex from
the brain's frontal poles extending back to, but not including, the motor association cortex, where motor plans are
formed. Also included are the basomedial portions of the
frontal lobes, that is, the base or underside of the frontal
lobe just above the eyes and the strip of frontal cortex on
the medial or inside of each brain hemisphere. These basomedial areas of the prefrontal lobe are closely associated
with emotion. The prefrontal lobes are the most recently
evolved part of the mammalian brain; relative to other pri-
mates, humans have large prefrontal lobes. From birth,
connections between the prefrontal lobes and the upper
part of the brain stem and thalamus allow the state of alertness and therefore the attentiveness of the individual to be

controlled. But the rich connections between the prefrontal cortex and all the other lobes in the posterior part of the brain—the parietal, temporal, and occipital lobes—develop more gradually and in the human do not reach full maturity until the late teens or early twenties. It is these connections that permit the prefrontal lobes to formulate, modify, plan, organize, and execute purposeful, goal-directed, appropriate behaviors based on the complex and integrated sensory information received from the outside world via the posterior cortex.

For this reason modern neuropsychologists have labeled the prefrontal lobes the *executive lobes*—the CEO of the thinking brain, where the highest and most complex cognitive activities take place. A person with frontal lobe damage who is involved in a well-learned, highly structured, concrete task will probably experience no difficulty. If the task is new, unstructured, and requires planning a strategy to initiate and complete the task, or if it involves thinking in terms of abstract concepts, then the person with frontal lobe dysfunction may well show deficits. Some neuropsychologists who work with children have even suggested that teenagers suffer from a type of inbuilt "frontal lobe syndrome" because their frontal lobes have not reached maturity and their behaviors at times reflect this! Gaining an understanding of how the frontal lobes work and their slowness to mature might help parents and teachers empathize with teenagers and cope with their behaviors more effectively and with less stress on both sides. Aggressive, impulsive, risky, and thoughtless behaviors, emotional swings, poor planning, and a careless disregard for consequences are all classic frontal lobe—and teenager—symptoms. In most cases, as long as teenagers and young adults can avoid real frontal lobe damage from closed head injuries—which, ironically, are common at this period of their lives in part because of their immature frontal lobes—their frontal lobe CEO will soon come fully on line and they will develop into sensible, healthy adults.

Executive thinking impairments are more common than any other type of cognitive problem following brain damage and brain disease. These problems may be mild to severe, and different combinations of deficits occur in different patients. Patients are said to have the frontal lobe syndrome based on the presence of a recognized pattern of neuropsychological and behavioral impairments, not on neuropathology. Although brain imaging of patients who display a severe frontal lobe syndrome may show a large area of damage in both frontal lobes, sometimes there is no obvious damage. In addition to patients whose frontal lobes have been damaged by a tumor, stroke, a penetrating object like a bullet, or, as in Phillipa's case, an assault with an iron bar, frontal lobe executive problems are common in alcoholics and people who sustain closed head injuries or have various forms of dementia, including Alzheimer's, Parkinson's, and Huntington's diseases. Thus assessment of frontal lobe functioning is as integral a part of a basic neuropsychological assessment as is the assessment of verbal and visuospatial abilities and memory functions.

Phillipa's left prefrontal lobe was removed surgically because it was so severely damaged that it was no longer functional, and if left to "mend" itself, the extensive scar tissue would almost certainly cause severe epilepsy. This reason for removing this part of the brain is very different from that of decreasing psychiatric symptoms, which has been used to justify the surgical removal of healthy prefrontal lobes. Such *psychosurgery* has a rather black history. In the 1930s and 1940s, a *frontal lobotomy*—the removal of the prefrontal lobes or their disconnection from the rest of the brain—was a relatively common treatment for some psychiatric disorders. But it soon became apparent that for many patients the results of the lobotomy—usually a passivity and the destruction of the ability to think creatively—were worse than the disorder it was meant to alleviate. Although psychosurgery for the purpose of alleviating psychiatric symptoms decreased substantially from the 1950s on, a modified procedure called a *leucotomy*, where the frontal lobes are partially disconnected from the rest of the cortex, is still carried out in some centers. These operations are reported to provide relief from some psychiatric symptoms, such as severe, intractable depression, with minimal frontal lobe symptoms.

*****

It was impossible to predict how Phillipa would react to anyone who came to see her, whether they were health professionals or family and friends. So when I returned to her bedside alone, I was relieved when she expressed enthusiasm to take part in my research; she thereafter greeted me with delight whenever I appeared. In fact, if I went into the room to see one of the other patients, she would yell across the room at me, demanding that I come and see her. Phillipa's university degree in English literature provided strong grounds for an estimation of a superior verbal intelligence prior to her brain damage, and her conversational language was certainly still fluent, although she did have a word-finding problem, common after any significant damage to the left hemisphere, often characterized as being dominant for language.

"I can't think of the word," she would complain, but then she might try some *circumlocution*, a roundabout way to describe the much simpler word she couldn't find. On one occasion she was feeling hot. "Can you open the...that...I can't think of the word, that clear stuff you look through and see things on the other side!"

So I gave her the initial "wi" sound, and her response was immediate.

"Window!" she exclaimed, giggling.

Executive impairments can result in problems in most areas of cognition, including memory. On some of the standard tests of general verbal intelligence assessing vocabulary, comprehension of language, and general knowledge, patients with frontal lobe damage may not be significantly impaired. This is due to the overlearned nature of the material in these tests. The problems arise when patients must master novel tasks that require the executive functions of organizing, planning, or thinking abstractly or "outside the box." When understanding the subtle connotations of language and behavior is important, numerous problems emerge. Before her brain damage, Phillipa would have had no trouble providing the metaphorical meaning of a proverb, but now she had difficulty not only with giving abstract definitions for proverbs but also in thinking creatively or "laterally" in normal conversation. Take, for example, this exchange.

> Jenni: Do you think you're getting a lot of support from your family and friends while you're here in the hospital?
> Phillipa: [*laughing*] Don't be an ass. What do you think this is that I'm lying on? It's a bed, silly. That's what supports me. Can't see Larry and the kids lying down on the floor so I could lie on them!
> Jenni: OK. But there is another meaning of support, like to care about someone and help them by caring. Do you see that?
> Phillipa: Well, "caring" means looking after, and "support" means support, and so they can't be the same.

Phillipa also demonstrated another common symptom of frontal lobe damage, *perseveration*: the stereotypical repetition of a sound, word, or action. After I read her the form that described and requested her consent to participate in my research project (as she insisted she didn't care what was in it), she took it from me and signed it with a flourish, roughly on the line where I pointed. She then proceeded to sign her name three more times up the left side of the page "just in case the first one isn't good enough." Fortunately, she was strongly left-handed, so her right-sided weakness did not prevent her from writing. In another example, when I asked her to copy me after I tapped out simple rhythms on the table with my fingertips, she quickly picked up the first rhythm, but when I changed to a new rhythm, she replied, "Right you are, boss" and continued to tap in the original rhythm. This time she added her voice, "ta ta ta taaa; ta ta ta taaa," in time with her tapping. Even when she managed to change the rhythm briefly, she would quickly revert to the first rhythm. She also perseverated on a memory test requiring her to learn pairs of words, correctly producing the word "cries" when given the word "baby," but then going on to give "cries" as the response to "obey," "school," and "fruit."

My research focused on hemineglect, the strange disorder where a patient ignores the side of space opposite to the brain damage (see Chapter 3). Although hemineglect is more common after right parietal lobe damage, it can also occur after frontal lobe damage, and Phillipa did not disappoint. On a number of simple paper-and-pencil drawing tests, she demonstrated clear right-sided neglect, but in addition, and unlike the patients with parietal lobe damage I had examined, she was also apt to embellish her drawings. For example, she drew only the left side of a daisy she was asked to copy and then added a butterfly! Her copy of a complex pattern (called the Rey Complex Figure) also demonstrated neglect and sported various embellishments (see figure 4.1). When asked why she had made these additions, she replied in a very teacher-like tone, "Well, the whole purpose is to draw something interesting, I have always believed!" Thirty minutes later, when

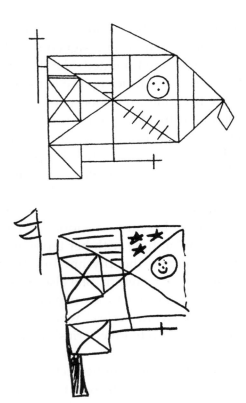

FIGURE 4.1
When Phillipa copied the model of the Rey Complex Figure (top), she embellished her drawing with stars and flags (bottom). (Reprinted from Ogden, J. A. 2005. *Fractured Minds: A Case-Study Approach to Clinical Neuropsychology, 2nd Ed.*, p. 167, with kind permission from Oxford University Press, New York.)

asked to draw the pattern from memory, she appeared to have no idea what I was talking about, but cheerfully drew some random squiggles and said, "There you are, that should be good enough even for you!"

Her rule-breaking behavior, typical of executive dysfunction, was dramatically displayed when I attempted to assess her on a *tactile neglect* task. The equipment for this test included an upright wooden frame 15 inches on a side with a curtain hanging from it. Phillipa was asked to put one hand through the curtain to manipulate the magnetic shapes and letters distributed along a metal strip on the other side of the curtain and therefore hidden from her view. She was then asked to pick from a second group of shapes, using first touch and then sight, the shapes she had previously manipulated along the strip. Tactile neglect would be demonstrated if she did not identify the shapes that had been on the rightmost end of the strip. Unfortunately, I was unable to discover whether Phillipa had tactile neglect because she insisted on using her other hand to pick up the curtain so she could peek under it. Telling her not to do it made absolutely no difference. She would verbally agree not to do it but then would go ahead and lift the curtain. I tried holding her free hand to stop her, but her response was to lean forward and peer over the top of the curtain. By this time, I had abandoned the original aim of the test and was more intrigued by her rule-breaking behavior. I offered her a chocolate biscuit if she did not try to peek behind the curtain (she had developed an insatiable appetite for chocolate and sweets since her head injury). She immediately agreed, but as soon as I placed her right hand through the curtain and guided her hand to a shape to feel, her left hand whipped out and lifted the curtain. Changing hands made no difference, and she managed to lift the curtain even with her weak right hand. I then tried yelling "Stop!" as soon as she began to lift the curtain, but this only had the effect of increasing her speed. She was unable to explain why she could not stop herself and found the whole thing very amusing.

Frontal amnesia is a term often applied to people who do not suffer from "true" memory impairments. That is, their poor memory is not a consequence of difficulties with taking in new information and later recalling it, a process that requires a number of mental steps. Rather, their "memory" problems arise because frontal lobe damage reduces the ability to form the plans required to complete the memory process successfully.

Working memory, the ability to hold information in a short-term store while manipulating it or working on it in some way, is susceptible to frontal lobe damage and may underlie other executive deficits, such as an inability to plan ahead. Planning ahead requires holding and manipulating in working memory current plans, tasks to be performed to work out the best future plans (such as checking out various travel options), and possibly memories of past activities if their success or failure is helpful in planning future activities. If the efficiency of this system is impaired by frontal lobe damage, planning and organization will certainly suffer.

Learning and later recalling new material—*long-term memory*—can also be compromised. Given a list of words to learn, the frontally impaired patient may be unable to organize the words to be learned in a logical way, such as building associations between words so that during recall one word cues another word. Providing the patient with external structure in the form of arranging the words in categories such as "fruits" and "clothes" and pointing out how one word within a category can lead, by association, to the next, can improve performance. In contrast, providing these sorts of external structures and cues to patients like HM (see Chapter 7), who has a true inability to memorize new material as a result of bilateral temporal lobe lesions, will not help them learn or recall word lists.

A difficulty with *prospective memory* is one of the most annoying memory problems for the patient with frontal lobe damage. The best way to describe this impairment is that the person "forgets to remember." For example, when asked to walk to the corner shop and buy the newspaper and a loaf of bread, she is likely to arrive at the shop but forget what she came for. The newspaper on the counter might cue her memory and she will purchase the paper but still forget the bread. Of course, as many healthy elderly people can attest, forgetting to remember can, at least in a minor way, become a frustration for anyone over the age of about 60. The complaint of the retired baby boomer who walks into a room to get the car keys, only to exclaim, "Damn, what did I come in here for?" is a common one. Aging appears to affect our prefrontal lobes relatively early.

Focusing and sustaining attention are other important functions of the prefrontal lobes. It proved impossible to assess Phillipa's ability to learn new verbal material using standard memory tests, because her attention was hard to capture for more than a few minutes at a time and her motivation to perform "boring" memory tests was poor. Her everyday memory for faces was good and she remembered me without difficulty, but her memory for new names was variable, again possibly the result of poor attention and motivation. Her memory for past events was hard to assess but Larry said she seemed to recognize various past occasions that he talked about, and she sometimes made comments suggesting that she remembered them reasonably well. When her children came to visit, she often asked them questions about their activities and clearly remembered, for example, that her ten-year-old son played football and her daughter loved ballet.

Most of the time, Phillipa had little insight into her condition, yet another common problem following frontal lobe damage. When asked why she was in the hospital, she was usually able to explain, "I was bashed over the head, and then had a brain operation." But when asked if she had any problems as a result, she would reply, "No, none that I can see and none that you can see." When asked about her family, she talked about them with little indication that she was concerned about her children or how they were managing without her. She would occasionally demand to go home, insisting that she needed to return to her position as a schoolteacher because the children would be getting lazy about their homework without her to push them, but she was easily distracted onto another subject. On other occasions she would make up stories, or *confabulate,* when asked about her current situation and how she came to be hospitalized. She would spin a tale about coming down to Auckland for a visit and taking time off for a rest before she returned to her busy life up north. One theory is that frontal amnesia encourages the patient to confabulate to fill memory gaps. The patient appears to have no awareness that these stories are incorrect or will be viewed as lies by the listener.

During the four months she spent in the hospital, Phillipa rarely seemed depressed, although on a few occasions she was found sobbing uncontrollably. One of these times was precipitated by the nurse's taking a bar of chocolate from her. She had developed a voracious appetite for sweets and was rapidly gaining weight. The dietitians had put her on a diet, and Phillipa was unconcerned by this as long as she couldn't see the chocolate or sweets denied her. On this occasion, she cried for ten minutes or more, and no one could calm her. She finally seemed to run out of energy, and when asked what had upset her, she had no idea.

*****

The most famous case of a person with a frontal lobe, or *dysexecutive,* disorder, is that of Phineas Gage, an efficient and capable foreman, who was injured in 1848 when a tamping iron was blown through the frontal lobes of his brain. Although he physically recovered well from this horrific accident, he suffered a significant and permanent personality change. The wonderfully evocative description written by his physician, J. M. Harlow, in 1868 captures the dramatic changes that follow the destruction of the executive seat of the human brain. As you will see, Phillipa and Phineas have a great deal in common.

He is fitful, irreverent, indulging at times in the grossest profanity (which was not previously his custom), manifesting but little deference to his fellows, impatient of restraint or advice when it conflicts with his desires, at times pertinaciously obstinate yet capricious and vacillating, devising many plans for future operation which no sooner are arranged than they are abandoned in turn for others appearing more feasible. His mind was radically changed so that his friends and acquaintances said he was no longer Gage.[1]

The healthy adult frontal lobes keep us on the straight and narrow. They inhibit us from doing things that would embarrass our parents. When we get drunk, our frontal lobes are temporarily impaired, and as a result we may well say and do things that we will be embarrassed about when we sober up the next morning. The neuropsychological term for this is *disinhibition*, and this is probably the personality change after frontal lobe damage that families have the most difficulty dealing with. Phillipa swore and undressed in front of strangers, and Phineas Gage demonstrated disinhibited behaviors when he was "irreverent, indulging at times in the grossest profanity (which was not previously his custom)."

People whose prefrontal lobes are not working properly—whether from permanent damage or alcohol intoxication—also lack insight into their problems and the effect they are having on others. When friends suggest to a drunk person at a party that he should have nothing more to drink, he laughs, or becomes angry, or simply ignores their advice. Once he is drunk, telling him to stop will have no effect. He has little insight into his intoxicated state, in spite of the fact that he is slurring his speech, knocking

[1]Harlow. J. M. 1868. Recovery from the passage of an iron bar through the head. *Publications of the Massachusetts Medical Society (Boston)*, 2, 327–346.

over drinks, and stumbling rather than walking. Phineas Gage also had "but little deference to his fellows," and almost certainly had no awareness of his problems. This lack of insight means that patients often have trouble recognizing their problems and learning from their mistakes, making successful rehabilitation extraordinarily difficult. A lack of insight is probably also related to another group of symptoms that includes a diminished sense of responsibility, little concern for the future, impulsiveness, mild euphoria, a tendency to make inappropriate and childish jokes, and an impoverished ability to initiate activities or to act spontaneously.

Other frontal lobe difficulties experienced by Gage include a poor ability to plan and follow through a course of action, and an inability to take into account the possible consequences of actions. Gage was often "devising many plans for future operation which no sooner are arranged than they are abandoned in turn for others appearing more feasible." Patients with executive problems also demonstrate a tendency to behave in an inflexible and rigid manner, seeming incapable of changing their behaviors or opinions even in the face of clear evidence that they are no longer correct or appropriate.

*****

While she remained in the hospital, Phillipa's primary rehabilitation was physical therapy. This was a frustrating exercise for the therapists. She seemed incapable of carrying out even the simplest exercise on her own and required the continuous presence of the therapist to show her repeatedly what to do. Over four months her right-sided weakness resolved somewhat, but according to her therapist this improvement did not result from an improvement in Phillipa's motivation. Rather, it was due to passive exercise—the therapist's moving her limbs—and some spontaneous recovery of both her limb weakness and her tendency to neglect or ignore the right side of her body.

Four months after the accident her husband elected to take her home, with nursing support and home help. After gamely struggling with a disinhibited, totally dependent woman who bore little resemblance to the wife he once knew, he finally succumbed to the necessity of placing her in an institution. For him, the final straw was when he arrived home from work one day to find that his two children had run away (to the shed behind their scout den), leaving behind a note that read: "We're sorry to leave you, Daddy, but Mummy doesn't want us anymore, and she needs you more than us. Please look after Bluey [their pet parakeet] for us." The note was completed by stick drawings of two children holding hands with tears running down their faces and of a bed with another stick person lying on it with a downturned mouth and one arm and fist raised. The home helper told Larry that she had come in from the garden on hearing shouting and swearing from Phillipa and had caught her in the act of throwing her full bedpan at her son and screaming at him to "get out." The home helper did her best to calm everyone down and did not realize until much later that the children had disappeared. They were found that evening, cold and frightened, and Phillipa was placed in a private psychiatric hospital two days later.

She has remained in psychiatric nursing homes ever since, and her husband and children (now adults) visit her about once every three months. It took many months of psychotherapy before any of them could put their guilt behind them and get on with their lives. As Larry told me when I spoke to him years later: "Phillipa is exactly the same as she was when she left the hospital. She appears to enjoy our visits and never seems to realize how long it has been since we last saw her. She seems to have no concept of time. If we stay too long, she starts yelling and swearing, and within minutes of us leaving the nurses say she has completely forgotten we were ever there."

*****

Frontal lobe damage and the impairments it causes can range across the entire spectrum from behaviors that are so subtle that it is difficult to tell if they are even abnormal to the extreme behaviors exhibited by Phineas Gage back in 1848 and Phillipa today. For people who suffer less severe frontal lobe damage, the impact of impaired executive functions on everyday activities is often much more debilitating than their formal test performance would indicate. Planning, preparing, and serving a relatively simple meal can become impossible. Shopping for groceries may be successful only if a list is constructed that groups food types together in the order in which they appear along the aisles of the supermarket. Even then, if each item is not crossed off as it goes into the cart, our shopper might wind up buying two of some items and missing others completely. Given that relatively simple and immediate tasks are difficult for people with executive problems, it is easy to understand why they find their businesses collapsing around them and are unable to plan for a family holiday.

Even quite minor frontal lobe damage such as that following serious alcohol abuse or moderate closed head injury can result in some disinhibition. In turn, this can render aggressive behaviors more likely and less predictable, especially for people who had a tendency toward violence before their brain damage occurred. Because acute alcohol intoxication affects the optimal functioning of the frontal lobes in people who are not alcoholics and have no frontal damage, it comes as no surprise that the consumption of alcohol by alcoholics or anyone with frontal lobe damage can, for a short time, increase their disinhibition, lack of insight, and aggressive tendencies to dangerous levels. In these cases, a family waiting in fear and apprehension for the father (or sometimes mother) to return home after a regular drinking session is a common scenario.

Frontal lobe damage must never be used as an excuse for violent behavior; rather, in cases where violent behaviors increase following frontal lobe damage, rehabilitation strategies must be put in place that include clear, concrete, frequently repeated rules of behavior, unambiguous boundaries of acceptable behavior, and immediate repercussions for unacceptable behaviors. It is important to be aware that frontal lobe damage per se is not invariably accompanied by an increase in aggressive behaviors. In many cases the reverse occurs and the patient becomes more passive. Indeed, passivity was one of the primary behavioral changes sought by psychiatrists when they referred their patients for frontal lobotomies.

After extensive bilateral frontal lobe damage such as that sustained by Phillipa, rehabilitation may prove impossible and institutionalization inevitable. In such tragic cases, family members probably suffer much more than the patient, who is spared by a lack of insight. Perhaps this is the mind's way of coping: severely disabled people who retain their insight may exist in a private hell and face years of psychotherapy and medication to alleviate their depression. In a case like Phillipa's, where psychotherapy falls on barren ground and depression is not a concern, the best a therapist can offer is grief counseling for the family along with therapy to help them move on with their own lives free of guilt.

■ Further Reading

Macmillan, M. 1996. Phineas Gage: A Case for All Reasons. In: C. Code, C.-W. Wallesch, Y. Joanette, and A. R. Lecours, eds. *Classic Cases in Neuropsychology* (pp. 243–262). Hove, East Sussex, UK: Psychology Press.

Ogden, J. A. 2005. The impaired executive: A case of frontal-lobe dysfunction. In: *Fractured Minds: A Case-Study Approach to Clinical Neuropsychology, 2nd Ed.* (pp. 158–170). New York: Oxford University Press.

5 ■

The Man Who Misplaced His Body

"Have you seen a case of Gerstmann's syndrome?" a neurologist asked me one day when she met me on the ward where I was assessing patients for a postdoctoral research project.

"No," I answered, trying to remember exactly what Gerstmann's syndrome was, but already feeling the anticipatory buzz that invariably accompanied the possibility of discovering for myself a "new" neuropsychological disorder.

"Well, you might like to check out a man who was admitted last week with a left parietal tumor of some sort. He's very alert and has no language problems, but he has left–right confusion, he can't write or calculate, and he gets his fingers muddled up."

I grinned at the neurologist. "I'd better read up about it first, but I'd love to assess him."

"Thought you might! Don't wait too long. I've put him on steroids, so his symptoms might disappear in a few days as the swelling goes down. I think he's got apraxia as well, so you'd better add that to your reading list."

I thought I'd introduce myself to the patient first and see if he were willing and well enough to carry out a few basic tests. Then I'd spend the rest of the day, and into the night if necessary, in the university medical library, reading everything I could find on Gerstmann's syndrome and apraxia. I flicked through the patient's medical file to check his admission details and read what the neurologist and nurses had written about him. Julian was a 59-year-old automobile and boat mechanic who lived with his wife, Anne, in a small seaside town in the sunny far north of New Zealand. He spent his spare time fishing and boating, and it had been after a weekend sailing trip that Julian had first noticed that his right arm was weak. He put this down to tiredness and advancing age, but soon after, Anne became concerned when she noticed he was having difficulty writing. Then he had two minor car accidents when he veered to the right, and within three months his right arm weakness had spread to his right leg until he was unable to stand alone. He was also becoming increasingly confused. Anne finally managed to get him to see his local doctor, and that same afternoon Julian found himself on a flight to Auckland. On being admitted to the Auckland Hospital neurology and neurosurgery ward, he had a computed tomography (CT) scan of his brain. This revealed a large, well-defined cystic tumor with surrounding swelling in the left parietal region of his brain, displacing the corpus callosum (the large fiber tract joining the two hemispheres) to the right.

The neurologist had noted that on admission, Julian demonstrated a right visual field deficit and had a mild weakness of his right arm and leg but no loss of tactile sensation. His comprehension seemed unimpaired and his speech was fluent and normal. He had difficulty telling his left from his right and was unable to subtract 7 from 100.

He was strongly right-handed, so not surprisingly his writing with his left hand was clumsy, but in addition his spelling was shockingly bad, whereas his wife said he had been a good speller previously. When the neurologist tested Julian's ability to identify his fingers by asking him to close his eyes and name the finger she was touching—little finger, index finger, and so on—he made a number of errors. In the light of his left–right confusion, *acalculia* (inability to calculate), *agraphia* (inability to write), and *finger agnosia* (inability to "know" and therefore name his fingers), the neurologist had queried Gerstmann's syndrome. She had started Julian on a course of steroid medication to reduce the swelling around the tumor.

The nursing notes were also interesting. When Julian was admitted, he had great difficulty putting the correct arms and legs into his pajamas, even when the garments were held in place for him. He became quite frustrated and told the nurse that he seemed to have "lost his marbles." His problem sounded like *dressing apraxia.* Apraxia is the inability to carry out, on command, learned skilled movements such as waving, brushing one's hair, or, as in Julian's case, dressing, despite good comprehension, full cooperation, and intact—or reasonably intact—motor and sensory systems.

Armed with the neurologist's and nurses' notes and my basic neuropsychology tool kit, I went to see Julian, who was sitting up in bed with his weak right arm propped on a pillow but was looking quite chirpy. I explained that I was keen to assess him for research purposes, and he said he would be delighted to "have a go" at my tests; he was bored already stuck here in the hospital when he could be out in his boat. I began with some of the standard tests of vocabulary, comprehension, and general information and found he had no problems at all with these. To assess visual neglect, a disorder where the patient does not attend to the space and the objects in it on the side opposite to his or her brain damage (see Chapter 3), I gave Julian five simple paper-and-pencil tests. He showed a mild right-sided neglect on only one. He did show symptoms of right-sided body neglect (another type of neglect where the patient is not interested in body parts opposite to the brain damage), which probably exacerbated the appearance of weakness of his right arm and leg. For example, although his right arm lay motionless at his side most of the time, when he was asked to concentrate on moving that arm or grasping my hand with his right hand, he could do so with near-normal strength. Another symptom of right-sided neglect was his request that people stand on his left because he did not like them standing on his right.

I asked him to point to his left ear. He looked confused and then, using his good left arm, pointed to the right side of his neck. This was a surprise, as I had been expecting left–right confusion but not body-part confusion. So I did some further spontaneous testing and quickly discovered that he really couldn't seem to locate the different parts of his body, or indeed the different parts of my body. At that point Julian's lunch was delivered, and I sat with him for a while, observing that by holding his fork in his left hand he managed to spear the food on both sides of his plate— cold meat, beans, and tomato sections—and deliver it to his mouth successfully. This was another sign that he didn't have significant visual neglect. I left him in peace, promising him I'd be back first thing next morning, and made a beeline for the medical school library.

In 1984 there was no rapid Internet providing electronic access to every journal article at the touch of a computer button. So when I got to the library I began my research by pulling out heavy neurological tomes and reading the classic descriptions of disorders. Next I checked for research articles under topic titles by going through card files stacked in the thousands in filing cabinets. Once I had a list of article references scribbled on my pad, I climbed down into the library basement, which housed most of the journals I would need—some over sixty years old. It was a dusty treasure trove of rolling shelves, and I could spend hours sitting on the floor between the shelves, a stack of dark green, blue, and black books of bound journals beside me, devouring the detailed descriptions of neurological disorders and syndromes written by the meticulous clinical researchers of the past. It always made me feel like a real researcher poised at the brink of an exciting new discovery. That "me" would never have believed that one day, only twenty years or so into the future, the contents of that entire archive of journals, extending back nearly a century, would be able to fit onto a single 100-gigabyte hard drive in a tiny computer which could sit on my desk! But for me that feeling of being part of the history of discovery—even if only on the very periphery—is not as acute when hundreds of research articles can be downloaded, categorized, and summarized in a flash without my needing to venture into the door of a real library or even take out a pen.

Sitting there on the library floor, along with reading about Gerstmann's syndrome and apraxia, I discovered some classic references to an even stranger disorder called *autotopagnosia*, which literally translated means "not knowing the topography of oneself." This very rare disorder was associated either with generalized brain damage or with lesions of the left parietal lobe. The main symptom was an inability to point on verbal command to human body parts, either one's own or those of another person (or a doll or picture of a human), although patients varied with regard to the exact symptoms they displayed. It took me quite a while to untangle the different hypotheses that had been postulated over the last sixty or more years to explain this strange disorder. In some cases the problem seemed to be a language-related impairment where the patient had lost the names of body parts but not those of other things. This made some sense, as the brain damage that gave rise to the disorder invariably included the posterior part of the left, "language" hemisphere. Then there were cases where the patient had a more general difficulty pointing to the parts of any objects, not just body parts. For example, a patient with this sort of problem, when asked, could point neither to a person's nose nor to the wheel of a car. This suggested that the disorder was at least in part a problem with the visuospatial system—a problem with locating object parts within a whole. This characterization also made "brain" sense, as the parietal lobe in the left as well as in the right hemisphere is associated with visuospatial functioning.

Having read everything I could find and having photocopied many articles, my next task was to come up with a battery of tests to assess Julian's many fascinating disorders—in particular, tests that would help me define the parameters of Julian's difficulties with pointing to body parts. Of course, as with all higher cognitive disorders, I knew that a complex disability such as autotopagnosia could occur for more than one underlying reason. Did Julian have a category-specific naming problem for body parts that prevented him from pointing to them on command, and if so did it extend to the body parts of other animals as well as humans? Perhaps his difficulty was more general, extending to a problem pointing to the parts of inanimate objects as well? Could he name body parts when shown them in isolation yet have difficulty locating them on a complete human body? There were no standard neuropsychological tests for this purpose; I would need to design my own. Given that Julian had already been started on steroids, time was of the essence; very likely his more dramatic symptoms would resolve as the brain swelling reduced. The other sad possibility was that his tumor might prove to be malignant and his condition could deteriorate. The chances of my ever having the opportunity to assess a patient with autotopagnosia again were very slim. There were very few cases reported in the literature, probably because patients with left parietal tumors or strokes large enough to cause autotopagnosia would usually have extensive language problems that would mask the more subtle symptoms of autotopagnosia.

*****

Julian did respond rapidly to steroid medication, regaining strength in his right limbs and becoming fully alert, oriented, and in his own words able to "think clearly" again. He underwent a biopsy of the mass in his brain seven days after admission to the hospital but had to wait a further week for the results. Happily, he always seemed delighted to see me and was eager to fill the long hours in the hospital doing the many tests I had waiting for him each morning. I kept him and Anne informed about my reasons for carrying out the various tests, and he frequently expressed amazement—and at times, amusement—at his own dramatic impairments. Although he sometimes became frustrated when he struggled with a test he knew he should be able to do easily, he quickly regained his good humor when we began the next task. In retrospect it seems strange that he was not more upset by his poor test performance, and it is impossible to say whether this signaled a poor understanding about his potentially serious brain tumor and the effect it was having on him, whether he was in denial, or whether his cheerful attitude was a reflection of his easygoing and practical personality. Certainly Anne believed Julian was under no illusions about his poor health and that he was exactly the same as he had always been—a man who just got on with life and enjoyed whatever it brought him. As she said, his favorite saying had always been "There's no point crying over spilt milk!"

In spite of my eagerness to assess his autotopagnosia, I forced myself to begin with some basic tests. Without understanding the limitations that sensory, motor, or more general cognitive deficits could place on my findings, it would be impossible to form or test hypotheses about the more bizarre disorders he displayed. Julian was strongly right-handed, as were both his parents, his three siblings, and one of his two children. As his wife was left-handed, it is likely that their left-handed child inherited her handedness from her. It was reasonable, therefore, to assume that Julian, like at least 92% of right-handers, was left hemisphere dominant for language. But a detailed aphasia assessment demonstrated that his conversation was intelligent, clear, and fluent, and he showed a readiness to initiate conversation. On tests of oral language comprehension, he scored easily within the normal range, and his comprehension was also good when it was assessed by asking him questions about a passage he had just read. He scored in the normal range when asked to tell a story about a complex picture, to read single words and complex paragraphs aloud, and to match written words with pictures and vice versa. When asked to pick specific objects from an array, he did so without hesitation or error. On naming tasks, he occasionally struggled to find the correct word, but he could describe the function or shape of the item he was trying to name. On an oral word fluency task, where he had to say in one minute as many words beginning with a specific letter as he could think of, he performed at the lower end of average range. This is usually considered a test of executive abilities, and Julian's reasonable performance in spite of his large posterior left hemisphere lesion indicated that the tumor was not affecting his prefrontal "executive" functions.[1]

[1] Phillipa, the patient described in Chapter 4, demonstrated a severe "executive syndrome" as the result of extensive damage to both her frontal lobes.

Given Julian's large left parietal tumor, it was surprising that he did not have significant language problems[2] and that he showed little generalized mental deterioration. This highlights the fact that every brain is unique in subtle ways—analogous perhaps to faces—and means that even when given detailed and accurate imaging of the brain and lesion, we cannot take for granted the pattern of abilities and disabilities a patient will exhibit. It is this variability—these individual differences—in the way each brain mediates behavior that makes neuropsychological assessment and research such an exciting challenge.

What of Julian's visuospatial abilities, which are usually impaired more extensively after damage to the right hemisphere but are also affected by parietal lesions generally, whether in the right or left hemisphere? On his sixth day after his admission, Julian could not copy a line drawing depicting a three-dimensional cube, suggesting he had mild *constructional apraxia* (an inability to conceptualize and construct objects as three dimensional, or draw them accurately), but by day 10 when shown models to copy he experienced no difficulties in using matchsticks to construct a diamond, a star, and even a three-dimensional house. But on the Block Design test, a task involving visuospatial conceptualization and construction, Julian had enormous difficulty even with the simplest items, and this had not improved by the time he was discharged on day 14. This test involves copying pictures of red and white patterns by putting together red and white blocks. Julian knew his attempts were incorrect, suggesting that his problem may have been related more to a difficulty with

[2] Irene, the patient described in Chapter 2, suffered a stroke that severely damaged the left side of her brain, including her parietal and temporal lobes. As a result she was unable to comprehend language and her spoken sentences were muddled. Mild to severe language difficulties are common following left hemisphere damage.

construction than with a pure visuospatial deficit. Many patients with *right* parietal lesions make significant errors on this task but because their visuospatial conceptualization ability is impaired often don't realize their attempts are incorrect (see Janet, in Chapter 3).

On memory tests, Julian demonstrated severe deficits in learning lists of words and recalling short stories (verbal memory) but was able to look at a simple pattern and draw it straight away from memory (nonverbal memory). One reason for this might be that his tumor was impinging on the left temporal region, important for verbal learning and memory.

I next assessed Julian's apraxia. Did the dressing apraxia and constructional apraxia he demonstrated on admission extend to other forms of apraxia? As the swelling around his tumor lessened, Julian's ability to dress improved, and by the 11th day after his admission he was back to normal. But in the first eight days, Julian displayed *ideomotor apraxia*—the failure to carry out a motor action on verbal command in spite of being able to perform it spontaneously. For example, the patient cannot poke out his tongue on command but licks his lips spontaneously. Julian could not wave, salute, or pantomime stirring a cup of coffee, brushing his teeth, or hammering a nail into wood with either hand when asked to do so, although he could accurately identify these actions when performed by me. He was often aware of his difficulties and made comments such as "How stupid I am. That is not a salute!" His ability to imitate these actions was slightly better but still clumsy. He also had *oral apraxia*, demonstrated by his inability to poke out his tongue, blow, or pretend to sip through a straw on verbal command, despite having normal spontaneous movements of his mouth and tongue.

He also occasionally showed elements of a much rarer form of apraxia: *ideational apraxia*, losing the idea of the use of an object. It has been described as an inability to handle real objects although the patient is able to pantomime how he would use the object. Ideomotor and ideational apraxia can overlap and are often observed in a mixed form in Alzheimer's disease patients. The best—and most amusing—example of Julian's ideational apraxia was captured on a video the neurologist and I had decided to make, hoping to archive his many rare disorders before they disappeared along with the swelling around his tumor. The neurologist and Julian sat facing each other, a small table covered with common objects between them. First the neurologist asked him to pick up a toothbrush from the array of objects and brush his teeth, whereupon Julian picked up the toothbrush and began shaving with it. The conversation then proceeded as follows:

> Neurologist: What are you doing?
> Julian: Well, I'm shaving, aren't I?
> Neurologist: What's that in your hand?
> Julian: [*looking at the toothbrush*] A toothbrush.
> Neurologist: What do you normally do with a toothbrush?
> Julian: Brush my teeth, of course!
> Neurologist: Where are your teeth?
> Julian: Where are my teeth? [*laughing*] Well, my teeth are in my mouth presumably!
> Neurologist: Show me how you would brush your teeth.

At this point, Julian once again began to shave with the toothbrush. He realized he was not doing it correctly and said, "Damn, I can't seem to do it." Julian then stiffly bent his right arm—he was still neglecting it—and held his palm upward at waist height, and with the toothbrush in his left hand made swiping movements across his right hand. We all began to laugh when it dawned on us that Julian had false teeth!

Next on my list to assess was *Gerstmann's syndrome.* This constellation of four deficits—agraphia, acalculia, right–left disorientation, and finger agnosia—was first described by Josef Gerstmann in 1930. I had learned that there was considerable controversy about whether this syndrome actually existed, given that the word "syndrome" suggests that the symptoms are tied to one another in some functional way, perhaps because they all share some underlying cognitive subcomponent. Quite often, however, patients demonstrated only two or three of the symptoms. Of course if Gerstmann's was a true syndrome a patient could show some symptoms and not others because certain symptoms require more severe damage to the underlying functional system[3] than others. But a more parsimonious explanation is that the four symptoms are simply mediated by anatomical systems physically close to one another and are entirely independent of one another, so that the term "syndrome" is misleading. This dilemma regarding syndromes is not uncommon and can be easily resolved if syndromes are simply viewed as descriptive terms without the necessity for explanations as to why those symptoms tend to occur together. One finding seems uncontroversial: When the four Gerstmann symptoms coexist, the lesion is almost always in the posterior left parietal lobe, often involving the junction between the parietal and occipital lobes.

Julian had clear evidence of all the symptoms of Gerstmann's syndrome, and these persisted throughout his stay in the hospital. At first, because of his right arm weakness and neglect, he was unable to hold a pencil in his right hand, but on the sixth day he demonstrated severe agraphia for both spontaneous writing and copying a printed

---

[3] A functional system refers to number of brain areas, often in different areas of the brain, working together to produce a complex behavior. See Chapter 1 for further explanation.

sentence when using his left hand. He had difficulty forming letters and would, for example, form a "B" instead of a
"J" and a "c" instead of an "a." He would often exclaim,
"That is not what I wanted to write. I wanted a 'J,' not a
'B.' " By the 10th day his right arm neglect had resolved
and he was able to hold a pencil in his right hand, but he
continued to make similar mistakes. When asked to print
the sentence "I will be very pleased when I can go home,"
he wrote in capitals "I WILL BE EVEY LLEASED WENW I
CAN GO HOEM." In contrast, when spelling aloud he got
18 of 20 words correct. These included both regularly
spelled words and irregular words such as "debt," "rogue,
"mortgage," and "subtle." His reading was also correct and
fluent, if rather slow. That is, he had *agraphia without alexia*
(reading impairment).[4]

Julian had unambiguous left–right confusion and was
unaware of his frequent left–right errors. This confusion
persisted even when his other deficits improved His acalculia was also clear and persistent. Although he could read
numbers and understood their value (e.g., "2 is a very
small number, 22 is much larger, and 100 is very large"), he
was unable to carry out even simple calculations other than
addition. For example, asked to subtract 6 from 10, he
tended to add the two numbers together. He was also
unable to multiply or divide. When given a string of two to
five numbers and asked to repeat them backward, he was
never able to get more than three, and usually only two.
"I can't go backward," he'd say, with a puzzled look. He
also sometimes had problems with simple logical–grammatical relationships. When responding to the command
"Place the pencil under the book," he was equally likely to
put the pencil on top of the book as under it, which suggests that his acalculia might have also been a problem

[4]The reverse disorder, alexia without agraphia, where reading is impaired but
writing is intact, is much more common; see the patient described by Oliver Sacks
in the Further Reading at the end of this chapter.

related to logical–grammatical relationships such as "take away" or subtract.

Finger agnosia is a strange symptom and not one that would be noticed without special testing. One can only wonder at the detailed assessments carried out by the neurologists of those early heady days when so many new things were being discovered about the cognitive brain; who knows what hypotheses motivated Gerstmann to test his patients for finger identity! I copied his examination instructions exactly and found that Julian could not name or number the fingers on either hand when I touched them, whether or not he was looking at them. He couldn't name my fingers either when I pointed to them. He was also given a non-naming test of finger agnosia by being asked, while blindfolded, to say how many fingers lay between two fingers being touched by me. He failed this as well.

At last I was ready to test Julian's autotopagnosia in detail. I had put together a number of tasks to test the various hypotheses about its underlying cause. Many of these tests used my children's books and toys: their "beginning reader" books with pages of animals and objects, to test Julian's ability to name specific objects; a rather grubby doll—the only one my daughter would let me borrow—to use when I asked him to point to different body parts; a teddy bear and other soft animals so I could see if Julian also had difficulty pointing to parts of other animals, especially given that some, like the teddy bear, had a similar shape to a human; and toy cars and trucks to see if Julian could point to named parts of these objects, I even commandeered "Mr. Potato Head"—a plastic potato with slots where plastic eyes, ears, nose, mouth, hat, and glasses could be inserted.

On the sixth day after Julian's admission, if I pointed to any body part, whether it was on his own body, my body, a doll's body, or a photograph of a man's naked body, he quickly and accurately named it. That is, his problem was not one of language or associating the body part with the correct label. In stark contrast, he made numerous errors when I named a body part and asked him to point to it. Even when he was correct, he was very slow. His strategy seemed to be to search the body until his eyes rested on the part for which he was searching. His search usually commenced somewhere on the upper part of the body, and if he did not happen upon the body part he seemed unaware that he should look lower down. When I asked him to point to specific parts below the waist, he would often look puzzled and comment, "I can't reach that" or "That part seems to have disappeared." On one occasion I was sitting directly in front of him with my hands on my knees and asked him to point to my hand. He looked all over my upper half, exclaiming, "Where's it gone?" At one point, he accidently touched my hand with his but still was unable to point to it. He clearly realized he should have been able to locate body parts and often laughed at his own inability to find them. He would sometimes indicate body parts above the waist correctly, apparently as a result of his eyes falling on the part during his search, but even in these cases he often expressed uncertainty. He would often indicate the wrong part, for example, the wrist for the elbow, or, on command to point to the elbow, he would touch the shoulder and then gradually move his hand along the arm until he reached the elbow and then say, "It's about here."

On days 10 to 12 after admission, I carried out a more systematic research test where Julian was first asked to name body parts I pointed to on him, on myself, on three dolls (my daughter had softened, and consented to my borrowing two more of her favorites) and on a photograph of a naked man. In total I pointed to 78 body parts, and Julian correctly named all of them. He was then asked to point to named body parts on the same bodies (124 commands in all). He was also blindfolded and asked to point to named body parts on himself (30 commands in total). Throughout testing he was asked to use his right hand—which he could now use quite well—for half the responses and his left hand for the other half. He made numerous errors, an approximately equal number with each hand. He showed no ability to discriminate right from left. Disregarding these numerous left–right errors, Julian was unable to correctly locate body parts 45% to 61% of the time on other people's bodies (mine, the dolls', or the photograph) while able to see and 28% of the time on his own body with his eyes open as well as while blindfolded. Strangely, when I asked Julian to point to items of named clothing on himself or me (nine commands), he was quick and accurate, although he still demonstrated left–right confusion; for example, for "left shirt cuff" he pointed to the right shirt cuff.

When he was presented with an array of pictures of isolated body parts and asked to point to specific parts on verbal command, he responded without difficulty, demonstrating again that his comprehension of body-part names was normal. To ensure that his difficulty was indeed unrelated to a language comprehension deficit, I also gave him a nonverbal test of locating body parts. I showed him pictures of the front and back of a naked man, with numbers on different body parts. I then asked him to point to the part on his body that corresponded to a specific numbered part on the drawing. He was able to point to the numbers correctly, but in 12 responses he made 6 errors when pointing to the corresponding body part on himself (excluding left–right errors). Thus he still demonstrated autotopagnosia even when comprehension of body-part names was not required.

The way Julian went about performing the tests along with his comments—the *qualitative* data—was very helpful in understanding his deficits. For example, when I asked him to point to a doll's stomach, he looked puzzled and moved his finger up and down the doll saying:

"Where has the stomach gone to? It seems to have disappeared. How silly!" Later, when asked to point to the doll's elbow, he pointed to its stomach and said, "Here is her elbow; it is probably a bit further up." When asked to point to his own eyebrow, he pointed to his eye and said, "It is about here; the eyebrow might be a bit further up." On being asked to point to the doll's armpit, he pointed to its groin. When I pointed out his error and asked him to tell me why he thought he went wrong, he said, "I start at the bottom and then seem to get lost in space from where I am." Julian's comments and methods of finding body parts seemed to indicate that he had difficulty remembering exactly where they should be in relation to the body.

When asked to draw a stick figure of a man, Julian did a reasonably accurate drawing. I then asked him where the foot would go. He pointed to the arm, drew a stick at the end of it, and said, "It would go here on the end of the leg." I then asked him where the hand would go, and he pointed to the "foot" he had just drawn on the end of the arm and said, "His hand would go here on the end of the foot—no, that's not right, the hand goes on the arm." I then introduced him to Mr. Potato Head. I removed its features while Julian watched and then asked him to put them back. He named each feature correctly as he picked it up but put the ears where the eyes should go, the eyes where the ears should go, the mouth on top of the head, where a hat was meant to slot in, and the nose in the correct place. He went to put the spectacles on and said, "They won't fit, the ears are in the way!" He then attempted to put the hat on top of the head and found the mouth was in the way. At this point he realized there was something wrong. A few days later, when videotaping him, I asked him to do the task again, and this time he was able to place the features correctly. When I asked him if he remembered how he had done it previously, he was greatly amused and said: "I had things everywhere! The mouth on top of the head and the eyes and ears mixed up!"

Julian's problem was not caused by his perception and identification of body parts in isolation. When his attention was drawn to a particular part on a body or when he was given a picture or model of an isolated body part, he could always name it accurately. He also knew the function of the parts, but when he was asked to describe the location of body parts, he had some difficulties. For example, when asked what a mouth was for, he replied it was for eating, drinking, and talking. When asked what a foot was for, he replied there were two of them and they were to stand on and walk with. When, however, he was asked where his left foot was he replied: "My left foot is down underneath my left boot. At the end of my left leg." For "right thigh" he answered: "Opposite side to my left thigh. It is a thick and heavy piece, around my middle." His description of the location of his right elbow was "About the middle of my body. Just below my right elbow bone." He said his ear was "underneath my eyebrow" and his mouth was "in the middle of my face—between my two nostrils, underneath my eyes."

His deficit was not part of a more generalized inability to analyze wholes into parts. In contrast to his difficulties in locating human body parts, his ability to locate parts of objects and animals was normal. For example, on a toy truck he pointed quickly and accurately on verbal command to the driver's seat, front wheels, flashing light, steering wheel, headlights, engine, passenger's seat, and the door to the driver's seat. On a real vase of flowers, he pointed on command and without hesitation to a petal, a leaf, the vase, water, and a stem, and on a picture of an elephant, he pointed to the mouth, eye, toes on the foreleg, tusk, tail, back leg, and ear. He could also put labels with the names of New Zealand towns in the correct places on an outline map of the country, and he put the parts of a story—Little Red Riding Hood—into the correct sequence.

To explain this pattern of findings, I needed to come up with a new hypothesis. Perhaps for some patients with auto-topagnosia, including Julian, the inability to point to human body parts is the result of a disruption of a discrete body image mediated by systems in the region of the left parietal lobe. The concept behind this is that when we look at a body, to know how it fits together, we compare it with a mental picture of the human body that we carry on a "scratch pad" in our mind—seemingly in the left parietal lobe. Thus if the scratch pad is damaged and we lose the ability to evoke the body image, we lose the template that tells us where, on a real body, body parts are located relative to the rest of the body. This implies that humans have a human body map hardwired into their brain, an intriguing concept![5]

At last my assessments were complete and the neurologist and I had documented Julian's many fascinating impairments on video, which, with Julian's permission, I used for teaching purposes for more than twenty years. My postgraduate neuropsychology students never failed to be amazed by his strange impairments, amused by his wisecracks, and moved by his lovely and generous personality, which turned what could have been a somber story into an uplifting one.

All the while I, along with the neurologist, had been hoping that the tumor would be treatable; the best guess from its appearance on the CT scan was that it was a low-grade astrocytoma, a slow-growing tumor that could be debulked—have some of the mass cut away—and perhaps not cause further significant problems for many years. But sadly this was not to be. The tumor proved to be an unusually large metastatic carcinoma, and further CT scans of Julian's body revealed a primary tumor in his lung, almost certainly a

[5]My findings on Julian, along with my suggested hypotheses for explaining them, are published in my 1985 article listed in the Further Readings at the end of this chapter.

consequence of his long history of smoking. Metastatic brain tumors are highly malignant, with a survival rate after diagnosis of often a matter of months. The large size of Julian's tumor and the three-month history of symptoms suggested that it had grown very rapidly and that Julian's condition would probably deteriorate quickly, even with the reduction of swelling afforded by the steroids.

Yet within a couple of days of being told his diagnosis, Julian seemed to come to terms with it. His daughters traveled to Auckland to be close to him, and they had more difficulty than their father accepting the terrible news that he had only months to live. But they took their cue from Anne and struggled to hide their feelings and take on Julian's adage to make the most of every day. This had always been his way. Although his symptoms had been causing him difficulties for some months before his admission to the hospital, he had not allowed them to influence his life much. In part, this may have been the result of a psychological denial mechanism sometimes observed in patients with a relatively slow onset of symptoms. Fear of a serious illness can underpin a delay in seeking medical help for both sufferers and families, and it is not particularly uncommon for patients to experience a debilitating leg weakness or an inability to use an arm for several months before they see a doctor. In some cases this apparent unconcern may in itself be a result of brain dysfunction, especially following right parietal lobe or bilateral frontal lobe damage. Both Janet, with right parietal damage (Chapter 3), and Phillipa, with bilateral frontal lobe damage (Chapter 4), deny their very severe problems. But in Julian's case, a psychological explanation for his denial—if that's what it was—seems more plausible.

A delay in diagnosis and treatment can have serious consequences in the case of a secondary metastasis in the brain. Julian's tumor had grown unusually large by the time it was diagnosed, reducing the chance of successful treatment by surgical removal, radiotherapy, or chemotherapy. He was offered radiotherapy, but he made a lucid and understandable decision to decline any further treatment other than steroids. This decision was based partially on his dislike of Auckland and a yearning to return to his quiet and beautiful seaside village to spend the remaining months of his life among his family and friends. In any case, given the very high malignancy and large size of Julian's brain tumor and the primary tumor in his lung, it is debatable whether his life would have been prolonged significantly if he had remained in Auckland a further four to six weeks for radiotherapy. There seems little doubt that the quality of life he was able to enjoy for a few more weeks was vastly superior to the quality of life he would have had to endure by remaining within the hospital system, away from the people and environment he loved.

Feeling comfortable with a patient's decision to refuse treatment is often difficult for medical professionals and therapists, perhaps because they believe it is their duty to provide the patient with every reasonable option for survival. The knowledge that in rare cases the growth of even malignant tumors such as Julian's can be significantly slowed by aggressive treatment, potentially adding quality time to the patient's life span, no doubt puts pressure on many doctors to encourage treatment. It is impossible to predict how an individual patient will react on being diagnosed with a terminal illness. Some continue to fight for their lives long past the time the medical profession has given up, and others continue to deny their terminal condition and that nothing more can be done for them even when they are totally dependent on others for their care and their quality of life seems abysmal to everyone around them. A few, like Julian, seem able to make a clear decision to live what remains of their life as well as they can, without looking for miracle cures.

The important lesson for the doctor or therapist is that whenever possible, the final decision should lie with the patient. In such a case, the most valuable contribution the medical professional can make is to give the patient as much information as possible about the prognosis and the pros and cons of available treatments both to fight the illness and to relieve the symptoms. Counseling can be offered to assist the patient—and often family members as well—in making these decisions and to facilitate coping with grief, loss, and dying. When the patient and family feel they have got as much out of counseling as possible, the professional's role is over, and all that remains is to feel at ease with the patient's decision.

On returning home, Julian continued to "mess about in boats" until he became too disabled to walk. His ability to speak and understand speech began to deteriorate six weeks after his discharge from hospital, and he spent his final three months in his own bed in a room with a view of the sea he loved so much. He was nursed by Anne and his daughters and seemed to enjoy brief visits from his grandchildren. Anne felt he was at peace with himself and his world when, surrounded by his family, he sailed into the sunset for the last time.

■ Further Reading

Ogden, J. A. 1985. Autotopagnosia: Occurrence in a patient without nominal aphasia and with an intact ability to point to parts of animals and objects. *Brain, 108*, 1009–1022.

Ogden, J. A. 2005. A body in the mind: A case of autotopagnosia. In: *Fractured Minds: A Case-Study Approach to Clinical Neuropsychology, 2nd Ed.* (pp. 99–112). New York: Oxford University Press.

Sacks, O. 2010. A man of letters. In: *The Mind's Eye* (pp. 53–81). New York: Knopf.

6 ∎
The Mind-Blind Motorcyclist

Michael was a motorcycle maniac. Like many a 24-year-old male in exuberant health and with a heady zest for life, whenever he could he leapt on his motorcycle and made for the open road. He often rode with one or more of his army mates, but sometimes he rode alone. So on a beautiful day in 1986 it was a stranger who came upon the horrific scene of a motorcycle wrapped around a tree and a crumpled and very still body lying under it. Michael was still alive—just—and was rushed to the critical care unit (CCU) of Auckland Hospital. He was in a deep coma and had multiple fractures where the left side of his body had been crushed by the heavy motorcycle. Even more worrying was the computed tomography (CT) brain scan showing swelling of the right hemisphere of his brain, caused when the right side of his head hit the ground. This dangerous swelling was treated with a drug (mannitol), and his many orthopedic injuries were pinned and set. Within days of his admission, the doctors gave up on trying to save his badly crushed left arm, and it was amputated.

Michael's mother, Joy, almost lived at his bedside, sure that he would know she was there, even although he showed no signs of regaining consciousness. The doctors tried to prepare her for the almost inevitable; that he would very likely die, and if he didn't he would almost certainly be left with severe brain damage and a crippled body from his horrendous orthopedic injuries. Michael's father had died years before and his one older brother lived hundreds of miles away, so Joy was pretty much alone as she struggled to keep up her spirits and her belief that her son would come back to her. Michael's mates and immediate superiors in the army visited for brief periods but could not wait to get out of the CCU, where machines breathed spookily for their silent victims, reminding the shocked observers that accidents do happen, especially to testosterone-fueled young men.

Two weeks after his admission, the doctors were able to tell Joy that Michael would probably survive. The swelling in his brain had subsided and he had made it through the worst. Secretly they thought it would have been better if he had died at the time of the accident; they knew only too well the agony and despair that lay ahead for Joy and her son. But Joy was true to her name, and the day she was told that Michael was out of immediate danger of dying was one of the happiest of her life. The doctors didn't try and curb her spirits; they knew she needed this hope to sustain her over the next weeks, months, and years. A few days later Michael's CCU doctor gently explained to Joy that Michael might not regain consciousness for a long time and she should prepare herself for the long haul—perhaps just come in and see him for thirty minutes every other day. Joy nodded and thanked him, and continued to spend hours every day at her son's bedside, talking to him and holding his remaining hand. Five weeks after his accident he opened his eyes, and when the relieved doctor asked Michael to squeeze his hand, he did so. With all his tubes removed and breathing on his own, he was transferred to an orthopedic ward, where he remained for another 11 weeks.

Once Michael had left the CCU his head injury was virtually ignored while the surgeons grappled with his severe orthopedic injuries. In an acute hospital where wards and medical services are physically divided according to types of illness or damage, it is often difficult to decide where a patient with multiple injuries should go. In Michael's case he clearly needed extensive orthopedic surgery and specialist care, and as he could by this time talk normally and seemed cheerful and even "chirpy," no doubt the staff were lulled into thinking he had recovered rather well from his head injury. In any case, there was clearly nothing further to be done for his brain either medically or surgically. Even with all the hard work put in by the orthopedic surgeons, the fractures in his left leg resulted in a twisted foot and a severe limp (which would be partially corrected seven years later by foot surgery).

In 1986 the assessment of head-injured patients was very limited, at least in New Zealand. Neuropsychologists were considered an expensive luxury in a stretched public health system, and so it was an occupational therapist who first tested Michael's general functional abilities a month after he had been transferred to the orthopedics ward. Joy had suspected Michael was blind from the time he regained consciousness at five weeks, but the occupational therapist thought that at times he seemed able to look at an object and recognize it. The therapist agreed, however. that his sight was very impaired. A neurosurgeon who was asked to check him over at one point wrote in his notes that Michael had double vision (*diplopia*). This led to a referral to an ophthalmologist ten weeks after the accident, and for the first time Michael's sight was properly assessed. Joy was right all along; her son was blind. But he was *cortically blind*: his loss of sight resulted from damage to the visual cortex of the occipital lobes rather than to his eyes or the optic tracts. It seems almost incomprehensible that Michael's blindness was not picked up by the medical staff for five weeks after he regained consciousness, but it was of some comfort to Joy to know there was nothing they could have done even if they had noticed his blindness earlier.

Strangely, Michael seemed unconcerned by his poor vision as he lay in bed. His optimism and good verbal communication skills perhaps fooled the medical staff into thinking his brain damage had not impaired his cognitive abilities very seriously. Given his right hemisphere swelling on admission to the hospital, it is likely that his lack of concern or even failure to recognize his blindness was a denial of his problems (called *anosognosia*), a not uncommon finding following right brain damage. On discharge from the hospital 16 weeks after his accident, Michael had mild spasticity of his remaining right hand (his dominant writing hand), and his speech and comprehension of language seemed normal. The New Zealand Foundation for the Blind assessed him as totally blind and enrolled him in their full-time, live-in rehabilitation program.

Twenty-one months after Michael had his accident, he suddenly noticed the moving lights of other cars when he was traveling as a passenger in a car at night. He also began to notice movement on the television. His rehabilitation therapists, excited by this, began an intensive program to improve his vision. Over the next four months, he progressed from being unable to read letters or words to being able to trace the outlines of letters and then recognizing them. At this stage he was able to read short words, such as "it" and "the," but he was completely unable to recognize any objects or people on sight. After a further three months of intensive rehabilitation, he could recognize numbers, use a telephone, and locate his ashtray. He could read simple booklets and his digital watch. When shown a real object or a line drawing or photograph of an object, he could not recognize it, but he could describe the shape of the object and sometimes work out what it was from that description. His ability to recognize objects via touch, sound, or smell was completely normal. For example, if he was shown a bunch of keys, he had no idea what they were, but if the therapist picked them up and jangled them, or as soon as he held them in his hand, he could immediately name them.

His inability to recognize faces (*prosopagnosia*) did not improve, and until she spoke, he never recognized his mother when she visited him. Of course, since people usually speak as soon as they meet, often visitors and staff were unaware that their faces were just a meaningless jumble to Michael.[1] He certainly seemed to have no serious concern about this, and wasn't inclined to tell them. This is likely another aspect of his anosognosia. (Already we can see that anosognosia might be quite a useful disorder to have in these circumstances. Without it, I suspect Michael would have been very depressed and not the cheerful, motivated fellow he was.)

A further three years passed before I entered Michael's contained world. I received a telephone call from his Foundation for the Blind therapist, who had heard about my work with other head-injured patients. She asked for my help in assessing Michael, in the hope that this might

---

[1] Richard Power's novel *The Echo Maker*, listed in the Further Readings at the end of this chapter, tells the strange story of a man who suffered a traumatic brain injury and as a result developed a delusion called Capgras syndrome, causing him to believe that the people he knew well were imposters. One theory postulates that this is because the part of the brain that recognizes familiar faces has been severed from the part of the brain that responds emotionally to that familiarity: The patient feels nothing for the person standing in front of him and so believes the person must be an imposter or double.

suggest new rehabilitation techniques because, as she said, "Something incredible happened to him and he seems to be getting his sight back, but he still can't see!" She also told me that he and his mother were keen to find out more about his problems and would love to be involved in research. Already I was feeling the excitement: was this that jewel, an eager and bright research participant with a fascinating disorder and a stable brain lesion? I had worked with (and sometimes cried over) too many patients who had terminal brain tumors or neurological disorders that got progressively worse, so hearing that Michael was definitely not in that category was a very big plus.

*****

The therapist's description of Michael's visual problems—his inability to recognize what he was seeing—sounded like *visual object agnosia*, a disorder that has been known to neurologists for more than 100 years. Numerous accounts of it have been published in the neuropsychological literature since it was described in 1883 by the French neurologist Jean-Martin Charcot. Charcot was in fact the first to describe many neurological and psychiatric disorders, and has been dubbed the "founder of modern neurology." He was a staunch advocate of hypnotism as a valid medical treatment, especially in patients suffering from the then popular diagnosis of hysteria (primarily affecting women, and later dismissed as spurious), but was also well known because of his many famous students, including Sigmund Freud.

Agnosia means "to not know," and thus *visual object agnosia* means "to not know objects by sight in spite of adequate vision." The disorder is "modality specific" in that the patient can recognize the object via the other senses of touch or sound (or sometimes even taste or smell if the object is blue cheese!). It is not a disorder of naming, because patients have no difficulty naming an object they can recognize via a nonvisual sense. The agnosia family encompasses a wide range of "not knowing" impairments, many specific to a particular modality or sense. Thus there are not only visual agnosias, although they are the most common, but also auditory and tactile agnosias. Within each modality there are even disorders that can be discriminated from one another. For example, included within the auditory agnosias—inabilities to recognize sounds in spite of adequate hearing—there are patients who cannot recognize words but can recognize nonverbal sounds and other patients who cannot recognize various characteristics of music but can recognize other sounds, such as a car starting.

There have been descriptions of patients who have visual object agnosia because they cannot perceive shapes, and descriptions of patients who, despite being able to perceive lines and shapes, cannot integrate them into a meaningful whole—the highest form of vision,. The neuropsychologist's task is to try to tease apart which type the patient has, as this might be useful information when designing a rehabilitation program, even if only to understand what the patient will be capable of doing. As we shall see, Michael's visual agnosia was the "highest" type. That is, he could correctly name lines, triangles, squares, and circles but had no idea what a picture of a bicycle was. This type of agnosia is called *integrative agnosia*.

Michael's other strange problem, prosopagnosia, the inability to recognize faces on sight, is often found in the same patients who demonstrate visual object agnosia. In both disorders the damage is to the occipital lobes at the back of the brain. One possible explanation for this co-occurrence is that in some patients, both prosopagnosia and visual object agnosia are consequences of damage to the part of the visual system that represents spatial entities comprised of many interrelated parts. Mild damage to this system would result in a problem in recognizing faces, clearly a difficult task since faces are complex and differ in subtle ways. More severe damage to this system would not only result in prosopagnosia but also cause problems with recognizing complex objects. Because objects tend to be much less complex than faces and easier to distinguish from other objects, more severe damage would be necessary to cause visual object agnosia than to cause prosopagnosia. There are also cases of visual object agnosia associated with *alexia* (an impairment of reading) rather than prosopagnosia. In these cases the problem appears to be in a system that represents numerous discrete parts, such as letters that make up a word and discrete parts that make up an object.

Together, these findings suggest that different systems or pathways in the occipital lobes are concerned with different types of visual representation. Thus patients who appear to have damage in similar areas of the brain may actually have damage to different pathways. In fact, many patients who cannot recognize objects and faces have more damage to the right occipital lobe than to the left occipital lobe, and vice versa for patients who cannot recognize objects and words. This makes sense in that the right hemisphere is more concerned with spatial concepts and the global picture, and the left hemisphere is more concerned with the details that make up the whole rather than the whole itself.

*****

Today visual object agnosia is considered one of the "classic" neuropsychological disorders, and its study has told us a great deal about the complex higher visual processes we humans use in our everyday lives without so much as a thought. So why did the possibility of studying Michael thrill me? Surely everything that could be discovered already had been? But this is rarely the case in neuropsychology. Given that exactly the same brain structures and neurons are rarely if ever damaged in two humans, it is not surprising that the disorders that result are also unlikely to be identical. Added to this is the brain itself; no two human brains are exactly alike. Even the brains of identical twins will develop differently according to their life experiences. Thus even if it were ethical for a neuroscientist to cut out a piece of human brain or, using microtechniques, to cauterize or chemically destroy a specific set of neurons with great precision, it would still not be surprising if the resulting deficits shown by the human guinea pigs were subtly different. So although there had been many well-described studies on patients with visual agnosia before Michael came into my life, I was still excited by what I might find. Indeed, even if all I could find was a classic case of visual agnosia, that too would be fascinating, as Michael was the first person with this disorder that I had ever come across. Reading about these almost unbelievable disorders is one thing, but observing them for yourself is a whole different experience. This is the excitement that motivates postgraduate neuropsychology students and turns their interest in the subject into passion.

But there is a big caution here. Because special case studies like Michael do not come along too often in the working life span of a neuropsychologist, when they do they often become almost "professional subjects." It is obviously important for researchers to guard against exploiting these generous people, an obligation that becomes more difficult over time as a personal bond develops between researcher and participant. The result is that the participant feels reluctant to disappoint the experimenter. Apart from always being alert for early signs of "participant burnout," one way of trying to balance out this potentially exploitative relationship is for the researcher to use the results of the various investigations in an effort to improve the rehabilitation strategies used with the participant. In this way, the neuropsychologist can become a useful member of the rehabilitation team and perhaps contribute to small improvements in the patient's functioning and quality of life. Whether or not this is possible, the majority of research participants gain satisfaction from knowing they have contributed to research that might help others in the future. And last, but perhaps not least, of the benefits to patients of participating in research is the enjoyment they can gain out of doing something different and meeting new people—even scientists! Having a long-term illness or being "disabled" can be very isolating and horribly boring, especially if the individual feels well but is dependent on others. This was definitely part of the attraction for Michael, who had always been and remained a gregarious, chatty, and optimistic soul.

My initial excitement proved to be well-founded. As we will see later in the chapter, my assessments demonstrated that in addition to the classic disorders of visual object agnosia and prosopagnosia, Michael had a significant and very unusual memory impairment and a number of other disorders of higher visual cognition, especially those to do with color, dreams, and imagery.

*****

Following my telephone conversation with Michael's therapist, I arranged for her to bring him to the psychology clinic at Auckland University. Ten minutes before our scheduled meeting I was having a cup of coffee in the common room when one of my academic colleagues came in. On seeing me he remarked, "I just passed a man in the corridor who, from the look of him, was on his way to see you." When I left the room I saw a tall, well-built young man limping and swaying unsteadily along the corridor, apparently following the person in front of him. His right arm was held at an awkward angle to his body, perhaps in an attempt to steady himself or to protect his body from banging into the wall, and his left arm terminated at his elbow and was finished with a large hook. I greeted his companion (the rehabilitation therapist) and then greeted Michael. He looked for my voice in midair, as blind people tend to do, thrust his right hand out for me to grasp, and with a broad, engaging grin said in a delightful "Kiwi" drawl: "Gidday. Am I pleased to meet you!"

So began a friendship and a research relationship that continued for many years. Michael's eagerness to partici- pate in any new experiment I could think up, and his inter- est in his own performance and what it could tell us not only about him but also more generally about how the mind works, made him a delight to work with. He was one of my keenest students, and if it had been possible to replace the lost neurons and connections in Michael's brain so that he could function normally again, I would not have been surprised if he decided to take up formal neuropsy- chological studies.

Of course many neurological patients who have disor- ders almost as interesting as those demonstrated by Michael do not become long-term "special" cases. Sometimes this is because they are not interested and will- ing to participate in ongoing experiments, but more often it is because they have other problems that prevent their involvement. For example, the attributes that made Michael an excellent research subject included his youth, normal verbal intelligence, excellent attention span, and ability to concentrate for long periods. These are precious commodi- ties in a neuropsychological subject, as neurological patients frequently have impairments such as poor concen- tration or difficulty understanding or following instruc- tions, making them difficult to test. Many patients who would otherwise be good neuropsychological subjects tire quickly, but in test sessions with Michael I often tired before him! A final important attribute of his case was the unchanging, stable nature of his brain damage and his neuropsychological problems. Brain scans since his discharge from hospital over a 14-year period demonstrated that no obvious changes occurred in that time. Even after many years of rehabilitation, Michael remained unable to recognize most objects on sight and remained completely unable to recognize faces on sight. His largely unchanging disorders were disappointing for his rehabilitation but paradoxically valuable for the research. On the bright side—the side Michael invariably took—other rehabilitation strategies were successful: these were strategies to help him live a richer life in spite of his disorders.

*****

When I first saw Michael, he had undergone a CT brain scan when in critical care but had never had a magnetic resonance imaging (MRI) brain scan. MRI technology was still very new and expensive, and at that time in New Zealand the only way to obtain such a scan was to travel to Australia. I applied for a small research grant specifically for this, and Michael was very excited when the funds were forthcoming. He and his mother boarded the plane for Melbourne and returned after a few days with a beautiful picture of his brain (see Figure 6.1). I had seen many MRI brain scans before, but this was the first I had seen of one of my own patients. The detail was amazing after the CT scans that I was used to. Now, many years later, this scan still looks good to me even though the MRI scans of today are so much better.

Look at Michael's scan and imagine it is of a slice made horizontally through the brain above the eyes. The two hemispheres of the brain are like two halves of an apple split through the middle. The *frontal lobes* (one in each hemisphere, above our eyes) are at the top of the picture, and the *occipital lobes*, at the back of the brain, are at the

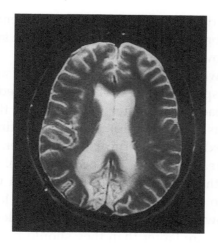

FIGURE 6.1
The magnetic resonance image of Michael's brain (with the right
hemisphere shown on the left side of the scan). It shows areas of damage
within the medial aspects of both occipital lobes (lower middle aspect of the
scan) affecting gray matter and subcortical white matter, with the damage
more prominent on the right. (Reprinted from Ogden, J. A. 1993. Visual
object agnosia, prosopagnosia, achromatopsia, loss of visual imagery and
autobiographical amnesia following recovery from cortical blindness: Case
M.H. *Neuropsychologia.*, *31*, p. 575, with kind permission from Elsevier
Science Ltd, Kidlington, UK.)

bottom. Between the two are the *parietal lobes*, and if you
could see a slice lower down in the brain, near the ears,
this area would be the *temporal lobes,* which lie below the
parietal lobes. Around the circumference of the brain you
can see the intricate folds of the gray matter of the cortex.
This is the outside layer of neurons of the brain; on an MRI
scan they look like white lines or creases. Michael's cortex
looks normal and healthy. Beneath the cortex is subcortical
white matter (which looks gray on this MRI scan). The
large white symmetrical areas in the middle of the brain
are fluid-filled spaces called lateral ventricles. The fluid in
these is cerebrospinal fluid (CSF), which is produced at the
rate of 600 to 700 milliliters a day within the ventricles,

flows out of them through other smaller ventricles lower down in the brain, and circulates around the surface of the brain right down into the spinal cord.

At the lower end of Michael's ventricles are two areas in a slightly splotchy white. This is an altered MRI signal indicating dead brain matter (*infarction*) on the inside, or *medial,* aspects of both occipital lobes, affecting both gray matter (cortex) and subcortical white matter. The area of damage is greater in the right occipital lobe. (Just to confuse things, the brain is usually reversed in CT and MRI brain scans so that the right is shown on the left of the picture.) The lower part of the lateral ventricles (called the *occipital horns*) are larger than they should be because they have extended into the space made when the brain tissue surrounding them died. These extended ventricles suggest that this damage has been there, unchanged, for many years. Other slices of Michael's brain showed that the forward-traveling neural pathways from the occipital lobes to the temporal lobes were damaged on both sides, and on the right side the forward-traveling pathways to the parietal lobe were also damaged. No other areas of significant damage can be seen within the brain.

Like Michael, most patients with visual object agnosia have damage to both occipital lobes—the visual lobes—at the back of the brain, although one lobe might have more damage than the other. The cortex of the occipital lobes is made up of the neurons involved in seeing (primary visual cortex), in visual perception (secondary visual cortex), and in visual knowledge (association cortex).[2] So we would expect patients with visual object agnosia to have damage to the secondary or association cortex, but that at least some of the neurons in the primary cortex would be intact

[2] See Chapter 1 for an explanation of the occipital lobes and how the different areas of cortex relate to the basic sensation of seeing, the next level of perceiving what the object is, and the higher level of knowing in more detail what one is seeing.

because if the primary visual cortex were completely absent, the person would not be able to see at all.

The next step after obtaining Michael's MRI scan was to assess how well Michael could see. The optometrist's findings were the same as his findings three years earlier: Michael's visual acuity was adequate and correctable to normal with glasses, but his visual fields were markedly reduced, leaving him with five- to eight-degree central fields in both eyes. What this meant is that Michael viewed the world down a tunnel. As long as the objects and pictures he was viewing were held at arm's length and were small, he could scan them and see them in their entirety perfectly well. This important fact allowed his impaired vision to be ruled out as the cause of his more complex, higher visual disorders: He was unable to recognize even the objects and faces he could see at the end of the tunnel. Michael was also found to have no color vision in his right eye and moderately impaired color vision in his left eye.

How his cortical blindness resolved at all almost two years after his head injury remains a mystery. Possibly some neurons in his visual cortex were disabled rather than permanently damaged at the time of his accident, and it took many months for the number of neurons necessary for useful sight to regain their function, perhaps via the formation of new neural connections. Another possible pathway for recovery is the formation of new neurons themselves, or *neurogenesis*. Contrary to what was once believed, we now know that neurogenesis can occur in the vertebrate brain: Rats exposed to an enriched environment both before and after a cerebral insult show enhanced neurogenesis and decreased cell death in the *hippocampus*, a brain area involved in spatial learning and memory. These same rats show improved cognitive performance, especially on tasks tapping those particular abilities. It also appears that the human hippocampal formation produces new neurons throughout adulthood. Although as yet there is no sound evidence that new neurons can form in the human visual cortex, perhaps some degree of neurogenesis was stimulated in Michael's occipital cortex by the intensive program to improve his vision instigated by his rehabilitation therapists when he first began seeing the moving lights of cars many months after his accident. But there is no evidence of any further increase in Michael's visual fields over the past 17 years, suggesting that the recovery in sight that did occur was time-limited.

Now that I had a detailed assessment of Michael's sight and knew where the damage was in his brain, I could try to tie up—or correlate—his behavioral deficits with his specific brain lesions, and I read up on similar cases to see if Michael's deficits and lesions matched them. Already I could see he was a "classic" case of visual object agnosia, and his lesions in the medial occipital lobe matched— roughly at least—the lesions of many other patients with visual agnosia. More fascinating were Michael's other disorders, some of which had not been reported before in connection with these rather well-defined bilateral medial occipital lesions. The detective in me was eager to get onto the case, and my keen assistant was Michael himself.

*****

To begin, I needed to know in general how he was functioning intellectually. Of course he could not be assessed on tests that required recognizing pictures and patterns, and his tunnel vision was too bad to permit assessing him on tests that relied on sight. But his performance on verbal tests was quite normal, falling easily within the average range. Even better, because he had been given the same tests three years earlier, I knew that his verbal abilities had remained unchanged over a three-year period, suggesting again that his brain damage was stable. He could repeat seven digits forward and five backward, demonstrating a normal attention span, an important consideration if a person is to be subjected to neuropsychological testing. He scored particularly well on tests of vocabulary and comprehension, a good indication of his pre-accident (or *pre-morbid*) verbal intelligence.

On tests involving the ability to think abstractly, Michael also performed well. Abstraction is one of the most advanced abilities humans possess, and is usually associated with the frontal lobes. For example, Michael had no difficulty giving the abstract meanings of proverbs such as "A rolling stone gathers no moss." Along with consistent evidence that his performance on other frontal lobe tests and his behaviors in a range of situations in daily life were generally appropriate, his performance suggested that his frontal lobe functions fell within normal limits. This is an important finding in a person who has sustained a severe traumatic brain injury, as frontal lobe damage is very common in this group. Even a CT or MRI scan that shows apparently undamaged frontal lobes is no guarantee that extensive frontal lobe damage has not occurred. Damage that involves shearing and tearing of the white matter tracts connecting the frontal cortex to the rest of the brain is often too diffuse to be visualized. Thus neurobehavioral assessment of frontal lobe dysfunction is essential given the subtle but significant influence of the executive deficits associated with damaged frontal lobes on a range of apparently unrelated abilities.

Michael's speech was fluent and his comprehension normal. He could point accurately on command to lower- and uppercase letters displayed randomly on a page. He could read fluently words in small print held at 1.5 meters to compensate for his tunnel vision. His writing and printing of individual letters, words, and sentences spontaneously and to dictation was slow but generally accurate, and he could read his own printing. His reading of handwriting was slower and less accurate than his reading of print. His ability to imagine letters was intact. For example, when asked to imagine a letter like a small "c" and decide whether it had curved or straight sides, he always responded correctly.

On tests of verbal memory and new learning, Michael demonstrated moderately severe deficits, suggesting that he had some temporal lobe damage, at least in the left, "verbal" hemisphere. Indeed, his MRI scan showed that the forward-traveling pathways from the occipital to the temporal lobes were damaged on both sides. It is important to note that his verbal memory deficit was not severe, as in the famous case of the global amnesic Henry Molaison, whose story is told in Chapter 7. For example, in contrast to his impaired scores on formal tests of new verbal learning, such as learning lists of unrelated words, Michael demonstrated good memory for conversations that held significance for him. He could recall the gist of conversations he and I had up to three years before and had apparently normal or near-normal recall of the names and other *semantic* (factual) information about people currently in his life. When I telephoned Michael on my return from a year long study leave overseas, on giving him my name he immediately responded by asking me how my trip was and what new tests and rehabilitation ideas I had discovered that might be helpful to him. Many years later I telephoned him "out of the blue" and he immediately recalled who I was. A long conversation about his life since we had last talked ensued, and he had no obvious difficulty with gross verbal recall. For example, within minutes of the beginning of our conversation he told me that Jill, his attendant caregiver, was there with him and that she was the same person who had been his attendant caregiver almost ten years previously, when we had been carrying out our original research. Michael probably also had some impairment of visual, nonverbal learning, but of course this could not be tested because he could not recognize visual patterns—other than simple shapes—or faces.

At last it was time to assess Michael on tests of visual object agnosia. A number of varieties of this disorder have been reported, and it was not a simple task to find out which, if any, fitted Michael best. Generally when assessing a higher cognitive disorder—that is, a disorder involving a deficit of thinking, whether conscious or unconscious—it is important to make sure that the lower levels of the skill are intact. I knew that Michael could see (the most basic sensory level), so I tested his visual perception (the next level in the vision hierarchy). He was accurate at discriminating line drawings of triangles with curved sides from those with straight sides, at pointing to the shortest and longest lines on pages of lines of different lengths, and at pointing to and recognizing different shapes (squares, rectangles, circles, hexagons, and so on). He could discriminate small from large squares and circles, and draw shapes accurately on command. But look at his copies of line drawings of a pig, a bird, and a turtle in Figure 6.2. He made these very slowly, hesitating frequently as he copied them line by line, admitting he had no idea what he was drawing. When asked what his copy of the turtle was, he said he didn't know, but perhaps it could be a bird. He wouldn't guess the identity of the bird.

These tests convinced me that Michael's visual perception was intact. He could not only physically see or *sense* drawings or objects; he could understand them at a basic level of lines and curves and size. But he couldn't put any meaning to what he perceived; he could not tell if the thing was an object or an animal or a scene. Over the years, he did learn to recognize a few objects that he used often, including his ashtray, eating utensils, and scissors. But even then he was very slow, especially if the object was out of context. The way he would go about it would be to describe the shape of the object out loud and then recognize from

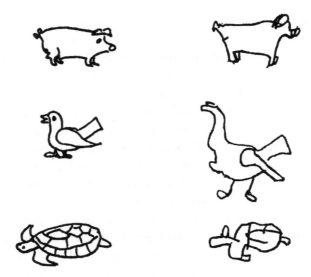

FIGURE 6.2

Michael's copies of animal drawings showing that he can copy the shape of the animals without knowing what he is copying. The models are in the left column and Michael's copies in the right column. (Reprinted from Ogden, J. A. 1993. Visual object agnosia, prosopagnosia, achromatopsia, loss of visual imagery and autobiographical amnesia following recovery from cortical blindness: Case M.H. *Neuropsychologia, 31*, p. 578, with kind permission from Elsevier Science Ltd, Kidlington, UK.)

his verbal description what it was. For example, he would say: "It is a long thin thing and has some thinner bits on one end. Aha, it's a fork!"

On a formal test where he was shown 30 real objects, he could recognize only eight, all of which he had been shown often as part of his rehabilitation program. He would describe each object to himself and then make a guess for every object whether or not he got them right. A yellow feather he called a "flower," a safety pin he called a "clothes peg," and a vegetable peeler he called a "razor." When shown a key, he described it thus: "A circle; there is a long, thin piece off one side; it is smooth on the top but seems to have a jagged edge on the bottom." But he could not recognize it. As soon as he picked it up, however, he recognized it instantly as a key. This was true for all the test objects. If the object could make a sound, he recognized it, and if he could feel it he knew what it was. His ability to recognize photographed objects, realistic three-dimensional paintings of objects, and line drawings of objects appeared slightly more impaired than his ability to recognize real objects. For example, he recognized a real telephone in four seconds (he often used a telephone), but he was still unable to recognize a line drawing of a similar telephone after 35 seconds of trying. I then said "ring, ring," and he said "Oh, is that what it is, a telephone!" One hour later, shown the same drawing, he was able to identify it correctly in five seconds.

He recognized two items, a house (eight seconds) and a spoon (six seconds), in a series of 20 black-and-white photographs of common items. He was shown 30 realistic colored paintings of common objects, animals, and people in context (e.g., sheep in a paddock, a baby eating from a bowl, apples on a tree, fruit in a bowl) taken from a series of books used for teaching words to three-year-old children. He was asked to name specific objects in each painting and was able to name only two items correctly, a pen and a person, and even those took him three and four seconds, respectively. He was unable to say whether the person was male or female, adult or child. He could identify some animals as animals after describing their form to himself, but he was not able to identify any specific animal correctly. In all the above experiments, he was given a minimum of 60 seconds—a very long time—before being permitted to give up, and longer if he thought he might be able to recognize the item given even more time.

Michael was also severely impaired in naming line drawings of single objects or living things. Of a series of 60 items, he named only three. Again, with repeated exposures over a short period he became faster at recognizing his own descriptions, but this did not indicate a true improvement in his recognition, as he soon forgot what his own verbal description was most likely to describe. For example, when first shown a line drawing of an elephant, he attempted to describe its shape but was still unable to recognize it after 30 seconds. He was then told it was an animal, but this did not assist him. He was then given the names of five animals and asked which one it was. He correctly selected an elephant and was able to point to the trunk. One hour later, he was shown the same drawing, and after nine seconds he was able to identify it as an animal "because it has four legs," but he could not be more specific. When shown the same line drawing two years later, he was once again completely unable to identify it or even correctly categorize it as an animal.

I gave the same 30 real objects used in the visual recognition experiment to Michael to manipulate with his right hand, his left arm having been amputated. I put large objects, such as a telephone, on a table in front of a blindfolded Michael, and placed his right hand on the object. Small objects like a key were placed in his right hand. He was free to manipulate the objects as he wished, and when necessary they were held steady while he explored them. He named all 30 objects correctly within one to four seconds.

While blindfolded, Michael was asked to name 20 sounds, such as water being poured from a jug into a cup, the rattle of a bunch of keys, the sound of rain outside the building, and scissors cutting paper. He named all sounds correctly within one second.

Just to be sure Michael didn't have a problem with knowing what an object or animal was in a more general sense (that is, not just via its appearance), he was given the name (e.g., "cat") or other identifying information (e.g., "something that goes 'meow'") about an object or an animal and asked to describe it. His performance was normal in almost all cases. When given the names, he was able to describe the function of the 30 objects used in the visual and tactile recognition experiments (e.g., he could say what a spade is used for). He was also able to describe living things and natural phenomena (e.g., trees, specific animals, clouds, mountains) and provide factual information about them. For example he said a cow provided milk and meat, a tree was a large plant that grew in the ground and provided shade on a hot day, and a cloud was a fluffy thing that floated in the sky and sometimes produced rain. In contrast, he was frequently unable to describe accurately the shape of the object or living thing. For example, when asked what a cup was, he said it was made out of pottery or china and was for drinking. When asked about its shape, he said that it was hollow with a handle to hold it. When asked if he could visualize a cup, he said he could not, but that he knew he picked it up by a handle to drink from, and it must be hollow to hold coffee. When asked what a canary was, he said it was a small bird that whistled, but he could not quite see its shape. He thought it had two legs. He did not know what color it was, but he thought it might be blue.

Michael could quickly and accurately draw from memory triangles, squares, rectangles, crosses, and circles. He could draw on command shapes of different sizes and lines of different lengths. For example, he responded correctly when asked to draw a line across the top of the page and underneath it a line of half the length of the first one. He could draw a large circle above a cross and a small circle below the cross. He could also draw on command some objects with simple shapes (e.g., a rugby ball, a basketball, a rugby field, an apple, a banana). He could draw in a simplistic fashion some more complex common objects on command. For example, he was able to draw a recognizable house and key (see Figure 6.3), but his drawing of a flower looked more like a palm tree and he drew a bed as a

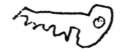

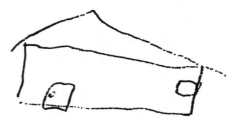

FIGURE 6.3
Michael's drawings of a key and a house from long-term memory. These
show that Michael can draw in a formulaic, nondetailed manner some very
common objects. (Reprinted from Ogden, J. A. 1993. Visual object agnosia,
prosopagnosia, achromatopsia, loss of visual imagery and autobiographical
amnesia following recovery from cortical blindness: Case M.H.
Neuropsychologia, 31, p. 580, with kind permission from Elsevier Science Ltd,
Kidlington, UK.)

rectangle with four legs. He would not even attempt more
complex or unfamiliar objects, such as a telephone or a
broom, because he said he could not think how they might
look. He was also unable to draw or visualize any specific
objects, such as the house where he grew up.

When asked to visualize and describe a surfing beach
where he had spent a great deal of time before his accident,
and which he had been to since, he said he could imagine
the waves and the sand and hear the surf, but he did not
describe the dramatic scenic surrounds of bushes, cliffs,
and rocky peninsulas. When asked the color of the sand,
he said it was pale, when in fact it is of a distinctive black
iron color.

It appeared, therefore, that Michael was unable to visualize or imagine objects and scenes from his long-term memory store, or, alternatively, that he had lost the visual memory "templates" (patterns of specific objects) themselves. The drawings he was able to do and his verbal descriptions of visual forms from memory were impoverished and nonspecific and probably represented stylized prototypes of general object categories. Michael also said he didn't have dreams, perhaps suggesting a loss of the ability to generate visual images.

*****

Michael had a total inability to recognize any faces on sight, and this has not improved over the 24 years since his accident. Practice and familiarity did not help; he never recognized his mother until she spoke although he saw her almost daily. He was unable to pick out any familiar face, including his own, in family photographs taken before and after his accident. I showed him a collage of photographs of faces of people famous and well known to him before his accident and faces of people he would never have seen. When asked to point to any faces that seemed more familiar to him, he said that none seemed familiar. When asked to describe verbally from memory the very distinctive face of a famous New Zealand prime minister who had been in the public eye for many years before and after Michael's accident, Michael said (accurately) that he had a lopsided smile. When he was then asked to guess which of the faces on the collage was this man's very distinctive face, he pointed to a man whose face he had never seen before.

Michael's ability to discriminate gender, age, and expression of faces was also greatly impaired. He would sometimes guess gender correctly by the length of hair, but when this was controlled for, he performed at chance levels. When asked to say whether a face looked happy or sad, he would rely on the shape of the mouth and made numerous errors. When asked how old the person in a photograph of a baby might be, he said it looked like an old man because it did not have much hair. When he was shown photographs of single faces and asked to match each one to the identical face in a pair of faces, he performed correctly on all eight trials, but took a long time, generally matching the face by the hairline.

Michael also had a problem with identifying colors, whether in isolation or in the context of an object. He commented that he saw everything as shades between white and black. When asked to name the color of tokens, he was correct only on white and black ones. All other colors he named either "white" or "pale," or "black" or "dark." Yellow was "white," and dark blue was "black." When asked to group tokens according to their color, he made two piles; one he called "dark," the other "pale." This loss of color perception is termed *achromatopsia*, and it results from bilateral lesions in the *prestriate visual cortex* extending to the temporal lobe, lesions that fit well with Michael's. When Michael was asked to give the colors of named (but not seen) objects, animals, or natural phenomena, he was usually correct with regard to natural phenomena that are frequently and stereotypically associated with their color names, such as blue sky, white clouds, blue sea, green grass, and white snow. He made numerous errors on most objects and living things. For example, he guessed a banana to be either green or blue, and although he described a strawberry as a small, sweet berry that grows on low bushes and is eaten with sugar and cream, he could not visualize its shape or its color. Toast was "dark" and an apple was "brown." He described a sparrow correctly as a small, common bird, but he was unable to visualize or remember its color. He guessed it to be blue, and when told it was brown, he said this did not enable him to visualize it. When asked what color his skin was, he first said it was blue; told that was wrong, he said pinkish white. This loss of the ability to visualize colors would probably impede his ability to remember or recall colors.

*****

Michael's loss of color memory was trivial compared with another of his memory problems. In apparent contrast to his reasonable verbal recall of life events since his accident, Michael had a striking loss of personal memories that extended back from his accident into his early childhood. His mother, other family members, and friends he knew in school and in the armed forces spent hours retelling Michael about his past. Michael would comment that he could not really remember a described episode, although he sometimes remembered it from having been told about it since. A striking example of this loss of all personal memories prior to his accident—*retrograde autobiographical memory loss*—was his forgetting of his 21st birthday, just three years before his accident. This was a large celebration remembered very clearly by his family and friends.

On a test of autobiographical memory where the individual is asked to describe facts (such as the address of the house lived in as a child) and personal events (such as an incident that occurred in primary school), Michael's score was well into the abnormally low range, more so for personal events and for events further back in time from his accident. He did retain some auditory memories from before his accident. While still a patient in the hospital he could recognize the horns of specific ships in the harbor close by; he had previously spent three years in the navy specializing in sonar. He was also able to recognize the voices of his friends, and even today he can still remember both the melody and words of some songs popular prior to his accident.

His severe loss of memory for personal events from before his accident is in dramatic contrast to his memory for personal events since his accident. Of course even his current memories don't contain any visual information. For example, he described a barbecue he had been to four days earlier thus: "I had a ball. It was a beautiful, sunny day after all that rain we've been having. They had some really good spicy sausages, and of course I got drunk later in the evening." He said he could recapture the sounds and tastes of the occasion in his mind and the good feelings he had, but he had no visual images or memories of the occasion whatsoever. Michael's memory loss for events prior to his accident is hard to explain when we look at his MRI scan. Occipital lesions do not result in amnesia, and although some pathways to the temporal ("memory") lobes were damaged, he had no obvious damage to the temporal lobes themselves. The only way to make sense of this deficit is to postulate that his autobiographical retrograde amnesia results from his inability to recall the visual components and visual images associated with his personal memories. Given that humans are generally very reliant on the visual aspects of their experiences, perhaps Michael's inability to recall or imagine visual aspects of objects, faces, and colors impoverishes his memories so much that it is as if he doesn't have any recall of an event. For example, even if Michael's recollection of his 21st birthday party could be activated by hearing a recording of a speech made at the party or by the music played, his reconstruction of the event would be so constrained by not being able to remember the dominant visual aspects such as peoples' faces, the room the party was held in, or his birthday cake that he might not recall the event at all.

*****

Michael's inability to recognize objects or faces is, in a sense, almost more debilitating than being totally blind. He is always striving to recognize what he sees, which can act as a barrier to learning how to cope without sight. Because he can read it is not necessary for him to learn braille; yet his tunnel vision makes reading extremely tiring. His problems in moving about due to his loss of one arm and his old orthopedic injuries are only exacerbated by trying to avoid objects that appear to loom up at the end of a tunnel and that he is not able to recognize. However, while he sometimes comments on his inability to make mental pictures and his loss of dreams, these impairments do not seem to worry him.

His mildly impaired ability to retain new information makes rehabilitation difficult at times. For example, learning how to cook with one arm and an inability to visually recognize a saucepan, carrot, or tomato requires that everything in the kitchen be kept consistently in the same place. Michael forgets what goes where and has difficulty remembering to follow simple but important safety measures when cooking. He cannot go out alone, because he cannot learn new routes as many blind people can and because his poor physical mobility makes it too dangerous.

His loss of pre-accident autobiographical memories does not seem to upset him unduly, perhaps because his mother and friends have spent many hours telling him about his past to help him gradually build up some sense of where he comes from. He remembers his old friends well (from their voices), but he cannot recall anything they did together. It is a credit to Michael's friendly and happy nature and great sense of fun that he has retained some good friends over the years since his accident. They still collect him and take him to their homes for a meal or party, where he enjoys drinking and socializing.

Given his many disabilities, it would be understandable if Michael often felt depressed and frustrated or became disenchanted with the ongoing grind of rehabilitation. Remarkably, this has not happened, and Michael consistently maintains his positive outlook. When asked how he does this, he replies that he is lucky to be alive and he could be much worse off. As he says, he has regained his sight, and his ability to walk about is improving, especially with the latest operation on his foot. He does not appear to harbor any underlying feelings of bitterness or anger about his fate, although he does, of course, feel depressed at times about the future. If he were always happy, it would indicate that he had poor insight into his problems and suggest that he had sustained some frontal lobe damage. Throughout his rehabilitation, Michael has generally maintained a high level of motivation, although he becomes frustrated with the slow pace of establishing the sequential steps needed to cope safely with activities of daily living.

After living in the Institute for the Blind, in his mother's home with a full-time caregiver and rehabilitation therapist, in a good friend's home, and in a home for young disabled people, six years after his accident Michael achieved, at least in part, his desire for independence. He moved into a rental apartment where he lived alone, but with an attendant caregiver, Jill, coming in daily to help him and accompany him when he wanted to go out. He learned his way around the rooms and became skilled at using the telephone and microwave oven, washing dishes, and cleaning. Jill has continued to come to his house for a few hours every weekday for the past 17 or more years. She is now a grandmother and she and her family have become Michael's close friends. As Michael joked, "Jill and I are like an old married couple, but without the sex!"

Some years after his accident Michael received from the New Zealand Government Accident Compensation scheme some belated compensation, which, with the help of Jill, he invested wisely for his future, but which also enabled him to follow some of his dreams. He purchased his own house and in 1999 he flew to the United States with Lou, a friend he made following his accident. Lou worked for an organization called Bikers' Rights and assisted motorcyclists injured in accidents. He and Michael became good friends, and Lou would often take Michael for trips in the sidecar of his Harley-Davidson. Michael has always loved motorcycles, and the accident that almost took his life and certainly changed it forever has not in any way diminished his passion. His total amnesia for the accident itself and his very hazy memories of the many months of operations and pain that followed was probably a significant factor in allowing his love of riding motorcycles to remain untarnished.

Michael had a dream to ride Route 66 in the US, and Lou said, "Why not?" Michael's mother was initially worried that he would end up in another accident, this time perhaps a fatal one. But his mother joined the dream-believers after thinking about Jill's wise comment that Michael could sit in his big leather chair in his safe house for the rest of his life, or he could follow his dream, even if the risks were great. After much organization and planning, Michael and Lou flew to Los Angeles from New Zealand, then to San Antonio, where they picked up a Harley-Davidson. They then proceeded to ride, with Michael in the sidecar, to New Orleans, Memphis— including Graceland—and Chicago, where they picked up Route 66 and rode to Los Angeles, Las Vegas, and back to San Antonio. In Chicago they fell off their motorcycle and Michael suffered a bad gash to his left leg, which had been severely fractured in his original accident. The Chicago surgeon who attended him was a motorcyclist himself, and stitched him in such a way that he could continue his journey across the States. As Michael told me later, "My leg was a mess when we got back to New Zealand, and I had to have more surgery, but man, it was worth it!"

When they returned, Lou made up a photograph album of their travels, but then realized that this wasn't much use to Michael. He then had the wonderful idea to put together a series of musical CDs to remind Michael of their trip. For example, the first CD includes "Leaving on a Jet Plane," "New Orleans," "Memphis, Tennessee," "Carolina Blues," "Miami Vice," "The Painted Desert," "Needles and Pins," "Grand Canyon," "Viva Las Vegas," "Tombstone," "Riders on the Storm," "Waltz Across Texas," and "Harley-Davidson Blues." Michael believes that he can remember parts of his trip, especially when cued by the songs on his CDs, which remind him of those locations or the music they enjoyed on their trip. Even if his memories of details of the trip are vague and nonspecific, the emotions and impressions of that trip—the feel and smell of the motorcycle and his leather gear, the wind on his face, the perfumes in the air, the music (often also linked to his past before he had the accident), and simply riding Route 66—are instantly and vividly brought to life for him by the music and of course by sharing stories with Lou, Jill, and his mother. With friends like Lou and Jill, who needs professional rehabilitation therapists! Michael's story is truly one of triumph over adversity, with a little help from friends.

Michael thinks he can "see" a little better now, and he and Jill sometimes even go to movies—although he admits that it is the sound track rather than the visuals that allows him to follow the plot. He thinks that he can recall autobiographical memories laid down since his accident that involve sound, tactile sensations, and emotions. Certainly, his spontaneous recall is clear for many of the tasks we did during the original assessments many years ago.

Michael's story not only teaches us about some fascinating neuropsychological disorders but also provides lessons in courage, stamina, determination, and an all-important ability to laugh at oneself when all else fails. These characteristics have enabled Michael to progress to a reasonably independent life despite minimal recovery of his visual and memory impairments. Now 48 years old, he has not been able to visually recognize his mother, friends, or the world around him for 24 years, half his life span. Yet he remains the positive, effervescent person I first met and continues to live life to the full. As he likes to say, "Well I can see a little, but can conceive of all!"

*****

For many clinical neuropsychologists, doctors, nurses, and rehabilitation therapists who work with patients like Michael, the theoretical insights provided by research studies are interesting but must take a backseat to the more urgent need to assist the patient to a state where he or she can regain a reasonable quality of life. To do so requires practical knowledge that often can be learned only by working with brain-damaged patients. Experienced rehabilitation therapists know, almost by intuition, when a patient can be pushed a little further and when it is time for a rest or a change of activity. They learn how to predict and prevent the sudden outbreaks of aggression that can happen to any patient as a result of frustration and fatigue, and they know when a touch of humor will lighten the situation and help the patient to laugh at himself or herself. They know when a patient needs to cry and to express anger or helplessness, and they learn how to listen to what the patient needs to help him or her at these times.

The rehabilitation therapist must have an abundance of practical knowledge, patience, stamina, determination, compassion, and humor. The rewards come from working with a person like Michael, who in spite of massive disabilities courageously continues to make small positive steps—and occasionally giant strides—while retaining his good humor and endearing himself to all who have the good fortune to come within his auditory or tactile orbit.

■ Further Reading

Ogden, J. A. 1993. Visual object agnosia, prosopagnosia, achromatopsia, loss of visual imagery and autobiographical amnesia following recovery from cortical blindness: Case M.H. *Neuropsychologia, 31,* 571–589.

Ogden, J. A. 2005. Vision without knowledge: Visual object agnosia and prosopagnosia. In: *Fractured Minds: A Case-Study Approach to Clinical Neuropsychology, 2nd Ed.* (pp. 137–157). New York: Oxford University Press.

Powers, R. 2006. *The Echo Maker: A Novel.* New York: Farrar, Straus and Giroux.

Sacks, O. 1970. The Man Who Mistook His Wife for a Hat. In: *The Man Who Mistook His Wife for a Hat* (pp. 7–21). New York: Summit Books.

Sacks, O. 2010. Face-blind. In: *The Mind's Eye.* (pp. 82–110). New York: Alfred A Knopf.

7 ■
HM and Elvis: A Special Memory

In August 1953, in a hospital in the town of Hartford, Connecticut, 27-year-old Henry Molaison lay awake on an operating table while a neurosurgeon drilled two 3.8-centimeter holes above his eyes with a hand-cranked rotary drill and inserted a spatula to lift up the frontal lobes of his brain, exposing the temporal lobes. He then proceeded to suction out—first on one side of the brain and then on the other—the seahorse-shaped brain structure called the *hippocampus* that lay within each temporal lobe.

When Henry died, aged 82, on December 2, 2008, extensive obituaries for him appeared in the *New York Times* and *The Lancet*, one of the world's best-known and respected medical journals. So who was this man, and why was he posthumously honored in this way? In the 55 years between that fateful day in 1953 and the day he died, Henry Molaison—for his protection known only as "HM" until his death—taught the world about memory. But he never received a Nobel Prize, and his fame did not come from his life's work as a medical or neuroscience researcher, vocations perhaps considered interesting enough to rate a *New York Times* obituary. No, he was just an average sort of fellow who worked on an assembly line in Hartford before his surgery. But his life's work after his surgery was anything but average.

The removal of the hippocampus on both sides of Henry's brain—an experimental procedure carried out in the hope of reducing the epileptic seizures he suffered—took away his memory. Fortunately for neuroscience, when his neurosurgeon, William Beecher Scoville, realized Henry was amnesic, he referred him to the eminent neurosurgeon Dr. Wilder Penfield and neuropsychologist Dr. Brenda Milner of the Montreal Neurological Institute. They had already begun memory experiments on two brain-damaged patients, but the extent and purity of Henry's amnesia, his intact intelligence, and the surgical precision of his brain lesions made him a perfect experimental subject. Thus Henry—HM—became the most studied and most famous medical case in history, mentioned in almost 12,000 journal articles. In between research sessions, usually carried out at the Massachusetts Institute of Technology (MIT), Henry lived incognito in a nursing home in Hartford, access to him denied to the media and restricted to fewer than 100 researchers among the thousands who would have loved to work with him.

Over more than half a century, researchers discovered that Henry's memory loss was far from simple. Not only was he unable to consciously learn or remember any new information after his surgery; he also suffered a memory loss for a period of 11 years before. In contrast, he did retain the ability to learn some new motor skills, but this learning was at a subconscious level. For example, he became faster at drawing a path through a picture of a maze, but he had no conscious memory that he had ever seen or done the maze test before. Even then, the number of errors he made did not decrease, showing that he could not learn the sequence of turns through the maze; he just learned to manipulate his pencil faster between the lines. In essence, until his death, Henry's conscious knowledge base remained as it was when he was a teenager, although his intelligence in other areas was largely unimpaired. It was as though time stopped for him around the age of 16 years, and from the day of his surgery forward he interacted only "in the moment" with whatever stimuli impinged directly upon him. For the last 55 years of his life Henry (shown at age 60 in Figure 7.1) was unaware of his priceless gift to humanity.

Suzanne Corkin, a professor in the Department of Brain and Cognitive Sciences at MIT, led the massive research program on Henry from the mid-1960s on and also acted

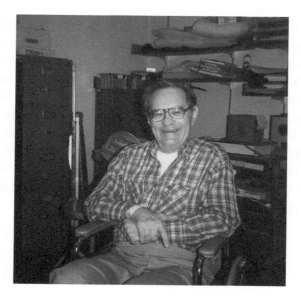

FIGURE 7.1
Henry Molaison, at age 60, in the neuropsychology test laboratory at the Massachusetts Institute of Technology, Cambridge, Massachusetts. (Photograph by Jenni Ogden, 1986.)

as his guardian and protector, carrying out this role with wisdom and compassion. Henry was a great favorite with researchers and clinical staff alike because of his endearing nature, sense of humor, and willingness to be helpful. The same experiment could be repeated time after time without Henry's showing any signs of boredom, because each time the experiment was new to him. Repeating the same experiment numerous times would certainly have become tedious for Henry's experimenters except for the delightful personality of their subject and the conversations and interactions that occurred during the testing session.

As a postdoctoral fellow in Professor Corkin's MIT laboratory, I was one of the fortunate few to meet and work with Henry, who was then 59.[1] In this chapter, as well as telling a brief version of the story of his life, I will try to paint a picture of Henry as a person, a view that is usually masked in the research literature by the technical descriptions of the experiment that is the focus of the article. In addition, I also hope to illustrate one of the most important aspects of studying a single case: how everyday interactions and behaviors as well as the quantifiable results of carefully designed experiments can feed into the hypotheses we propose and then test to develop theories about how the mind works. In Henry's case the primary focus was memory and its many facets, but along the way Henry provided many clues about how memory—or its absence—relates to other cognitive or thinking processes and influences most aspects of our psyche and our social world.

*****

Born in 1926, Henry had a normal, uneventful childhood until he was nine, when he was knocked down by a

[1] I am grateful to Brenda Milner and Suzanne Corkin for their permission to study Henry.

bicycle and became unconscious for about five minutes. When he was 10 years old he began having *absence seizures* (minor seizures involving only a small area of the brain and noticeable only by a brief loss of focus on a task), possibly as a result of this earlier minor head injury. He remembered suffering his first *generalized seizure* (a major seizure involving the whole brain and resulting in a loss of consciousness and often convulsions; previously called a *grand mal seizure*)[2] on his 16th birthday when he was a passenger in a car. He left high school because he was teased by his peers about his seizures, but he returned later to a different high school and graduated at the age of 21, having taken the "practical" course. He enjoyed roller-skating and hunting, and until his death often reminisced about these activities. After he completed high school, he was able to work for a while on an assembly line before his seizures became too frequent. Henry showed little interest in girls and never married or had a serious girl-friend. His lack of interest in sexual relationships or conversation about sexual topics didn't change after his operation, and there has been some speculation that the removal of his hippocampus exacerbated a preexisting hyposexuality, perhaps a consequence of his epilepsy or antiepileptic drugs.

From the age of 16 until his operation 11 years later, Henry had about ten absence seizures a day and one generalized seizure a week, and these seizures could not be controlled by large doses of antiepileptic medications. During minor seizures there were some generalized electroencephalography (EEG) abnormalities, especially in the temporal lobe regions of both hemispheres, and this presumably encouraged Dr. Scoville to perform a *bilateral medial temporal lobectomy* when Henry was 27. This means that the inside (medial) region of the temporal lobe, which

[2]See Chapter 8 for more detail on different epileptic seizure types.

constitutes most of the *hippocampus*, was removed (a lobectomy) on both sides (bilaterally).

Magnetic resonance imaging (MRI) scans many years later (see Figure 7.2) showed that Scoville had removed five to six centimeters from each hippocampus, leaving the

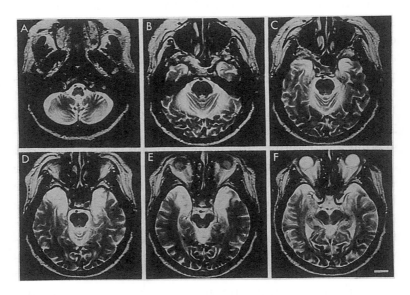

FIGURE 7.2

A magnetic resonance imaging scan of Henry Molaison's brain carried out when he was age 66. It shows T2 weighted axial (horizontal) sections through the brain (as if looking down on it). *A* and *B* are lower sections and show the two cerebellar hemispheres (primarily concerned with the coordination and fine tuning of movements) that lie below the two cerebral hemispheres. These have white areas (showing fluid-filled spaces) on Henry's scan indicating marked neuronal death (atrophy). In sections *E* and *F* the eyes can be seen at the top of the scans indicating the position of these higher sections through the brain. In sections *C* to *F* the temporal lobes can be seen clearly, following the outer curve of the lower part of each cerebral hemisphere. The white areas indicate spaces filled with cerebrospinal fluid where Dr. Scoville removed, on each side, the hippocampus lying within the temporal lobe, along with the amygdala near the end of each temporal lobe. (Reproduced from Corkin, S., Amaral, D. G., Gonzalez, R. G., Johnson, K. A., and Hyman, B. T. 1997. *Journal of Neuroscience, 17 (10)*, p. 3970, with kind permission of the *Journal of Neuroscience*. Copyright 1997 by the Society for Neuroscience.)

posterior two centimeters intact. Both the *amygdala* (a small blob of brain situated immediately in front of the hippocampus and believed to be connected with emotions and aggression) and other medial brain areas close to the hippocampus were also removed or damaged. The poles of the temporal lobes were cut away, but most of the *temporal neocortex* (the outside portion of the temporal lobe that can be seen on the lateral view of the brain) was left intact. The temporal lobe is especially important for auditory functions—hearing words (primarily the left temporal lobe) and tones (primarily the right temporal lobe)—and the posterior part of left temporal lobe includes an area called *Wernicke's area* that mediates comprehension of language, so the neurosurgeon knew that he must not damage these essential areas of brain. Scoville had previously carried out medial temporal lobectomies on 30 psychiatric patients, but the psychological assessment of those patients was very crude and only one patient showed obvious memory problems after the surgery. Thus in 1953 it was not yet known that the hippocampus was essential for making new memories.

Even Scoville admitted that the operation was "frankly experimental." It reduced Henry's generalized seizures to one or two a year and his absence seizures to about five a month, although he had to remain on antiepileptic medications for the rest of his life. But as Scoville carefully sucked out Henry's hippocampus, first on one side and then the other, he sucked out Henry's ability to form new memories as well. How Henry experienced this we will never know. As he lay there on the operating table, his skull numbed by a local anesthetic, perhaps he was trying to take his mind off the unpleasant sounds and smells of the activity going on at the top of his head by thinking about how his life might improve after the operation if his seizures were cured. And then at some point he must have lost his focus as his ability to tie his thoughts together over time vanished with his liquefied hippocampus. If Scoville had asked him at that point why he was having a brain operation Henry's answer might well have been "I don't remember," a phrase he would use more than any other over the next 55 years. Once the tragedy of Henry's memory loss became apparent, Scoville campaigned widely against performing bilateral medial temporal lobectomies on humans in the future.

Following his operation, Henry lived with his parents, attending a rehabilitation workshop daily for 10 years. After his parents died, from 1980 until his death he lived in a nursing home. He remained unsure about whether his parents were still alive. If asked, "Where are your parents?" he replied by giving the name of the town in which they lived. If asked more directly, "Are your parents living?" he replied that he was not sure. When asked where he lived, he often replied that he lived in a house with his mother, even 25 years after she had died.

Two or three times each year Henry stayed for one or two weeks at the Clinical Research Center at MIT to have a medical checkup and participate in memory and other psychological experiments. He seemed to enjoy his visits, greeting everyone with a smile and readily engaging in conversation. When asked if he would be willing to participate in an experiment, he always agreed immediately and was cooperative and pleasant throughout the test session. Over the many years that he came to the research center, he learned to associate the hospital environment with the university, and could tell you he was at MIT, always appearing pleased to have got this right. He knew he had a memory problem, although it is unlikely that he was aware of its extent or that he was the subject of a great deal of research.

I spent a considerable amount of time with Henry around his 60th birthday and did not meet him again until he was 66. In the intervening six years he had gained a little weight and was finding it increasingly difficult to walk, but otherwise he seemed exactly the same. His facial expressions, the sentences he used, the stories he told, and his mannerisms were uncannily identical to those I had witnessed six years before. My life had moved on, but Henry's had not.

*****

On the day before his operation, Henry was assessed on a general intelligence scale; his IQ was above average and would remain there for the rest of his life. But because there was no reason to believe that his memory would be affected by the operation, his memory abilities were not assessed. But after his surgery it quickly became evident that he had severe memory problems, and so began a new era of memory research.

Since Henry's operation, experiments on many brain-damaged patients have shown that impairments in new learning and memory can occur for verbal material (words) after damage to the structures—including the hippocampus—that make up the medial temporal lobe (MTL) of the hemisphere dominant for language (usually the left hemisphere). Memory for new nonverbal material (sounds, patterns, faces) is impaired to a lesser degree after damage to the MTL of the other hemisphere. Although either type of memory impairment can cause severe disability, the individual can usually continue to live independently, is well aware of the passage of time, and can often use intact memory abilities to compensate for those lost. For example, someone with a verbal memory impairment may not be able to recall a new name but will remember the person's face. Thus the problems these people experience are in no way as debilitating as the problems faced by someone with *global amnesia*, such as Henry. It seems clear that Henry had both verbal and nonverbal memory impairments because he had lost significant portions of the MTL structures of both hemispheres.

Global amnesia is global in the sense that it pervades every aspect of the victim's life. It includes an inability to learn or remember new personal experiences or facts from the time of the brain damage, whether verbal or nonverbal. The amnesic person can form no conscious memories of facts or events, whether they are experienced through the eyes or ears or by touch, taste, or smell. Global amnesics often also have a period of memory loss for events and facts that occurred before their brain damage. Henry's memory impairment encompassed all of these aspects.

Henry's case, since supported by experiments on other globally amnesic patients, demonstrated that such a dramatic loss of memory usually results from damage bilaterally to various structures, including the hippocampus, that lie deep within the brain. These structures form the *limbic system*, which is linked with emotion, motivation, and, as we now know because of Henry, memory. The disease herpes simplex encephalitis can damage the hippocampus on both sides of the brain and leave the sufferer with a global amnesia very similar to that shown by Henry. Korsakoff's disease, which is caused by a deficiency in thiamine—usually due to alcoholism—also results in global amnesia, but in this case different areas of the limbic system (namely the mammillary bodies and parts of the thalamus) are destroyed bilaterally. These brain areas along with the hippocampus are connected in a "C" shape, and work together to establish memories. The amnesia of Korsakoff's disease appears to be qualitatively different from the amnesia suffered by Henry. Henry's ability to store new information is severely curtailed, and therefore he has no information to later recall. In contrast, recall in people with Korsakoff's disease is aided by cues, which suggests that under some circumstances they can store new material and later retrieve it. Korsakoff's patients have great difficulty spontaneously using higher-order concepts to organize material to be remembered (for example, they struggle to group objects into categories like "items of food"), but when they are *instructed* to store them under category labels ("Remember these food items," "Remember these animal names"), a later reminder of those categories will improve their recall. Unlike Henry, Korsakoff's patients frequently *perseverate* (repeat actions or words) and *confabulate* (produce unconsidered, inconsistent, and sometimes exotic explanations, perhaps to fill memory gaps). These behaviors are also seen in people with bilateral damage to the frontal lobes, and in Korsakoff's patients perseveration and confabulation may be associated with frontal lobe atrophy resulting from alcoholism rather than with the lesions in the memory loop.

*****

In spite of all the cutting-edge technology neuroscientists now have at their fingertips, no machine has yet been developed that can take the place of careful "bedside" observations and descriptions of human behavior, the rock on which good medical and psychological practice and research is based. Of course technology gives us the means to expand and refine our theories far beyond simple observations, but both types of research are required for a full understanding of human behavior and cognition. In the rather personal view of Henry in this chapter, I have used transcripts of recordings of my conversations with him to illustrate some of his memory impairments. While carefully designed and controlled experiments are essential to obtain reliable information on memory, a simple conversation not only can give the real "flavor" of the memory loss but can reveal so much more about the person, for example, Henry's "in the moment" normal thinking processes and his sense of humor. In his gentle comments we can sense the sadness—perhaps quickly forgotten by Henry—of his lost memories. So often he said, sounding to me rather dejected, "See, I don't remember."

One way of understanding memory is to think of it as a process. It begins with taking in information through our senses and holding that information very briefly in short-term storage. This is called *immediate memory*, and humans have an immediate memory span of five to nine items of information. We can test this by giving a person seven digits to remember and then asking them to repeat them back immediately. This is how we hold a telephone number in our mind long enough to use it. If we are distracted, we forget it. Henry's immediate memory span for numbers was six to seven after his operation (and probably before it) but dropped a little to five digits as he aged (this is not unusual even for neurologically normal elderly people). He achieved similar results on a spatial immediate memory span task in which he first watched while the examiner tapped out a spatial sequence on a random arrangement of blocks, and then straight away tapped out the same sequence. So we know that the hippocampus is not necessary for these early immediate memory processes.

Henry also retained the next memory process, *working memory*. This refers to an active store where we work on material in our immediate memory, as when we are performing a mental arithmetic calculation. Working memory is really just another aspect of immediate memory. It is also an important aid for the next process—*consolidating* or turning into a lasting memory, the information we wish to retain or learn. One way we can do this is by repeating information over and over in our working memory or, even better, associating the information with other, better-known information to add richness to the memory. These strategies serve to consolidate the memory and allow it to be stored somewhere in the brain so that it can be recalled at a later time. At this point the memory is called *long-term memory*. Most of what we remember comes from long-term memory: the book we read yesterday, the person we met last week, and the holiday we enjoyed ten years ago. Because Henry was unable to consolidate or store the very brief and simple memories he could hold in his immediate memory, his long-term memory was severely impaired. It didn't matter whether the memory was visual, auditory, tactile, or olfactory, he still couldn't store it. And if he couldn't put it into long-term memory, he had nothing to remember or recall later.

Henry almost seemed to enjoy surprising the researchers who were always giving him things to memorize. One day he was given five digits to repeat and remember, and then the experimenter was called away. An hour or more later, she returned to Henry's room and on seeing her, Henry accurately repeated the five digits! At first the researcher thought Henry had shown some ability to put the number into long-term storage, but she quickly worked out how he had actually managed this unlikely feat. As he had been alone and not distracted, he had been repeating the numbers the entire time, thus containing them in immediate memory. Because time is measured by the memories that are laid down as it passes, Henry was presumably unaware of the time that had elapsed since the experimenter had left the room.

On another occasion Henry did appear to keep track of the time, much to my surprise. I told him that I would leave him alone for a period, and when I returned I would ask him to guess how long I had been out of the room. I left the room at 2:05 p.m., and when I returned at 2:17 p.m., I asked Henry how many minutes had elapsed. Without hesitation he replied, "12 minutes; got you there!" There was a large clock on the wall—forgotten about by me—and Henry had noted the time when I left and continued to rehearse it in his short-term memory while looking at the clock. When asked how many minutes had passed, he simply subtracted—in his working memory—the time he had been rehearsing from the time now shown on the clock. This anecdote illustrates not only Henry's intact immediate and working memory but also his sense of humor, his willingness to cooperate with anything researchers might dream up, and his good intellect. What it doesn't illustrate is an ability to estimate time without memories. Rehearsing a five-digit phone number and thinking about it in a way that enhances storage, perhaps by looking for familiar patterns in the sequence, allows people with normal memory abilities to retain the number in long-term storage and later recall it. But Henry could never go this next step. He could repeat a phone number over and over if not distracted, but he could never learn it.

So in contrast to his normal immediate and working memory, Henry's long-term memory for verbal and for nonverbal material, experienced via all his senses—vision, hearing, smell, taste, touch—was severely impaired. He couldn't learn stories, block patterns, songs, drawings, new vocabulary words, visual and tactile mazes, strings of digits, object names, object locations, faces, tonal sequences, new smells and tastes, and nonsense syllables. This list, which could be much longer, gives a hint of the enormous amount of research that Henry participated in over a half century. And he remembered none of it.

At first researchers thought Henry's long-term memory impairment was absolute, but as they came up with increasingly novel ways of "looking" for memories, they found evidence that he had a limited ability to store and use new information. This came from experiments using *repetition priming*, where prior processing of material enhances later purposeful performance. For example, without being told that he was to be given a memory test, Henry was shown a list of words in capital letters like "DEFINE," and to ensure that he had processed the words, he was asked to decide whether each word had the letter "A" in it. He was later given a word stem—"DEF-" in our example—and asked to complete it with the first word that came to mind. He usually responded with a word from the word list he had previously seen. People without memory impairments also show this priming effect. But unlike healthy people, Henry was unable to pick out from a new list of words the words he had been shown earlier. Similarly, if Henry was asked to draw a figure by connecting five dots in a matrix of nine dots and was later asked to draw the first pattern that came to mind on a matrix of nine dots, he responded by drawing the previously drawn figure as often as control subjects did. But if then shown the pattern he had drawn along with other patterns, he could not pick out his. His limited new learning was outside his conscious awareness.

Henry has a *declarative memory* impairment. Because he has no conscious recall of information and personal events, he can't "declare" the information. Most traditional psychological tests of recognition and recall assess declarative memory. But there is another type of memory called *nondeclarative* or *procedural* memory, and memories of this sort do not require the conscious recollection of previous experiences. The ability to learn new procedural skills—knowing how to do something—is included under this label. Procedural memory is the type of memory that allows us to ride a bike without consciously thinking about it. As I discussed earlier, Henry was able to learn some procedures, as evidenced by his becoming faster at the skill of drawing a pencil line through a maze. In fact, it was an early experiment on procedural memory, published in 1962 by Dr. Milner, that first made the neuroscience community sit up and take notice of Henry. She asked him to trace a line between two outlines of a five-pointed star, one inside the other, while he watched his hand in a mirror. Try it and you will discover that because the mirror reverses left and right, at first you make many mistakes, but with practice you get better and better, just like riding a bike. Given Henry's dramatic inability to consciously remember new information, Dr. Milner was surprised when Henry improved with practice. The only difference between him and control subjects was that every time he saw the mirror drawing test it was as if he had never seen it before, and the test had to be explained to him afresh.

Henry's almost normal ability to learn how to perform new tasks was evident in his daily routine. For example, at the age of 60 he broke his ankle and was obliged to use a fold-up wheelchair to get around. He learned how to open it and he also learned the most effective way to position himself to get into it from another chair. Later, when he advanced to using a walking frame, he acquired the procedure for dealing with that equipment as well. Although he used the walker with considerable skill, he could not remember why he needed it.

Yet another way of classifying memory is to consider the type of information to be remembered. We use *semantic memory* when we remember general facts that are available to everyone, such as the names of objects and capital cities. We use *episodic memory* when we remember personal experiences associated with a particular time and place. People with global amnesia like Henry have impairments of both semantic and episodic memory. An important episode from his life illustrates Henry's almost immediate forgetting of personal events. He was staying at MIT at the time of his 60th birthday, and the staff and researchers at the Clinical Research Center organized a birthday party for him. It was a very jolly occasion, and Henry clearly enjoyed himself. The next day I went to see him, sitting in his room surrounded by birthday cards.[3]

>   Jenni: Do you remember anything special happening to
>   you yesterday?

[3] All conversations between Henry and myself are verbatim transcriptions from audio recordings.

Henry: No, I can't say that I do.

Jenni: [*pointing to all the birthday cards on his table*] Look at all these. I wonder what they are here for?

Henry: They are birthday cards, aren't they?

Jenni: Oh, I wonder whose they can be?

Henry: [*grinning*] Well, they could be mine. Perhaps it was my birthday!

But when questioned further he clearly had no recall of the occasion at all.

Many studies assessed Henry's semantic memory by testing his knowledge about public events and figures. These studies demonstrated that he was severely impaired. But in 1988, the MIT researchers argued that those findings might be a result of the recognition or recall procedures used to assess new semantic knowledge: People with amnesia, including Henry, demonstrated learning only when it was assessed without the subject's conscious or declarative knowledge. The MIT group devised a way to assess new semantic learning in Henry using unconscious or nondeclarative measures of performance. They carried out a series of experiments using uncommon words and words new to the English language since Henry's operation. In one experiment, Henry and control subjects were taught definitions of eight uncommon English words, and learning was assessed by improved performance over trials with the same words. Subjects were never asked whether they had seen the words before. As expected given his verbal memory problems, Henry, unlike controls, was unable to learn the meaning of any word he did not already know.

A second experiment examined the possibility that Henry would learn new words better if they were presented in a real-life context rather than in the laboratory. He was tested on the recall and recognition of words that had entered a standard English dictionary between 1954, one year after his surgery, and 1981. All the words were commonly known to high school students and they were interspersed with similar, pronounceable nonwords (words like "bown" that could be pronounced like real words but were made up). Henry was asked to decide whether each letter string was a word or nonword and to give the meanings of the real words. He recognized and could provide definitions of real words that entered the English language before 1950, but he had only limited recall for words from the 1950s and was severely impaired on his recall for post-1950s words.

Another experiment examined whether Henry could recognize names of famous people when they were interspersed among names of nonfamous people. He scored normally on famous names from before the 1950s, was mildly impaired on names that became famous during the 1950s, and was severely impaired on names that had become famous in the 1960s to 1980s. This series of experiments provided good evidence that Henry had suffered a markedly impaired ability to encode (turn into a form that the brain can store) and store semantic information since his operation, and testing his memory using nondeclarative methods made no difference. But just occasionally Henry would recognize or recall a name or face of someone famous who had entered the political or entertainment arenas after the year of his operation. Two explanations have been proposed for this. The first is that because the posterior two centimeters of his hippocampus remained bilaterally, this spared tissue may have been sufficient to mediate some new memories. Alternatively or in addition, memory circuits that bypassed the hippocampus and amygdala may have been able to mediate new memories, albeit in a very impoverished way.

Often we see films or read books in which someone suffers some sort of physical or psychological trauma and as a result loses his memory for his entire past. In fact, to lose one's past memory under these circumstances is rare. Realistically these fictional characters should not be able to learn anything about their life *after* their trauma rather than forgetting everything *before* it. Some dementing conditions, such as Alzheimer's disease, do cause a gradual memory loss for the past, but until the disease is very advanced, people with dementia tend to remember their very early life but forget more recent events. When a memory impairment is the result of sudden brain damage such as a head injury, a very rapid disease onset as in Korsakoff's dementia or herpes encephalitis, or brain surgery, the consequent memory impairments can be very clearly separated into "before" and "after" scenarios. The term *retrograde amnesia* refers to a loss of "remote" memories that were learned prior to the incident that caused the amnesia, and *anterograde amnesia* refers to an inability to form memories after that incident. In Henry's case the incident was his operation; in a head-injured patient, the incident is the injury, and in herpes encephalitis and Korsakoff's dementia, the incident is the feverish disease that rapidly destroys specific parts of the brain.

A number of objective tests of remote memory given to Henry supported his having an 11-year period of retrograde amnesia. The tests used the recall or recognition of famous tunes, public events, and scenes taken from the 1920s to the 1960s. Henry's personal episodic memories were nearly all from the age of 16 years or earlier, also suggesting a loss of memories or inability to retrieve them for an 11-year period before his surgery. It may be that Henry's seizures and high doses of antiepileptic medications resulted in an inability to store new memories before his operation, and loss of his remote memories increased after the surgery because of impoverished rehearsal of them.

Henry could, however, retrieve some memories from the 11-year presurgical period, usually via a recognition or cueing procedure rather than via spontaneous recall. For example, if given the first two letters of the name of the surgeon who carried out his operation, whom he knew in the years immediately preceding the operation, he would quickly produce Dr. Scoville's complete name. He also occasionally remembered information he must have stored after the operation. For example, he knew that as a result of the surgery he had memory problems and that the operation has not been done on anyone else since. The remote memories from his first 16 years that were intact seemed reasonably clear, presumably because to Henry they were relatively recent memories that had not been contaminated by new memories. He couldn't place them in time, however, and these personal memories are better described as "gist" memories, or memories that reflect the general idea of events that probably occurred often. As we grow older and reminisce about our childhood, it is normal for those old memories to lose their specificity and become rather generalized descriptions, for example, a Christmas memory comprising a melding of Christmas gatherings. So from this point of view, perhaps Henry's remote memories were as good as anyone else's of a similar age.

When asked about various singers such as Frank Sinatra and actors such as Cary Grant famous during his childhood, Henry could often describe them and name the songs they sang and the films they were in, and who their costars were. He knew the names of the friends he had in second grade, remembered his first major seizure, and related pleasurable memories of hunting with his father and roller-skating. When I asked him when he was 60 about roller-skating, he said he gave it up about 13 years ago! He also related stories about his parents' families, presumably told to him by his parents when he was young. He spoke about his mother's trip to Ireland as a girl to be confirmed into the Catholic Church, and an aunt who emigrated to Australia. This latter story was often cued when I told him repeatedly that I came from New Zealand.

Constant retelling of old memories, whether they were factual or not, did not change them significantly for Henry, because unlike most of us, he was unable to update his memories and recall the slightly changed versions. As a result, the many researchers who assessed Henry can all repeat—with very similar words and intonations—stories Henry told. When Henry was distracted while telling one of his stories, he could be cued into retelling it a few minutes later and would repeat it using not only the same verbal expressions but also the same facial expressions and gestures. Occasionally he appeared to lose the thread of the story and inserted a different line, but he then quickly returned to the old story.

For example, when asked about his operation, he would usually launch into a story about wanting to be a brain surgeon. The following transcript of a conversation I had with Henry illustrates this. In this particular conversation, the first time he told the story he made some small changes (indicated by italics) to his usual way of wording it. Near the end of the story he forgot he had just been telling it but cued himself into telling it again, this time using the phrases he normally uses. This conversation also gives some insight into the way Henry thought about his own operation and its consequences.[4]

> Jenni: Do you know why you are here at MIT?
> Henry: I wonder at times, but I know one thing. What is learned about me will help other people.
> Jenni: Yes, it has helped other people.
> Henry: And that is the important thing. Because at one time that's what I wanted to be, a brain surgeon.
> Jenni: Really? A brain surgeon?

[4]This conversation and the ones that follow are reprinted from Ogden, J. A. & Corkin, S. 1991. Memories of H.M. In *Memory Mechanisms: A Tribute to G. V. Goddard*, pp. 201–205. Hillsdale, NJ: Lawrence Erlbaum Associates, with the permission of Taylor & Francis Group LLC—Books.

Henry: And I said "no" to myself, before I had any kind of epilepsy.

Jenni: Did you? Why is that?

Henry: Because I wore glasses. I said, suppose you are making an incision in someone [*pause*] *and you could get blood on your glasses*, or an attendant could be mopping your brow and go too low and move your glasses over. You could make the wrong movement then.

Jenni: And then what would happen?

Henry: And that person could be dead, or paralyzed.

Jenni: So it's a good job you decided not to be a brain surgeon.

Henry: Yeah. I thought mostly dead, but could be paralyzed in a way. You could make the incision just right, and then a little deviation, might be a leg or an arm, or maybe an eye too; on one side in fact.

Jenni: Do you remember when you had your operation?

Henry: No, I don't.

Jenni: What do you think happened there?

Henry: Well, I think I was, ah—well, I'm having an argument with myself right away. I'm the third or fourth person who had it, and I think that they, well, possibly didn't make the right movement at the right time, themselves then. But they learned something.

Jenni: They did indeed.

Henry: That would help other people around the world too.

Jenni: They never did it again.

Henry: They never did it again because by knowing it [*pause*] and a funny part, I always thought of being a brain surgeon myself.

Jenni: Did you?

Henry: Yeah. And I said "no" to myself.

Jenni: Why was that?

Henry: Because I said an attendant might mop your brow and might move your glasses over a little bit, and you would make the wrong movement.

Jenni: What would happen if you made the wrong movement?

Henry: And that would affect all the other operations you had then.

Jenni: Would it? How?

Henry: Because if that person was paralyzed on one side, or you made the wrong movement, in a way, and they possibly couldn't hear on one side, or one eye, you would wonder to yourself and that would make you nervous.

Jenni: Yes, it would.

Henry: Because every time you did you would try and be extra careful and you might be detrimental to that person; to perform that operation right on that time because you'd have that thought and that might slow you up, then, because you were making a movement and you should have continued right on.

Jenni: Do you remember who the surgeon was who did your operation?

Henry: No, I don't.

Jenni: I'll give you a hint. Sc—.

Henry: Scoville.

Jenni: That's right. [*laughing*] You got that fast.

Henry: Well, because I couldn't remember fully, but the little hint.

The most memorable aspect of Henry's memory impairment was his dense anterograde amnesia for nearly all episodic information since his operation. He could not say what he was doing five minutes ago; where he lived; whom he lived with; what day, month, year, or season it was; or what his age was. The following conversation between us illustrates his confusion about age.

Jenni: How old do you think you are now?

Henry: Round about 34. I think of that right off.

Jenni: How old do you think I am?

Henry: Well, I'm thinking of 27 right off.

Jenni: [*laughing*] Aren't you kind! I'm really 37.

Henry: 37? So I must be more than that.

Jenni: Why? Do you think you're older than me?

Henry: Yeah.

Jenni: How old do you think you are?

Henry: Well, I always think too much ahead in a way.
   Well, nearer, well, 38.

Jenni: Thirty-eight? You act 38! You know, you are really
   60. You had your 60th birthday the other day. You had
   a big cake.

Henry: See, I don't remember.

Henry did not recognize anyone he had met or seen
since 1953, and even after fifty years of returning to MIT
and being assessed every year by Professor Corkin, he still
demonstrated no real recognition of her, although when
asked he would sometimes say that he thought he knew
her from high school. As mentioned, he had no conscious
memories of public events after the age of 16 years, 11 years
before his surgery. For example, if he was asked about the
content and temporal context of public events, he had normal recall of events from the 1940s (compared with neurologically normal Americans of his own age) but impaired
recall for events, as well as famous people, from the 1950s
until his death. His occasional recall of people and events
that became famous after his operation in 1953 was spasmodic at best, and he tended to confuse those memories
with other events or confused them in time. In the following conversation I had with him in 1986, he confused Elvis
Presley's death in 1977 with the significantly earlier assas-
sinations of President John Kennedy and Senator Robert
Kennedy. The first time an Elvis Presley recording was
played on the radio was 1954, one year after Henry's
operation.

Jenni: Do you know who Elvis Presley is?

Henry: He was a recording star, and he used to sing a lot.

Jenni: What sort of things did he sing?

Henry: Jive.

Jenni: Do you like to jive, or did you like to jive?

Henry: No.

Jenni: [*laughing*] Why not?

Henry: I liked to listen, that was all.

Jenni: Do you think he is still alive, Elvis Presley?

Henry: No, I don't think so.

Jenni: Have you any idea what might have happened to him?

Henry: Well, I believe he got the first bullet, I think, that was for Kennedy, I think it was.

Jenni: You remember Kennedy?

Henry: Yes, Robert.

Jenni: What was he?

Henry: Well, he was the president. I think about three times. He was appointed to president too.

Jenni: He got a bullet. What was that all about?

Henry: Well, they were trying to assassinate him.

Jenni: And did they? Did they kill him or not?

Henry: No, they didn't.

Jenni: So is he still alive?

Henry: Yes, he is still alive, but he got out of politics in a way.

Jenni: I don't blame him.

Henry: No, guess not.

Jenni: How long ago was he the president, do you think?

Henry: He became the president after Roosevelt. 'Course there was Teddy Roosevelt. That was a long time before that.

Jenni: What is Franklin Roosevelt's wife's name?

Henry: I can't think of it.

Jenni: It starts with "E," I think—Eleanor. You were going to say that?

Henry: No, I wasn't. I was going to say Ethel. [Ethel was Robert Kennedy's wife.]

Henry spent much of his day watching television and reading the newspapers, so he heard, saw, and read reports of major news items many times over. It appeared that exposure to many repetitions of significant events made it more likely that Henry would recall them in part, at least over a period of days. After two weeks of massive media coverage of the explosion of the American space shuttle *Challenger* shortly after it was launched, Henry replied to my question, "What is a space shuttle?" with the following description: "Well, I think it is a spaceship they shot up and after it is shot up, then it turns itself on. And also there is another part to it that can be sent back. After they've shot off, and shot off the second one, they can return. They use part of it again." Further questions about specific details of the *Challenger* tragedy cued no clear memories, and when he was asked the occupation of the first American civilian to go into space, a female teacher, he replied, "I think of working for the army." This illustrates the dense nature of Henry's anterograde amnesia. Although he had some knowledge of the space shuttle program generally, his memory of the *Challenger* explosion specifically was at best fragmented and incomplete despite constant media coverage, which emphasized the tragic death of the civilian teacher.

Of course researchers don't always get it right, and the following story illustrates how good research practice can sometimes be overlooked in the excitement of the moment. At 9:30 a.m. on February 14, 1986, I went to collect Henry from his room. He was eating a large chocolate heart that had been given to him by the staff to celebrate St. Valentine's Day. He finished the heart, crumpled up the shiny red paper it had been wrapped in, and put the paper in his shirt pocket. He then came with me to the testing room, and for the next two hours we concentrated on various tests. At about 11:30 a.m., Henry put his hand into his shirt pocket to get out his handkerchief and pulled out the shiny red paper at the same time. He held it at arm's length and looked at it quizzically. So I asked him why he had the paper in his pocket. "Well," replied Henry, "it could have been wrapped around a big chocolate heart. It must be St. Valentine's Day!" I tried to contain my excitement over this evidence of recall of a personal episode that had occurred two hours earlier, and I told Henry to replace the red paper in his pocket. I took him to the lunchroom and then left to tell my story to John Gabrieli, an experienced tester of Henry. John said that Henry, being a true American, had been eating large chocolate hearts wrapped in red shiny paper every St. Valentine's Day since he was a year old. This was just an old, well-learned association and certainly not evidence of new learning and recall. I insisted that this was not so and took John to the lunchroom, where I asked Henry to look in his shirt pocket. He pulled out the shiny red paper, held it at arm's length, and looked at it quizzically. I asked him why he had the paper in his pocket, and he replied "Well, it might have been wrapped around a big chocolate rabbit. It must be Easter!"

*****

Neuroscientists by definition are fascinated by how the mind works, but when most people hear about Henry, the first questions they ask are "How did he cope with having no memory? Was he depressed? What sort of personality did he have?" For most of us, the thought of living in a timeless vacuum as Henry did is incomprehensible. Yet Henry's personality could best be described as placid and happy. One of his most striking characteristics was that he rarely complained about anything. To his caregivers, in some ways looking after Henry was rather similar to looking after a baby. They had to rely on their observations of his behaviors to sense whether he was feeling unwell, hungry, thirsty, or tired. But working out specifically what Henry was feeling was not as difficult as with a baby, because Henry responded to direct questions. If asked, "Where do you have a pain?" he usually wouldn't answer with a specific location but had to be asked, "Is it in your head? Your tooth?" and so on until the right body part was mentioned.

The inability to comment spontaneously on his state seemed to extend to Henry's tendency not to initiate new topics of conversation. Rather, he responded readily to a conversational opening from another person, and from then on the conversation was maintained and changed to different topics by the person talking with him or by Henry's cueing himself into reciting a story from his first 16 years of life. Impoverished conversational spontaneity is usually associated with bilateral frontal lobe damage, but frontal damage was not the cause in Henry's case, as both neuropathological evidence (CT and MRI scans) and behavioral evidence (his normal ability to perform tests of frontal lobe function) suggested that his frontal lobes were intact. Rather, Henry's amnesia probably made it impossible for him to prepare mentally and to retain the information and logical structure necessary to allow him to introduce a new topic of conversation.

It is surprising that Henry did not react with some degree of confusion, frustration, or anger from continually not knowing where he was, what year it was, what new type of technology or development he was looking at, or the identities of the people who were speaking to him. It is tempting to think that because he was unaware of what had just happened and was unable to think about what was about to happen, he had nothing on which to base feelings of anger or frustration. That is, it seems reasonable to suppose that an ability to remember is a prerequisite for strong emotional reactions. Other cases with amnesia nearly as dense as that suffered by Henry do not support this hypothesis, however. Clive Wearing, a noted musician and choirmaster from England, was left globally amnesic as a consequence of herpes simplex encephalitis. Clive was constantly angry, frustrated, and upset by his experience of living minute by minute in a world he would not remember, and he frequently complained that he had been dead and had just woken up this minute.

In the case of Henry, it may be that the removal of the amygdala from each hemisphere resulted in a severe dampening of his emotions. It is well established in the animal literature that the amygdala is associated with control of the expression of aggression. Henry's many years of antiepileptic medication may also have lowered his threshold for emotional arousal. Alternatively, perhaps he was just a contented and happy person by nature, and his personality had little to do with his epilepsy or his brain surgery and drug regimen. His father was apparently very similar to Henry: good humored and placid. On rare occasions, Henry did become briefly annoyed when provoked. He sometimes became angry when his mother "nagged" him when he lived with her, and apparently kicked her in the shin and hit her with his glasses on one occasion. He sometimes looked and sounded sad when he was told that his father was dead.

It has often been said that memory equates with consciousness or even "soul." In spite of the fact that Henry lived minute by minute with no conscious knowledge of his past beyond his childhood years or of what his future would bring, everyone who met him was impressed by his friendly conversation, his appropriate interactions, his sense of humor, and his intelligent problem-solving skills. Memory is clearly a critical part of our identity, but to me it seemed that Henry was conscious of himself as a whole person, even if that person had not changed for more than

50 years. That he had a "soul" was never in doubt in my mind.

*****

Henry's lost memory deprived him of his independence. From the onset of his amnesia, he was not able to go anywhere unaccompanied and often required assistance when making important decisions that affected his own life, although he was judged by a psychiatrist to be qualified to give informed consent for testing. As the world continued to change, Henry's knowledge of how to live in it became increasingly outdated. The world of the 21st century is very different from the world of 1942, the year that marked the beginning of Henry's retrograde amnesia. It is thus hardly surprising that he needed assistance with decisions. He seemed rather negligent about his self-care and required supervision to ensure that he washed, shaved, dressed, changed his clothes, and even ate. This of course may not have been negligence but simply a consequence of his amnesia. Without a sense of time of day, it must have been difficult to know when to wash and so on, and of course Henry could not remember when he last washed.

Henry spent his days doing crossword puzzles—which could have the answers erased so he could do them again!—watching television, and reading the newspaper. He was compliant with his caregivers and anyone else who asked him to do anything. He got up and retired to bed when he was told, ate when he was told, and would happily put away his crossword and go with a researcher to the laboratory—which he had no memory of ever seeing before—for an experimental session. He would go anywhere with anyone, and if he was asked to sit in a particular chair he would sit there all day without moving or complaining if not told otherwise. This vulnerability to others of course was why his identity was closely guarded during his life and why the scientists who were given approval to carry out experiments on him were kept to a minimum and were closely monitored.

Henry greeted everyone with warmth, and people who met him for the first time as well as those who spent years with him shared an uncanny feeling that he recognized them and was greeting them like an old friend. Yet when asked the question "Do you think you have seen me before?" Henry usually replied, "No, I can't say that I have," or sometimes, "Well, I don't remember, but as soon as you asked me that, I had an argument with myself. I think I might have met you before."

The many studies carried out with Henry have shown that we require at least one intact hippocampus to be able to encode, store, and recall new declarative information, whether it is episodic or semantic. Many epilepsy sufferers since Henry have had *one* hippocampus removed to reduce seizure activity, and their memory abilities remain largely intact, although they often experience specific memory problems in the modality associated with the hippocampus removed (e.g., problems with remembering names after their left hippocampus is removed). Thus one hippocampus can cope with the task of consolidating memories so they can be stored, but if both are removed, a global amnesia is certain. In contrast, the studies of Henry have shown that the hippocampus and other MTL structures are not required for nondeclarative memory, at least for motor or perceptual skills.

For half a century, Henry put enormous effort and time into memory research, and the fact that he had no conscious memory of that work does not in any way detract from the debt we owe him. He was and will continue to be famous throughout the psychological and neurological world; most first-year psychology undergraduates have heard about him and answered examination questions about him, numerous people have felt honored to be introduced to him, and a smaller group of people who have cared for him or worked with him, including me, came to think of Henry as a dear friend. The poignancy in this is that Henry was unaware of any of us as soon as our conversation with him ended.

*****

Two months after Henry's death in December 2008, Columbia Pictures and producer Scott Rudin acquired the rights to make a film based on a biography of him being written by Suzanne Corkin, who had been studying him for almost half a century. One of her final "HM" research projects was to organize MRI scans of his brain hours after his death so that neuroscientists could ascertain more precisely which areas of his brain were still intact and which were damaged. Then in December 2009, Henry's frozen brain became the focus of a brain-mapping project in which Jacopo Annese, a neuroanatomist at the University of California, San Diego, was filmed for a 30-hour live webcast while he dissected Henry's brain into more than two thousand very thin slices. The digitized images of the slices were then made available to scientists as a three-dimensional map that could be searched by zooming in from the whole brain to individual neurons. Scientists now and in the future will be able to reanalyze the behavioral, memory, and other cognitive information discovered about Henry during his life in the context of detailed information on the brain areas that were spared or damaged. The historic and tragically unique brain of Henry Molaison has been preserved for posterity.

■ Further Reading

Hilts, P. J. 1995. *Memory's Ghost: The Strange Tale of Mr. M.* New York: Simon & Schuster.

Ogden, J. A. 2005. Marooned in the moment: H.M., a case of global amnesia. In: *Fractured Minds: A Case-Study Approach to Clinical Neuropsychology, 2nd Ed.* (pp. 46–63). New York: Oxford University Press.

Sacks, O. 1970. The lost mariner. In: *The Man Who Mistook His Wife for a Hat* (pp. 22–41). New York: Summit Books.

Wearing, D. 2005. *Forever Today: A Memoir of Love and Amnesia.* London: Doubleday.

Wilson, B. A., and D. Wearing. 1995. Prisoner of Consciousness: A State of Just Awakening Following Herpes Simplex Encephalitis. In: R. Campbell and M. A. Martin, eds. *Broken Memories: Case Studies in Memory Impairment* (pp. 14–30). Oxford: Blackwell.

8 ∎

The Singer or the Song:
A Pact with Epilepsy

Melody's future was looking rosy. She was marrying the man she had loved for the past three years, her work was going well, and the jazz band she had been singing with for two years had signed a 12-month contract with the town's popular coffee club and bar, guaranteeing them a gig there on three Friday nights each month. She shared all her good news with her GP when she went in for her regular six-month checkup, and at first didn't quite take in the implications of the GP's query about her plans for having children, now that the marriage date was set. Of course, Melody knew there were some issues related to becoming pregnant when taking her antiepileptic medication; she had read about its contraindications when she had started taking it after her first flurry of temporal lobe seizures. That was eight years ago and now, at 25, she was an old hand at working with her seizure disorder so that it didn't disrupt her life too much. Somehow, in her excitement over her engagement, she had managed to overlook the problems that pregnancy would bring. She and Tim definitely wanted to have children, and the sooner the better. That was one of the reasons they had decided to get married.

"So, what will I do when I get pregnant?" she asked her doctor, hopeful that there would, by now, be a new antiepileptic drug that was safe for expectant mothers. Melody had experimented with reducing her medication in the past and knew that without it her seizures would increase to levels that would interfere with her work, her singing, and her social life.

"There's no easy answer to that, I'm afraid. But you should definitely not stop contraception until we have sorted out a solution," her doctor told her. "Is there any hurry? Perhaps after you've been married for a year or two we can explore possible ways you could start a family safely."

"I'd like to sort it out before we get married; there's six months to go before the wedding, so that would give me time to try out new medications."

"As far as I know, there are no antiepileptic medications considered safe to take during pregnancy, but the best idea is for you to see your neurologist. He'll be more up to date than I am on the latest drugs and other strategies you could look at."

"OK, I will. We really don't want to wait. We want at least four kids and I'm getting older by the minute!"

Unfortunately, crossing her fingers and praying that her neurologist would magically produce a new, safer medication made no difference. He suggested adoption, but Melody wasn't ready to consider that before even attempting to get pregnant. His next suggestion was even scarier. She could go off her medication at the point she and Tim decided to try for a baby, and stay off it until the baby was born. She might have to give up work if she found her seizures became too frequent and debilitating to cope with, but he didn't think she would come to any harm. Melody was silent for a long moment, and then shook her head.

"No, I don't think I could cope with those seizures again. I was having up to six a day when I tried reducing—and not even stopping—my medication a couple of years ago. And every time I have a seizure, I feel so tired afterward that I have to sleep, sometimes for hours. As soon as I wake up I have another one. It would be impossible." She couldn't stop her tears, and the neurologist handed her a box of tissues.

"Well, there is one other possibility. We did talk about it briefly before, but decided the medication was doing a good job keeping your seizures under control. I could put you on the waiting list for surgery to have the part of the temporal lobe where your seizures start cut out."

"I wondered if you would suggest that," Melody said, her voice very quiet. "It seems very drastic. Is it really the only way?"

"I think it might be the best solution for you, although you would need to undergo a lot of assessments first before we could decide if your case were suitable. It's a big decision, and the first step is for you to read up about it and talk to Tim. Then we can discuss it in detail and I can answer your questions."

"Yes, I want to do that if it's the only way. And if it works I'll be able to go off medication for good and not have to worry about getting pregnant as often as I want?"

"That's the spirit, and yes, that is possible. We've had many patients in our epilepsy surgery program who have been able to completely give up medication after a year or so following their surgery."

"So long? I'd better get onto it fast."

"You need to realize that sometimes it is not possible to give up medication completely if you want to be free of seizures. But even if all the surgery does is reduce your seizures considerably rather than cure you completely, that would enable you to go off medication for the duration of your pregnancy. Take this information pack away with you and come back and see me when you're ready to discuss it. Bring Tim with you on your next visit."

"Thank you," Melody said as she took the thick bundle of paper. "I'll be back to see you next week!"

*****

Epilepsy, an umbrella term for a range of disorders of the central nervous system that include seizures as a symptom, is a common disorder, affecting about five in every 1000 people. There are a number of different types of epilepsy, the most disabling being *generalized tonic–clonic seizures* (sometimes called *grand mal seizures*). Victims often cry out and lose consciousness as their bodies convulse violently, usually for two to five minutes. Breathing stops or becomes shallow, the victim froths at the mouth, and there may be a loss of bladder or bowel control. On regaining consciousness there is a period of confusion and no memory of the seizure. Deep sleep often follows, as well as nausea, headache, and vomiting on awakening. Generalized seizures involve the whole brain, and the treatment is usually antiepileptic medication, although in extremely severe cases where medication is ineffective and the seizures are constant, surgery is performed in a final attempt to reduce the seizures. The most successful operation involves cutting the *corpus callosum,* the large fiber tract connecting the two brain hemispheres, thus preventing the seizure spreading from one hemisphere to the other. If the seizures are a result of a severely damaged hemisphere, in very rare cases the entire damaged hemisphere is removed—a *hemispherectomy*—and this sometimes stops the seizure activity. Kate, the woman described in Chapter 9, underwent a hemispherectomy with remarkable results.

At the other end of the spectrum are *petit mal*, or *absence, seizures*, where there is a transient and very brief lapse of consciousness, often barely perceptible to an observer. Absence seizures tend to be restricted to the childhood years, and if frequent can result in significant learning difficulties at school.

Melody suffered *temporal lobe seizures*—also called *complex partial seizures* or *psychomotor seizures*—which are the most common type and fall around the middle of the epilepsy spectrum. The sufferer often experiences an "aura" preceding the seizure, which might be an unpleasant smell, a feeling of fear, or a visual hallucination, and during the seizure may perform purposeless movements such as lip smacking or picking at clothing. Hallucinations, perceptual distortions, alterations of mood, or obsessional thinking are also common. These seizures usually arise in a seahorse-shaped brain structure underlying the temporal lobe, called the *hippocampus*. This structure is best known for its role in the formation of memories. The exact neural mechanisms triggering seizures are not known, and researchers interested in the causes of seizures are continually exploring new hypotheses and refining old ones. In simple terms, brain functioning can be conceived of as the outcome of electrochemical impulses that travel along neural pathways and are directed and coordinated by a complex process in which some neurons are excited by an impulse and others are inhibited by it. If, perhaps because of brain damage, the balance between excitatory and inhibitory neurons is disrupted and more and more neurons become excited without being counteracted by inhibitory activity, the storm of electrical activity in the brain results in a seizure. This usually causes some transient alteration in consciousness—from a comatose state to a brief period of confusion—accompanied by motor, sensory, cognitive, or emotional changes that together make up the seizure event. Any damage to the brain can become a focus for seizure activity, but many cases of epilepsy are *idiopathic*; that is, no cause can be found for the seizures.

Seizures can be debilitating or embarrassing and in some cases may indicate or cause brain damage or dysfunction that can result in cognitive and personality disorders or impairments. Thus almost everyone who suffers from epilepsy seeks a cure. For some a cure occurs spontaneously, but for most the best they can hope for is good control via medication that does not otherwise significantly interfere with their lives. Unfortunately, the antiepileptic medication can itself result in lowered or slowed cognitive function and can restrict lifestyle choices. For example, as Melody discovered, pregnancy is inadvisable for a woman on antiepileptic medication. If antiepileptic medication fails to control frequent seizures, in the case of temporal lobe epilepsy, where the seizures begin in a specific part of the brain that can be removed without drastic consequences, a *temporal lobectomy* may be an option. Although in Melody's case medication was quite effective, reducing her seizure frequency to around one a week, surgery provided the best hope of permitting her to stop her antiepileptic medication without increasing her seizures, thus giving her the opportunity to become safely pregnant.

*****

True to her word, Melody returned to the neurologist's clinic the very next week, this time accompanied by Tim. They had read the information thoroughly, discussed the pros and cons of going ahead with a temporal lobectomy with Melody's parents and siblings, and were determined to begin the necessary assessments immediately. Unfortunately, there was a long waiting list for temporal lobectomies, and the best the neurologist could do was add her name to it, with the caution that she might have to wait a year or more for surgery if her case proved to be suitable. However, he was able to get the assessments under way, and Melody was booked for an magnetic resonance imaging (MRI) brain scan. A previous MRI scan at the time of her initial diagnosis had shown that her right hippocampus was smaller than the left, and that the rest of her brain was normal. The neurologist was fairly certain that the shrunken hippocampus was the cause of her seizures, as this was a common finding in people with temporal lobe epilepsy. The latest MRI confirmed that Melody's brain was normal in appearance except for the shrunken right hippocampus.

Melody's next appointment was with me. My first task was to carry out a psychological assessment to determine whether Melody had the right personality to undergo such a potentially life-changing operation. For most people being cured of epilepsy is wonderful, but a few have difficulty adjusting to a future where they are expected to be independent and take full responsibility for all aspects of their lives. I also wanted to explore Melody's ability to cope with the disappointment if, after going through the trauma of brain surgery, she continued to have frequent seizures.

Melody told me that she was the youngest child in a family of four children, and until she experienced her first seizure, enjoyed a happy and healthy childhood. She performed at a comfortably average level at school, excelled at swimming and gymnastics, and was always passionate about music. Her mother was a music teacher, and Melody began music lessons almost before she could talk. By the age of five she could sing in tune, play simple melodies on the piano, and play the ukulele. On her eighth birthday she was given her first guitar, and from that day on, the guitar was her favorite instrument. She became the star performer at school concerts and family gatherings, first singing folk songs and then blues and jazz. At 15 she and her all-girl jazz band won a national talent quest and she decided that she would do whatever it takes to become a professional jazz musician.

Looking back, she thinks she probably had quite a few seizures in her final year at school without understanding what they were. She was 17, and was smoking her first—and last—marijuana joint at a party. "I felt weird, and then heard a female humming voice going up and down a minor scale. Of course I know now that it's my aura, but back then I thought it was the marijuana. The humming is seriously spooky and it always sends shivers up and down my spine," she told me. "I never touched drugs again after that. But over the next few days I had a few more episodes just like that one, and I thought I'd damaged my brain."

"Not possible, I shouldn't think, from one joint," I commented. "So how did you discover you were actually having seizures?"

"My mother noticed I was acting strangely—not that that was very difficult, because after I have the aura of the woman humming, I put my left hand up and cup my left ear and shake my head. I'm unaware of doing that, and apparently I act confused for a few minutes although I can hear people speaking to me and I answer them in a vague sort of way. Then all I want to do is lie down and sleep for hours."

"So that is always what happens when you have a seizure?"

"As far as I know."

"And what happened after your mother became concerned?"

"I told her about the marijuana, and she took me to the doctor. He told me it sounded like I was having small seizures and perhaps the marijuana brought it on that time, but there was no way it could have caused the underlying problem. Then I went to the neurologist and had an MRI and EEG [electroencephalograph]. It all showed that I was having complex partial seizures, and I was diagnosed with temporal lobe epilepsy."

"That must have been frightening."

"Yes, it was, but I got over it, and when I started having seizures every other day, I went onto medication. That made a huge difference."

"No side effects?"

"Not too bad after the neurologist had changed the dose a few times until I was having just enough to keep the seizures at a low level without making me feel like a zombie."

"Did it change your lifestyle in any way, for example, what you did when you left school?"

"Actually, I think it might have a bit. I used to think I'd go to university and do a music degree, but I decided not to. It seemed too much bother, and I wasn't all that smart. I would have had to work awfully hard."

"So do you think that was a result of the antiepileptic medication or your seizures?"

"Both, really. The medication does make me a bit unmotivated, and I find it a struggle to concentrate sometimes. Also, I still have a flurry of seizures every month, just before my period, even on medication, and if I am stressed I have seizures—like when I broke up with my boyfriend when I was 20, the doctor had to increase my medication for a while."

"That sounds very typical. Unfortunately antiepileptic medication is not yet the perfect treatment. Have you ever had other sorts of seizures, like a generalized seizure where you lose consciousness?"

"No, thank goodness. I have a friend I met through the Epilepsy Association who has grand mal seizures, and it is awful. She convulses and wets herself, and it is so embarrassing for her. Her boyfriend decided he couldn't cope after seeing her have a seizure, and dropped her; good riddance, I say."

"That's sad. There is still so much ignorance in the community about epilepsy. Have you experienced any prejudice?"

"No, I've been lucky. My employer is very understanding. I sometimes need to take a couple of days off when I get those seizure flurries, but that's about all really."

"Tell me about your work."

"I love it. I work in a retail music store and get to listen to music all day as well as getting discounted CDs! I give private guitar lessons to kids after school three days a week as well; I leave the store early on those days. And I have my singing, and the jazz band. Not the all-girl one any longer. I'm the only female in this one! But it's my singing that really matters—well, that and Tim of course," she said, grinning.

*****

I had on file the results of a neuropsychological assessment Melody had when she was 19, a few months after she began her antiepileptic medication. I repeated most of the tests, giving her parallel versions (i.e., the same tests but with different items) where possible, although after a six-year gap she would be unlikely to recall enough to inflate her scores. If she now performed at a lower level than previously, that would indicate that either her epilepsy or her medication was having a deleterious effect on her cognitive abilities and add to the reasons for going ahead with a temporal lobectomy. More importantly, I wanted to ensure that her pattern of cognitive strengths and deficits was consistent with right temporal lobe damage and rule out damage to other brain areas. For example, given that Melody was strongly right-handed and from a right-handed family— and therefore it was likely that her left hemisphere was dominant for language—I would expect that she might have some problems with nonverbal memory but not with verbal memory. If she had significant problems with verbal memory, this could indicate that her left as well as her right temporal lobe was compromised, even although it appeared normal on the MRI scan. In that case, if the surgeon removed her shrunken right hippocampus along with part of the right temporal lobe, Melody could be left with a poorly functioning left hippocampus. The sad case of HM, described in Chapter 7, taught us that removing both hippocampi leaves the patient with no ability to make new memories. In contrast, thousands of unilateral (one-sided) temporal lobectomy cases have proven that as long as the patient is left with one "good" hippocampus and temporal lobe, whether the right or left ones, memory functions are preserved at about or just below the level they were at prior to the surgery.

Overall, the results of Melody's neuropsychological assessment showed little change from her assessment at age 19. She was of average intelligence, consistent with her school history, and she had an immediate memory span of seven digits forward and five backward (i.e., recited in the reverse order from which they were presented), attesting to normal attention and concentration and good working memory. Her performance on all the tests of verbal memory— learning word lists, recalling short stories, and recognizing previously seen words—fell within the average range, sup- porting the conclusion that she had a healthy left temporal lobe. In contrast, she was moderately impaired on nonverbal memory tests, including recalling a complex figure she had previously copied and recognizing photos of 50 faces she had seen briefly minutes before. She also demonstrated a mild impairment on a test of psychomotor speed where she was asked to scan a series of numbers and copy from a table above, the symbols that were paired with each number. Being slower than normal on tests like this is not unusual for people on antiepileptic medication, as the medication "dampens down" or slows thinking processes. So far, so good; Melody's pattern of results was entirely consistent with an epileptic focus in the right temporal lobe and hippocampus, where nonverbal, visuospatial memory is mediated.

I considered giving Melody some musical ability tests but decided against it, as both she and her mother said that her musical skills were as good as always; neither of them had noticed any problems in the years since her seizures had started. In fact her mother said her singing voice had never been better and that she had received only praise from the parents of her guitar pupils. I asked Melody whether she had noticed any problems learning new songs—in particular, new melodies rather than lyrics. She didn't think so; she had an excellent ear for music. Her method was to listen to a recording of the song and sing along with it until she learned it. Then she would add her own style. Although she had learned to read music as a young child and could sight-read, she also played by ear. In fact, one of her "party pieces" involved someone humming or singing a song—any song—whereupon Melody would play it on the piano or guitar, improvising as she went. She also wrote her own songs, mainly for her own entertainment, although the band she sang with did include two of her better ones in their repertoire.

Six weeks after her neuropsychological assessment Melody was admitted to the hospital, taken off her medication so that her seizures would increase, and monitored by EEG while being videotaped for 12 hours. When she felt an aura coming on she would press a button so that her behavior on the video could be synched with the EEG recording. The result was clear; the onset of each seizure was correlated with epileptiform activity (electrical impulses typical of seizures) arising from the vicinity of the right temporal lobe. Equally important was the finding that there were no epileptic foci in other areas of the brain.

After a meeting of all the health professionals involved in the temporal lobe epilepsy surgery program, including the neurosurgeon who would perform the operation, it was agreed that Melody was an excellent candidate for the surgery. I had one concern, however. Melody's music was very important to her, and if her right hippocampus and most of her right temporal lobe were removed she might struggle to learn new melodies, just as people whose left temporal lobe is removed sometimes have a small drop in their ability to learn new verbal material. The fact that her aura consisted of a woman's voice humming a scale was also of concern; perhaps this indicated that her right hippocampus and temporal lobe played a part in her ability to sing.

The research literature on this was absent or inconclusive. In most people the left hemisphere is dominant for language, and the right hemisphere—especially the right temporal lobe—for music. Some musicians, however, especially those who have been learning music from a very young age, appear to use both hemispheres when listening to—and possibly when performing—music. It has been suggested that they analyze music like a language rather than simply listening to it as a pattern. Given Melody's very early start to her musical education it was entirely feasible that she had developed a "musician's brain," with some of the more analytical aspects of her musical perception and performance being mediated by her left hemisphere. There was another reason to hope that a right temporal lobectomy would not affect her music: Perhaps, given her shrunken right hippocampus—which may have been atrophied years before she began experiencing seizures—her musical perception and musical memory had been taken over by her left temporal lobe and hippocampus.

The epilepsy team decided that apart from giving Melody a Wada test—in which (usually) the right hemisphere of the brain is temporarily "inactivated" to check that the left hemisphere is dominant for language and can form new memories without the right temporal lobe—there was little they could do to reassure Melody that her musical abilities would be unaffected. She would have to decide for herself whether she wanted to take the risk. If she chose to go ahead, a Wada test would be scheduled for the day before her surgery.

By the time Melody heard the epilepsy team's decision, her wedding was fast approaching, and after two counseling sessions with me where she fluctuated between going ahead with the surgery and hoping for the best, and giving it up and her dream of having her own children with it, she decided, very sensibly, to put a decision on hold until after the wedding. In the meantime she would concentrate on self-care strategies to reduce the likelihood of stress-related seizures in the run-up to the wedding. She decided to reduce her coffee intake to one cup in the morning, give up alcohol, drink lots of water, exercise regularly, eat lots of fruit and vegetables, get lots of sleep, and ban any talk about future temporal lobe surgery until well after the wedding. When she left the clinic after that counseling session she was smiling and already looked less stressed.

She looked even happier in the wedding photos she e-mailed me when she returned from her honeymoon, and three months after that she made an appointment to see me. We met the next day and she began by showing me more photographs of her wedding. Then she told me that she had made a decision. "I had to decide whether it was the singer or the song. Tim and my dad thought I should have the surgery because then I might be able to go off medication completely and my life would be so much better, and best of all we could start a family. My mother understood my feelings more. She knew how frightened I was that I would lose my music, but as she said, it was only a possibility that I would, not a certainty. And even if I did, as you explained before, it is likely to be a problem with learning new songs, not remembering old ones. I thought I could learn as many new songs as possible now, while I'm waiting for the operation."

I replied: "Also, we'll do that test I told you about, the Wada test. It might give us more information if I gave you one or two extra tests where you need to recall songs."

"Yes, I want that. So that's what I've decided. I want the operation—at least if the Wada test doesn't show anything too awful—and if I lose my music or some of it, I'll deal with it. I'll be too busy having children anyway to have time to sing!"

Six months later Melody's name reached the top of the surgery waiting list and she was admitted to the hospital. The day before her operation was scheduled, she underwent the Wada test, named for the man who developed it. In this test a drug, sodium amytal, is injected into the internal carotid artery of one hemisphere of the brain—the hemisphere that is going to be operated on—while the patient is awake. This anesthetizes that hemisphere for about five minutes, causing the patient to become paralyzed on the opposite side of the body. The aim is to test the other, "awake" hemisphere to see if it can speak and comprehend language and memorize objects and sentences without the help of the other hemisphere. If it can, this is good evidence that removal of the temporal lobe in the anesthetized hemisphere will not cause serious disability.

Unfortunately no standard tests have been developed within the Wada protocol to test for musical ability and memory—skills more difficult to assess in a very brief period than language and verbal memory—so all I could do was add a couple of items to the usual test procedure. With the help of Melody's mother, I selected a number of classical pieces (melodies without lyrics) and folk songs that were familiar to Melody. I also had to be able to hum the first few bars of four of these melodies. Immediately before the sodium amytal was injected, I gave Melody the standard Wada baseline tests of speech, object naming, and remembering objects and sentences. I also hummed the first bars of one of the classical melodies and one of the folk songs and asked Melody to name them. She did, without hesitation, which was a relief, as I was unsure whether my renditions would be recognizable! I then asked her to hum the first bars of two tunes: again, one a classical piece without lyrics and the other a folk song. Her right hemisphere was then anesthetized, and her left arm and left side of her face became paralyzed. She performed well on my rapid tests of speech, naming, and memory, confirming that she was left-dominant for language and could remember objects and sentences with only her left hemisphere and hippocampus working. I then asked her to hum again each of the two songs she had practiced before the injection. She did this perfectly. Next I hummed the first bars of two new songs, one classical and the other a folk song, and told Melody to remember them. After the anesthetic had worn off she correctly recalled both of the songs I had hummed before she was given the sodium amytal, but of the two songs I had hummed after her hemisphere was anesthetized she could recall spontaneously—that is, without a cue—only the folk song. When I gave her the names of three classical pieces, however, she was able to tell me which one I had hummed, demonstrating that she could recognize the classical melody. Her performance suggested that her left hemisphere was capable of storing melodies but that it was able to recall tunes that are usually associated with lyrics more easily than tunes never associated with lyrics. This makes sense, since the left hemisphere is the expert on lyrics. Overall we were pleased with the Wada results, and although they didn't provide certainty that Melody's musical memory would be unaffected following a right temporal lobectomy—for example, the anesthetic didn't last long enough to enable me to assess her ability to learn new songs—they did suggest she would retain her ability to sing in tune and her memory for songs she already knew.

In the near future, musical abilities will probably be able to be assessed using functional MRI (fMRI). In specialist epilepsy centers where it is available, fMRI is used to directly visualize the origin of the seizures, and it is increasingly taking the place of the much more invasive and less reliable Wada test for safely and reliably assessing the lateralization of language. This is an important consideration when there is a possibility that the patient is right-dominant for speech and language, for example, when the person is strongly left-handed and comes from a family of left-handers. If the epileptic focus is located in the left temporal lobe but the fMRI studies show that the right hemisphere is the active one during speech tasks, then removing a part of the left temporal lobe will be less risky. Sometimes the seizure focus is very close to the motor or sensory strip, and in such a case fMRI can map the motor or sensory cortex so that the surgeon knows which parts of the cortex can safely be removed without causing a disabling paralysis or a loss of sensation.

But at that time, we had to make do with the Wada. Melody was comforted by the results, as before going ahead with the test she had decided that if it indicated that after the surgery she could still sing in tune and remember old songs, she would be happy. After all, she already knew hundreds of songs. The next day she was anesthetized again, but this time it was a general anesthetic, and she knew that when she woke up a part of her brain would be gone forever, and hopefully her epilepsy with it. The neurosurgeon cut away the temporal lobe four centimeters from its tip and removed most of the shrunken hippocampus. This was a smaller resection than he usually did, as he wanted to remove the seizure focus but protect as much of Melody's musical ability as possible. On waking from the anesthetic, she performed adequately on the simple speech and verbal memory tests I gave her, but she would not have a full follow-up neuropsychological assessment for another year, to give her time to recover from the surgery and return to her normal life.

For six months after her surgery Melody remained on medication, and then, because she had had no seizures, it was gradually reduced. A year later she was drug- and seizure-free, and she returned to see me for a follow-up psychological and neuropsychological assessment. Arriving with Tim at her side, she looked well and very happy. She had returned to her job at the music store and was teaching the guitar again. She had left the band just prior to her surgery and hadn't taken that up again—they had a new singer—but she didn't seem concerned about this. When I asked if she missed it, she answered: "A little, I suppose, but I'm not keen on late nights in a bar anymore; I'd sooner spend my evenings with Tim. And anyway, we're trying for a baby now that I'm off all my medications. Once she"—she grinned at Tim—"or he is born, I won't have time to sing in a band!"

She hadn't noticed any problems with her memory, and Tim reported that her singing and playing were even better than before. Melody didn't entirely agree with this and said she was getting a bit rusty, but that was only from lack of practice. She told me she had tested herself on learning some new, quite difficult jazz numbers, and found this more of a challenge than in the past. "It just takes me a lot longer, but I get there in the end. And once I have learned a new song, I don't forget it."

I repeated the neuropsychological tests I had given her prior to her surgery, and to her delight she performed at a higher level on the psychomotor tests—almost certainly a consequence of stopping medication—and she said that she did feel much more "with it" and "alive" now that she had stopped her medication. "I think it really was slowing me down," she explained. "I noticed when my neurologist first reduced my dose that colors seemed brighter, and when people were talking their voices seemed louder—too loud at first until I got used to them!"

Her verbal memory had also improved slightly, again probably a consequence of being taken off medication. On the nonverbal memory tests she showed no change.

"Well, you are definitely a success story," I told her, as delighted as she was. "It took courage to go ahead with the surgery knowing you might lose some of your musical ability. You truly deserve this wonderful outcome."

"Yes, it was a hard choice, the singer or the song. But as it turned out it was the singer *and* the song!" She leaned over and kissed Tim on the cheek. "And now all we need to complete our little family is a baby."

"Or two," said Tim, smiling at her.

*****

For a healthy person, major neurosurgery may appear to be a rather extreme measure to contemplate simply because of focal seizures, but for people who suffer from frequent debilitating seizures despite trying various antiepileptic drugs, the chance of a permanent cure for their epilepsy often makes even such nonreversible measures seem worthwhile. In fact, the Wada procedure and temporal lobectomy do not carry significant risks, and it is uncommon for patients to suffer major long-term problems as a result of these procedures. For some, the chance to have this operation becomes the most important aspect of their lives, and when the operation is successful (as in the vast majority of cases), many view it almost as a miracle. With ever-improving and safer assessment techniques such as fMRI, along with more accurate and safer microsurgical techniques, surgical intervention for epilepsy is becoming more attractive. As research studies find out more about possible long-term negative as well as positive outcomes from surgery and weigh these against the negatives and positives of drug therapy for focal seizures, it may well be that in the future, surgery will become the best option even for those people for whom drug therapy works reasonably well.

The evolution of the treatment of shortsightedness perhaps provides a good model. Fifty years ago shortsighted people wore glasses, and then, as the technology improved, more and more took to wearing first hard, then soft contact lenses. These tiny bits of plastic gave their wearers freedom and a new appearance, but on the downside contact lenses and their cleaning agents were expensive, they were a nuisance to put in and take out, and minor eye infections were common. Then came laser treatment, and with this a long-term cure. It seemed like a miracle after such a small operation to be able to look up at the night sky and see bright pinpricks of light rather than fuzzy saucers! At first the operation was seen as a risky and very expensive procedure, but today it is possibly less risky and less expensive than a lifetime of wearing contact lenses.

I predict that in the not too distant future, for sufferers of temporal lobe epilepsy, temporal lobectomy—perhaps a much more individually tailored and "smaller" operation than currently possible—will be the treatment of choice when compared with a lifetime of antiepileptic drugs. Drug treatment may come to be viewed as more expensive and likely to result in more medical, psychological, and cognitive problems than a one-off surgical operation to remove an area of cortex that is already compromised and causes more problems than benefits to its owner.

*****

As happens in a busy hospital world, Melody disappeared from my life after that final assessment, a sign of her return to a full life with no more need for doctors and psychologists.

So when, many years later, we bumped into each other after a concert, it took both of us a few moments to place the other's face and connect it with a name. In fact, Melody realized who I was before I retrieved her name. Perhaps her recognition for face–name combinations had improved as mine diminished with age! Over a cup of coffee she caught me up on what had happened in her life in the years since we'd last met.

"Tim's at home looking after the kids; that's why I'm concert-going with my girlfriend," she explained.

"So you did have children; I'm so glad."

"Yes, I was pregnant within two months of my last assessment with you. Priscilla's just had her sixth birthday, so it must be seven years since we last saw each other. And Todd is four. They're both beyond cute!"

"I can imagine," I laughed. "And are they musical?"

"Priscilla is well on her way to becoming a professional ballerina, and Todd is a drummer. But my mother teaches them piano and I teach them guitar, so hopefully they'll both have musician's brains!"

"And your music? Are you as involved as ever?"

"Not quite yet. I've been too busy being a mother. But my mother looks after the kids a couple of afternoons a week, so I was able to start teaching the guitar again last year. And one day I think I will see if I can start up a new jazz group—or join one—just for fun. I'm still passionate about singing."

"And you've had no more seizures?"

"Not a one. Drug-free and seizure-free! The singer, the song, the husband, and the babies—all intact!"

We parted ways a little later, and I haven't seen her since. But thinking about her always brings a feeling of satisfaction. I still find it just a little mysterious that the removal of a large part of the human brain can result in such a positive life change, leaving the singer whole and happy and her song still sweet.

■ Further Reading

Ogden, J. A. 2005. Out of control: The consequences and treatment of epilepsy. In: *Fractured Minds: A Case-Study Approach to Clinical Neuropsychology, 2nd Ed.* (pp. 64–82). New York: Oxford University Press.

Sacks, O. 2008. *Musicophilia: Tales of Music and the Brain. Revised and Expanded.* New York: Vintage Books.

Stein, G. 2005. *How Evan Broke His Head and Other Secrets.* New York: Soho Press.

9 ∎

The Amazing Woman: Half a Brain
Will Do the Job!

Joseph missed Franklin D. Roosevelt's historic speech on December 8, 1941, delivered to the nation the day after the Japanese flew their deadly bombers into the Pacific fleet in Pearl Harbor. Perhaps it was just as well that there was no radio in the waiting room of the hospital in small-town Massachusetts where Joseph paced back and forth, every fiber of his body zinging with anxiety and hope as his wife panted and pushed nearby in the "fathers not admitted" birthing unit. Joseph and Isobelle already had five healthy sons, ranging from two to 12 years old, and all fingers and toes in the family were crossed for the long-awaited daughter. So when the baby arrived, a robust nine pounds with a lusty cry, their joyful celebrations were barely dampened when it dawned on them that their newest family member had been born into a country at war. As for Isobelle and her parents, the infant's innocent sweetness filled a corner of the gaping hole torn in their hearts by the news that Kane, Isobelle's only brother, and a seaman on the USS *Arizona*, would never meet his small niece.

A big hole for a little girl to fill, but fortunately Kate—the girl's name closest to Kane that they could find—was up to the challenge, and by the age of ten months she had every member of her extended family wrapped firmly around her chubby finger. Sparkling blue eyes, golden curls, and a sunny personality were just part of her charm; she had already made it clear that the normal developmental stages were child's play as she galloped past them at an astonishing rate, crawling almost as fast as her three-year-old brother could run and pulling herself up on the furniture in her eagerness to keep up with him. But how fragile a thing happiness is; for the second time in a few short months, this family was to learn that in a breath our lives can change.

Ten-month-old Kate, waking from her afternoon nap and hearing her brothers playing outside the window, somehow managed to pull herself up the sides of her cot, where she must have teetered and fallen, slamming her golden head on the hard floor below and lying still, without even a cry. How long she lay there before her mother found her when she peered in to see why her baby was sleeping so long, they would never know. Would the consequences have been less horrifying if she had been found straight away? Why didn't they have a thick rug on the floor under her cot? So many questions for Isobelle and Joseph to punish themselves with as they struggled—in those days with no help from counselors—to come to terms with their tragedy. But their guilt had to take second place to their daughter's more urgent needs, and perhaps that saved their sanity and possibly even their marriage.

Kate was taken by ambulance to the hospital where she was born such a short time ago, and taken care of behind closed doors while her parents kept vigil in the waiting room, only allowed to see her for ten minutes, four times a day. At home the children's grandparents did their best to answer the questions put to them by Kate's five brothers and distracted the children and themselves with picnics in the country and games of baseball on the back lawn. Kate slowly regained consciousness and two weeks after her fall opened her bloodshot blue eyes and looked at her mother. The next day she curled the still-chubby fingers of her left hand around her father's finger, and he believed he could see a glimmer of a smile on her now pale little face. When the doctor told them he thought she was out of danger and could probably return home in another week, they were so relieved they didn't fully grasp the implications of his next pronouncement.

"I'm afraid she might never regain the use of the right side of her body," he told them.

"What do you mean? Surely she'll get better in time?" Joseph said, grasping Isobelle's hand.

"I think further significant recovery is unlikely, although not impossible given how young she is. Kate suffered a severe head injury and as a result she is paralyzed on her right side. That's why she can't move her right arm and leg and why her smile is lopsided; the right side of her face doesn't move properly anymore."

"But why? What happened to her brain?" Isobelle managed to ask.

"Movement of the right arm and leg is controlled by the left side of the brain. That hemisphere of her brain must have been badly damaged when she hit her head. That's the most likely cause of her paralysis."

"But how will she manage? Will she have to be in a wheelchair all her life?" asked Joseph, his voice breaking.

"Why don't you cross that bridge when you come to it," the doctor suggested. "She has youth on her side; young brains are more flexible than old brains. And her left limbs are not affected at all. With lots of physical therapy she could well learn to walk with a walking frame or even a brace and walking sticks. She'll be able to learn to use a pencil and do everything with her left hand."

"Poor little Kate," said Isobelle. "She was so bright, and now she has this to bear."

"The fact that she's so bright will help her make the best of her life," the doctor said gently. "But I do have to tell you about one other problem she might have. The left hemisphere of the brain is also the language hemisphere. It's where our speech and comprehension of language comes from. I'm afraid Kate may have trouble learning to speak."

"My God, that's worse than not being able to walk!" Isobelle cried.

"Yes, I realize that. But again, she is very young and perhaps her brain will be able to adapt, and hopefully the essential language areas haven't been badly damaged. But it might be necessary for her to have special help with learning to talk later on, and I didn't want you to be thinking she might start talking at the usual time."

"And there is no way you can look inside her head to see what's damaged?" Joseph asked.

"Not without opening up her skull, and we don't want to do that just to see what has happened to her left brain; that would be a very dangerous operation to do on such a little person. Hopefully, one day we will have some sort of X-ray that can see inside the head and visualize the brain itself, but until then we can only surmise what the damage is from her symptoms and rate of recovery."

*****

The next months were a nightmare of sleepless nights and exhausting days for Isobelle. Her heartache for little Kate, her promising future lost, when added to Isobelle's still-raw grief for her brother, was almost too much to bear.

But she struggled on, trying not to neglect her five sons while caring for a baby now more needy than a newborn and worrying about her parents, who had aged ten years overnight. Joseph, a lawyer, had no choice but to return to his law practice; the family would need every dollar he could earn. Joseph's mother was a lifesaver for Isobelle, coming in daily to help her, and both grandfathers spent as much time as possible with the five boys. And as the months wore on, Isobelle's mother found it easier to put Kane, her lost son, out of her mind for a few moments as she watched her grandsons playing gently with their lopsided little sister.

With intensive physical therapy twice a day, Kate's useless right leg gradually gained strength, and by 15 months she was crawling again, pulling herself along by her left hand, her right arm bent uselessly under her but her right leg mostly managing to keep up with her strong left leg. The weakness on the right side of her face had resolved, and her smile, although not so frequent as before, now brought forth dimples in both cheeks. By two years she could say a few words and pull herself up on the furniture. Six months later she was walking in a small walking frame made to support her right side, and by her fourth birthday she was walking with a leg brace. The speech therapist's tests showed that Kate's speech and language comprehension were equal to those of the average three-year-old.

Life was finally getting easier for Isobelle with all five sons at school, and the family had almost forgotten there was anything wrong with Kate as she spent more and more time outside, her golden curls constantly in a tangle as she threw herself into her brothers' rough-and-tumble games. On the dark side, she was prone to dreadful tantrums, which if anything had been getting worse since they first became a problem when she was two. But Isobelle and Joseph put these down to her frustration with her clumsy leg brace and her paralyzed right arm, which she now held bent at the elbow and curved into her body. When they gently tried to straighten it her screaming would start, and they soon decided it wasn't worth the stress.

Not long after her fifth birthday, Kate tumbled from a swing suspended from a branch of an old apple tree. Her brother was pushing her high in the air, and suddenly at the top of the arc she catapulted off, landing, once again, on the left side of her head. By the time the ambulance arrived she had regained consciousness but was still drowsy, and after a night in the local hospital she was transferred to Boston Children's Hospital. To her parents' dismay, a lumbar puncture revealed blood in the cerebrospinal fluid (CSF), indicating that she had suffered a brain hemorrhage. Her CSF gradually cleared and she became fully alert, but an investigative electroencephalogram (EEG) showed some seizure activity in the left occipital area of her brain typical of petit mal, or absence, seizures where there is a transient and very brief lapse of consciousness, often barely perceptible to an observer. Her parents took her home a week later, with instructions to watch her carefully to see if she lost focus or looked "absent" from time to time. Absence seizures are often difficult to detect, but in schoolchildren they can be a serious block to learning. With every seizure the child stops attending for a second or two and loses track of what is going on, especially if there are many of these seizures in a day or sometimes even in an hour. If this began to be a problem for Kate, already clearly disadvantaged by the earlier damage to her left hemisphere, she would need to be started on antiepileptic medication.

Kate began attending a special school when she was seven. By then her spoken language and comprehension were quite good, and she managed physically surprisingly well, walking with a limp but without a leg brace or sticks. Her right arm remained spastic and flexed, with severe muscle wasting. She continued to have tantrums and was frequently violent toward the other children at school and her brothers at home, hitting and biting them. She was a slow learner, with a short attention span, in part probably as a result of absence seizures. Although she learned to write rather clumsily, her reading and spelling were poor and she had difficulty with even simple arithmetic. She even disliked art, and spent more time tearing up her art paper—as well as the artworks of other children—and throwing paints and pencils across the room than concentrating on her drawing or painting.

When she was nine Kate began to have generalized seizures where she lost consciousness and convulsed violently. A primitive radiographic test called a pneumoencephalogram was performed and showed an enlarged left lateral ventricle (one of the compartments in the middle of the brain filled with CSF) and extensive air between the left hemisphere and the membrane called the *arachnoid mater* that covers the brain. The interpretation of this finding was that the left hemisphere had almost totally atrophied. Many antiepileptic medications were tried, with little success, but in spite of frequent seizures every day, Kate continued to attend school intermittently and managed to complete the eighth grade, although her schoolwork remained well below the average standard for her age group.

Kate's behavioral and emotional problems worsened in adolescence. She was difficult to manage at school and at home and frequently behaved aggressively, rudely, and inappropriately. As a result of her behaviors and her frequent seizures, her social development was stunted, and she had no friends. By the age of 15 she was having twenty-five seizures a day, and an EEG showed seizure activity in every lobe of her brain, but especially in the left temporal and occipital lobes. So her parents made the difficult decision to go ahead with a radical brain operation—a *hemispherectomy*—in a last-ditch attempt to reduce her seizures.

Neurosurgeons at Boston Children's Hospital had performed a number of these operations on children who had an atrophied brain hemisphere and disabling seizures untreatable by antiepileptic medicine, and in many cases the patient's seizures were significantly reduced. This risky operation involved removing the atrophied and useless brain hemisphere so it could no longer spark off seizures. The theory was that this would prevent the spread of seizures to the other, "good" hemisphere via the *corpus callosum*—the thick fiber band connecting the two hemispheres and allowing them to communicate. Not all hemispherectomies were successful, and some children died as a result of complications of the surgery, one being the collapse of the remaining hemisphere into the space left by the removal of the atrophied hemisphere.

Fortunately this didn't happen to Kate when, at 15, she had her first two operations. Most of her left hemisphere was dissected away, and to everyone's relief, her seizures decreased dramatically. But sixteen months later her seizures increased again and she had a third and final operation. A large cyst that had formed and took up most of the space in the hemisphere was removed along with almost of all the remaining left brain tissue, leaving only the inside—medial—surface of the left occipital lobe. But it wasn't until Kate was 44 that a computed tomography (CT) scan of her brain was carried out and the dramatic results of the hemispherectomy could be clearly seen (see Figure 9.1). The CT showed a large space, filled with CSF, on the left side of the brain where most of the left hemisphere had been removed. The right hemisphere appeared intact, although the lateral ventricle was enlarged.

Kate's disruptive behaviors prior to her first operation had caused numerous problems for the hospital staff, and they were surprised to find her quiet and compliant in the days following her surgery. Initially they put this new docile behavior down to her tiredness after the operation,

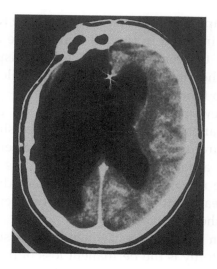

FIGURE 9.1

A CT scan of Kate's brain taken when she was 44 years old. The left side of the scan shows the fluid-filled space where most of the left hemisphere was removed. All that remains is the medial—inner—surface of the occipital pole. The remaining right ventricle is dilated. (Reprinted from Ogden, J. A. 1988. Language and memory functions after long recovery periods in left-hemispherectomized subjects. *Neuropsychologia, 26,* p. 649, with kind permission from Elsevier Science Ltd, Kidlington, UK.)

but when her energy returned it became apparent that she had undergone a dramatic personality change. The new Kate seemed to be a reasonable and perfectly pleasant teenager! Joseph and Isobelle were amazed and delighted by this unexpected bonus, and the neurosurgeon told them he had seen this phenomenon in other patients following hemispherectomy. One possible explanation was that before her atrophied left hemisphere was removed, Kate experienced massive seizure activity in both hemispheres of her brain much of the time, even when she wasn't having an observable seizure. Her bad behaviors were possibly a consequence of this ongoing disruption of normal brain function. For example, disruption of her healthy right prefrontal lobe would have prevented her from inhibiting inappropriate behaviors.[1] Because Kate's seizure activity was initiated in the left hemisphere and traveled to the right, the removal of the left hemisphere would have freed the right hemisphere from epileptic activity, allowing it to function more normally.

Kate's new personality proved to be a permanent change, and after her final operation when she was 17 she became seizure-free, a remarkable result given her twenty-five seizures a day prior to her surgery. As a preventive measure, she remained on antiepileptic medications for a number of years, but she was weaned off them completely by the time she was 21.

The main negative consequence of a successful left hemispherectomy is the permanent loss of the right half of the visual field (a right *homonymous hemianopia*.) This is an unavoidable consequence of removing the occipital (visual) cortex along with the visual pathways on the left. As a result, when Kate looked straight ahead, she saw only the left side of the "view." But like most people with visual field defects, she quickly adapted to this by moving her eyes or her head to the right, allowing her to scan both sides of the world. In fact, Kate seemed unaware that she had any restriction of her field of view. Fortunately she had no desire to drive a car!

Following the hemispherectomy, Kate's language abilities remained the same, she continued to walk unaided but with a limp, and she still held her wasted right arm in the flexed position. This lack of change was because Kate's right hemisphere had taken over as many of the physical and cognitive functions as it was capable of long before her surgery—probably by the time she was 12 years old, when it is thought that language abilities become set. Her left hemisphere had contributed nothing but seizures and

[1] Read the description of Phillipa's case in Chapter 4 for examples of inappropriate behaviors resulting from severe prefrontal lobe damage.

unhappiness to her life. Imagine how wonderful it must have been for Kate to wake every morning looking forward to a life where she could do whatever she desired without being shot down by a seizure. The stigma attached to the sort of seizures Kate had, where sufferers fall to the ground convulsing, incontinent, drooling, and with their eyes rolling up, was much greater in the 1950s than it is today. It was hardly surprising she made no friends.

It is to her great credit that she wasted no time in making the most of her new "normality." In this she was fortunate in having a supportive family who, rather than protecting her, went out of their way to introduce her to new people and situations, encouraging her to explore her independence. Of course this didn't happen overnight, but day by day her life improved. She made a number of friends and began to enjoy going to movies, parties, and even family picnics. Over the next few years she learned how to socialize and took on some voluntary part-time jobs, such as putting flyers in envelopes for charities and assisting with filing and other office tasks. When she was 23 she began her first full-time paid job—in charge of the photo-copying machine in a library—which she held until she was 50. She retired at that point, not because she could no longer perform well but because she wanted time to spend on other leisure activities. Outgoing and sociable, Kate has lived independently all her adult life, enjoying a reasonably good marriage for a number of years before she and her husband obtained an amicable divorce.

Kate continued to have medical follow-ups at Boston Children's Hospital, and when she was 45 and I was a research fellow at the Massachusetts Institute of Technology (MIT), I asked her doctor to pass on to her my invitation to participate in a research project. I was delighted when she accepted, and she enthusiastically agreed to come to MIT so I could carry out a detailed assessment of her cognitive abilities. On our first meeting I couldn't believe that Kate was the owner of the CT brain scan I had seen, taken just the previous year. The scan showed a massive space where the left side of her brain should be, and here she was, walking unaided (so much for the right leg's being controlled by the left side of the brain), talking fluently and rapidly (so much for the left hemisphere's dominance of language), and conversing, discussing, and joking appropriately and delightfully (so much for the theory that major frontal lobe damage causes inappropriate behavior)![2] So I was excited about assessing Kate in considerable depth to see if there were cognitive abilities that were more difficult for her. Surely her remaining right hemisphere couldn't do everything.

*****

Many neuropsychologists believe—and this is backed up by numerous studies—that in infancy, the two brain hemispheres are *equipotential* for language; that is, both hemispheres are capable of developing language up until about the age of 12 years. By this age the *plasticity* of the brain (allowing some brain areas to take on functions they do not normally support) has been greatly reduced. By early adolescence, in 96% of right-handers and 70% of left-handers who have healthy brains, the left hemisphere has become strongly dominant for language and verbal memory, and the right hemisphere more weakly dominant for visuospatial functions and nonverbal memory. Because Kate's grandparents, parents, and five siblings were all strongly right-handed, I made the assumption that she too would have been right-handed if her right hand had not been paralyzed as a consequence of her head injury when

[2] Since assessing Kate I've assessed five other adults who have undergone hemispherectomies because of severe seizure disorders caused by massive damage to one hemisphere in infancy, and all of them have had normal social and conversational skills.

she was a baby. Thus when she was born, Kate's brain would almost certainly have been biologically programmed to develop language in the left hemisphere. My hypothesis was that as Kate's right hemisphere had taken on the left hemispheric language abilities, some of the usual right hemispheric visuospatial abilities might have been "crowded out" entirely or only poorly developed.

I tested Kate over two days, and we both enjoyed the experience.[3] Her long medical history had made her somewhat skeptical about the medical profession and its fund of knowledge—or lack of it—about the brain. After all, she could perform many tasks that she had been told she would never be able to do. So she was highly motivated to try my tests and prove that she wasn't such a "dumbo" after all. Her delightful sense of humor and down-to-earth assertive manner ensured that there wasn't a dull moment, and during our breaks I discovered she had strong opinions on any number of topics.

I already had copies of Kate's previous cognitive assessments from her medical file. Before her hemispherectomy—at the age of 14—her cognitive abilities fell in the "dull normal" to "borderline" range, but after her final operation, most of her scores had steadily climbed into the average range for her age, and they had remained stable since the age of 33. I extended the assessments to look in more detail at her strengths and weaknesses.

Kate's scores on tests of vocabulary and comprehension confirmed that she was of average verbal ability. Her spoken language was entirely normal, both rich and expressive, and her comprehension was good. For example, if asked to pick up a pencil and draw a circle on a

---

[3]Kate, under the initials KOF, has featured in a number of scientific articles, including Cavazutti and Erba (1976), Corballis and Ogden (1988), and Ogden (1988, 1989, 1996), that discuss the abilities and impairments of hemispherectomized people. The full references can be found in the Further Reading section at the end of this chapter.

piece of paper, then put the pencil down, pick up a dime, and give it to me, she could perform without hesitation or error. I also assessed her on some more difficult language tests that other researchers had reported were impossible for people with left hemispherectomies. These required the comprehension—shown by pointing to the correct picture—of difficult "passive negative" sentences such as "The truck is not pulled by the car." Kate had a perfect score when she read the sentences for herself rather than having them read to her. It is likely that to successfully complete tasks like these, Kate needed more time than a normal person to think things through, and reading the sentences for herself gave her this time. So having half a brain appears to increase the time it takes to think (understandably so, because any type of brain damage has the potential to slow thinking processes) but not necessarily the ability to carry out a task if given sufficient time. It is important therefore to separate out these two factors if we wish to discover what the brain can do rather than how fast it can complete a task.

As speech and comprehension are more important for communication than reading and spelling and would have developed earlier in evolution, I was intrigued to find out whether the right hemisphere could also take over these less essential "left hemisphere" language functions. Kate, it turned out, could write spontaneously, copy writing, and write to dictation. She could also read slowly but fluently, although at 45 she did not read books for pleasure, in spite of working in a library all her adult life. This was possibly due in part to the intermittent schooling she had had because of her seizures and behavior problems; reading and spelling were also not a priority in the special school she attended. On discovering during our sessions that she could read quite well, she began to read light novels, and I carried out more detailed reading and spelling tests six years later, when she was 51.

During this assessment Kate performed normally when asked to read extensive word lists, including regularly spelled (e.g., "dump"), irregularly spelled (e.g., "womb"), concrete (e.g., "table"), and abstract (e.g., "happiness") words. She could also spell most of these categories of words reasonably well, especially given her poor schooling, but had difficulty spelling some irregular words, a common problem for people with limited formal education. She also had marked difficulty reading and spelling nonwords (e.g., "dat"). The fact that she couldn't sound out nonwords as well as words that she didn't know suggested that although she had a normal left hemisphere lexicon—a "list," stored in her memory, of all the words she had learned—and could recognize these words from their visual forms or when she heard them, she had not developed the phonological, "sounding out" route to reading and spelling. The phonological approach to reading and spelling is typically mediated by the left hemisphere, so it appeared that Kate's isolated right hemisphere had not been able to take over this function.

On a word fluency test where she was given one minute to say as many words starting with a particular letter as possible, she performed at the level of a 10-year-old. This is a task requiring the formation and initiation of a successful strategy—an "executive" ability—and is considered a test of left prefrontal lobe function. Kate's impaired performance indicated that her right prefrontal lobe was not able to mediate all executive functions at a normal level. Kate also struggled with visuospatial tasks, normally the strength of the right hemisphere. She couldn't match complex shapes or carry out mental problems involving spatial relations, such as imagining turning a picture of an abstract shape or an elephant around in her "mind's eye." Copying a cube or a five-pointed star was a challenge (see Figure 9.2), and her copy of a complex figure was severely impaired (see Figure 9.3). In neuropsychological jargon she

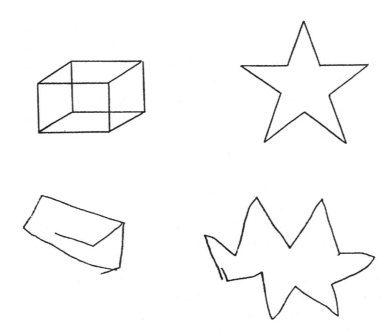

FIGURE 9.2
When asked to copy the drawings of a cube and a star at the top, Kate produced the drawings on the bottom. (Reprinted from Ogden, J. A. 2005. *Fractured Minds: A Case-Study Approach to Clinical Neuropsychology, 2nd Ed.,* p. 355, with kind permission from Oxford University Press, New York.)

had *constructional apraxia,* the inability to perform tasks involving the manipulation of objects—or pencil lines—in space. Her executive difficulties exacerbated her visuospatial problems, as shown by her lack of planning a logical approach when copying the complex figure.

But Kate had developed and retained some very important right hemispheric functions in spite of the "space" the language functions had taken up. An important right hemispheric ability that we take for granted is recognition of familiar faces, and certainly in everyday life Kate experienced no difficulty with this. In fact, when shown 50 photos of new faces, followed by 50 pairs of faces comprising one face from the 50 just seen and a new face, she

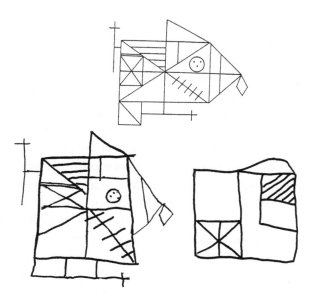

FIGURE 9.3
When asked to copy the Rey Complex Figure (top), Kate drew the picture
on the lower left. Forty-five minutes later, she drew from memory the
picture on the lower right. (Reprinted from Ogden, J. A. 2005. *Fractured
Minds: A Case-Study Approach to Clinical Neuropsychology, 2nd Ed.,* p. 356,
with kind permission from Oxford University Press, New York.)

could point to the more familiar face in 46 of the pairs.
Even on a difficult face discrimination test where faces
photographed in various degrees of shadow have to be
matched with the same face under different lighting conditions, she obtained a normal score.

   She also performed normally on some visuospatial
tasks that are usually mediated by the left hemisphere.
These included telling left from right and following direc-
tions ("Turn second left and then first right") in order to
draw a pencil line through a simple map. *Personal
orientation* and knowing her *body schema* were other left
hemispheric functions that Kate was good at. She could
accurately point to her own body parts and match them

with the body parts of a drawing of a person facing the same or opposite way from her.[4] But Kate was severely impaired on a test of *extrapersonal orientation* where she had to walk a path between nine circular markers according to a visual map indicating the path to be followed, with "north" marked on one side of both the map and the markers,. On this test she was also worse than some much younger left-hemispherectomized people assessed in other studies, so perhaps aging accounted for her poor performance.

Almost any sort of arithmetic calculation had Kate completely stumped. She could add or subtract two numbers under 10, but any sort of division or multiplication above the "2 times" table was beyond her. This disorder is called *acalculia*. Calculation—because of its logical and sequential requirements—is primarily a left hemispheric ability, but because of the spatial aspects of many mathematical problems (e.g., carrying figures across columns) the right hemisphere also makes a contribution. Mathematics is one of the many abilities that supports the finding that in the healthy, fully functioning brain, it takes two hemispheres to tango.[5]

An adequate memory is essential to living an independent life, so I expected Kate would demonstrate quite good memory abilities on formal tests. She had a normal immediate memory span—she could repeat six numbers or words—and her scores on tests of learning new verbal information were impressive—above normal and above the level I expected given her average verbal abilities. Comparisons with her assessments over past years showed that her verbal memory had improved steadily between the ages of 33 and 45, but a further assessment when she was 51 showed a moderate drop in her scores, although

[4] Read the case of Julian in Chapter 5 for descriptions of rare left hemispheric body schema disorders.

[5] You can read about Janet's right hemispheric calculation difficulties in Chapter 3 and Julian's left hemispheric acalculia in Chapter 5.

they were still in the normal range for her age. As most people in their late fifties and older can attest, an increasing difficulty with verbal learning and memory—such as remembering names—is common as we get older. But this memory decline is not as precipitous as Kate's. It may be that aging affects memory functions more rapidly when memory is mediated by only one hemisphere than it does in people with normal brains.

In all the assessments she underwent, Kate's nonverbal memory—often involving visuospatial concepts—was usually worse than her verbal memory. Take a look in Figure 3.3 at her drawing from memory of the complex figure she had copied 45 minutes earlier. Remembering such a detailed picture seems difficult to most people when they first see it, but this is one of the most common visuospatial memory tests in the neuropsychologist's test library. Kate's score on this memory test was much lower than the scores of large groups of women of her age, ethnicity and verbal ability, averaged across the group (called *normative scores*). Fifteen years after her hemispherectomy, when she was 32, Kate recalled 55% of the figure 45 minutes after copying it, but by the time she was 45 she could only recall 25%. Of course, her difficulty in copying the figure in the first place would have affected her ability to store it for later recall, but even taking this into consideration her recall was very poor, always falling into the lowest 10% of scores for normal adults of her age. The presence of a visuospatial memory impairment was supported by Kate's poor performance on a number of simpler visuospatial memory tests, on all of which her scores declined even more rapidly between the ages of 45 and 51, when I last assessed her.

Producing and comprehending emotional tone in speech—*prosody*—is thought to be a right hemispheric ability, so I was keen to assess Kate on this, although in everyday conversation she definitely had no problem with appropriately expressing her emotions in her voice. I asked her to identify the tone of voice when hearing the sentence "I am going to the movies" recorded on tape by the voices of a man, woman, and child. Each voice said the sentence in six different tones—happy, angry, disinterested, sad, surprised, and tearful. Kate was also asked to repeat the sentences in the same tone for each of the voices and to say the sentences with the six different intonations on command. In addition, she had to visually identify my facial expressions as I attempted to convey the same six emotions, copy these expressions, and make the facial expressions on command. Kate performed perfectly on all these tests of prosody. Clearly this right hemispheric function is not disadvantaged by the development of language in the right hemisphere, perhaps because prosody and facial expression are so intimately tied to speech. This makes evolutionary sense given that words and congruent emotional expression each contribute to clear communication.

*****

Few other hemispherectomized people have verbal abilities as remarkable as those demonstrated by Kate. It is therefore likely that she would have been of superior intelligence had she not suffered damage to her left hemisphere as a child. Her father and her five brothers all had university degrees, so this assumption is certainly supported by her genetic heritage. Although Kate's performance on several higher cognitive tasks remains compromised, her life does not seem to be unduly affected by this. Perhaps it's a case of "what we don't know, we don't miss," or as Kate remarked one day, "Half a brain will do the job!"

Kate's attitude toward health, hospitals, and researchers was influenced by her experiences; she had a healthy if rather cynical approach to medicine and science, and when she needed to see a doctor she was assertive about her needs and her right to information. She enjoyed assisting in research projects if they fitted within her social schedule, the research was fully explained to her, and she was provided with the results of the studies she had been involved in. She was justifiably proud of her achievements, and she delighted in the enthusiastic, often incredulous comments of researchers about her abilities.

So what have we learned about the human brain from Kate and other people who have had one hemisphere of their brain removed after severe damage in infancy? Comparisons between left and right hemispherectomized people have informed us about the equipotentiality at birth that the two halves of the brain possess for the development of particular functions and about the time frame—the *critical period*—the brain has to realize this equipotentiality before it loses its plasticity. One notion is that in the normal brain, basic language abilities develop early in the left hemisphere and more complex language functions develop later on as the brain matures. We know from studies of people who had their left hemispheres extensively damaged after the age of 12 and suffer severe language deficits with minimal recovery that our brains are fairly "set"—at least with respect to language—by adolescence. This is not to say that intensive rehabilitation programs for language loss in adults following a left hemispheric stroke (or other type of damage) cannot result in some improvements; there are numerous examples of people who have regained considerable language function. But it must be remembered that strokes and other forms of damage rarely destroy all of the left hemisphere. In massive strokes where language impairments are still severe after the damaged brain has had time to recover from the immediate effects of the stroke, lost language functions are unlikely to recover.[6]

[6]Luke and Irene's struggles with aphasia in Chapter 2 tell both sides of this story.

Comparisons of right and left hemispherectomized patients strongly suggest that early extensive damage to one hemisphere results in the remaining hemisphere's developing language functions first and nonverbal, visuospatial functions second. If the left hemisphere is the intact one, language skills develop at a normal rate and nonverbal visuospatial skills are disadvantaged. If the right hemisphere is the intact one, as it was for Kate, language abilities again develop first, but the more subtle and complex aspects of language develop more slowly or not at all. Moreover, some nonverbal visuospatial skills do not develop or are degraded as a result of the right hemisphere's involvement in language; they are "crowded out" by the language functions. Because visuospatial functions are so poorly developed, they may be the first to suffer from the effects of aging.

It can be hypothesized that the cognitive functions taken on by a single, isolated hemisphere will be those most important for living an independent life. At the top of this tentative hierarchy of functional importance are those abilities that Kate and others like her do best. They include production and comprehension of speech, including prosody, and of emotional expression generally; language comprehension; verbal memory; left–right discrimination; personal orientation; and face recognition. Many of these are usually left hemispheric functions, but some of them, such as prosody and face recognition, are typically associated with the right hemisphere. Lower in the hierarchy, and therefore more poorly developed or absent, are more complex language functions and many visuospatial functions, including memory for complex patterns. And according to my studies of six hemispherectomized patients, mathematical skills are at the bottom of the pile when it comes to living a happy and independent life!

Looking back, I am grateful that I met Kate relatively early in my career as a neuropsychologist. This amazing woman showed me that the human brain could adapt to early severe damage to an extent that previously I would not have believed possible, and these revelations changed forever the way I thought about the brain. Kate's story typifies the courage and sheer determination that so many of the patients I have met over the years have displayed as they worked, year after year, to overcome their disabilities. But it is rarely only about the patient. Most of these triumphant success stories are stories of family and the power of love and hope. In the 1940s and 1950s, a middle-class family like Kate's would have been expected to place a child as severely brain-damaged as Kate in an institution. In time, as her seizures and behaviors worsened, she would almost certainly have ended up in a psychiatric hospital—horrific places back then—where she would have been condemned to a life of pain, misery, and emotional isolation. It is likely that she would have been subjected to numerous—perhaps hundreds—of electroconvulsive therapy treatments, in those days given inhumanely and indiscriminately to patients with any one of a wide range of psychiatric or behavioral problems.

But Kate's family didn't take that road. They kept their very difficult daughter within their large family, got her through school, and made the courageous decision to go ahead with the hemispherectomy, praying it would give her the best chance of finding some relief from her seizures. It is unlikely they could have imagined in their wildest dreams just how successful that operation would be, giving their blue-eyed, golden-haired, sunny little girl, born on the day the US entered World War II, another chance at happiness.

■ Further Reading

Cavazutti, V., and G. Erba. 1976. Deficit mnestici dopo emisferectomia totale sinistral in pazienti con emiplegia spastica infantile. *Rivesta Sperimentale di Freniatria, 20*, 585–612.

Corballis, M. C., and J. A. Ogden. 1988. Dichotic listening in commissurotomized and hemispherectomized subjects. *Neuropsychologia, 26,* 565–573.

Ogden, J. A. 1988. Language and memory functions after long recovery periods in left-hemispherectomized subjects. *Neuropsychologia, 26,* 645–659.

Ogden, J. A. 1989. Visuospatial and "right-hemispheric" functions after long recovery periods in left-hemispherectomized subjects. *Neuropsychologia, 27,* 765–776.

Ogden, J. A. 1996. Phonological dyslexia and phonological dysgraphia following left and right hemispherectomy. *Neuropsychologia, 34,* 905–918.

Ogden, J. A. 2005. A whole life with half a brain: Kate's story. In: *Fractured Minds: A Case-Study Approach to Clinical Neuropsychology, 2nd Ed.* (pp. 348–361). New York: Oxford University Press.

10 ■

Just a Few Knocks on the Head: The Concussion Conundrum

This is a tale of two teenage boys who lived in the same large city but came from very different backgrounds. Jason was the eldest of two sons and lived with his well-off, white, professional parents in a large house in one of the wealthiest suburbs of Auckland. He attended a private boys' school and at 16 was already looking forward to university in two years. Howie, also 16, was the third eldest in a family of eight children and lived in a three-bedroom state house in one of the poorest suburbs of Auckland. His Maori mother worked as a cleaner and his white father was unemployed. Howie attended a large coeducational state school where most of the pupils came from poor families and where few of the pupils went on to university.

Yet these two boys had one very important thing in common. They were both mad about sports, and in particular rugby, New Zealand's national game. What's more, as a result of their passion they were both up-and-coming sports stars in their schools. In fact, as I later discovered, Jason and Howie had met each other on quite a few occasions on the rugby field and at parties after school matches. Their schools may have been miles apart in their educational standards and the discretionary funds they had to spend on extras for their pupils, but they were neck and neck when it came to rugby. One year the top team—the First Fifteen—in Jason's school would win the annual secondary school rugby competition, and the next year the honor would go to the First Fifteen in Howie's school. Of course some years neither school would win, but invariably both would be in the top six. At 16, Jason and Howie were young to be in their schools' First Fifteen teams; most of the players were 17 or 18 and in their final school year. Perhaps it was their physiques—Both boys were tall and strong for their age—that prompted their premature selection for the top team. Certainly their size was one of the factors that made them good "locks," the rugby position they both held and that exposed them to more risk of head injuries than many other positions on the field.

Like every boy in every First Fifteen, Jason and Howie fantasized about a career as a professional rugby player. But in reality they knew that this was a long shot, and Jason had a backup plan, to obtain a master's degree in sports psychology. Howie's backup plan wasn't quite so ambitious: he thought he'd try to get an apprenticeship as a mechanic at the local garage. Messing about with vehicles was his other passion.

Sadly, for these two boys the chance of being selected for the All Blacks—New Zealand's famous rugby team—was stymied. Before they reached their 17th birthdays they were to discover they had one more thing in common—brain damage. Of course, nobody in their families thought of it as brain damage. For many months the boys and their parents, and even their teachers and sports coaches, looked upon the mild difficulties Jason and Howie were having as unfortunate but temporary consequences of "just a few knocks on the head."

*****

Jason's mother, Becky, was a "mature" student in the large undergraduate "Introduction to Clinical Psychology" course I taught at the university. I knew her by sight, as she always sat in the front row of the lecture theater and often came up after the lecture to ask me a question. So when she knocked on my office door I assumed she was there to talk about her upcoming essay assignment. But after a brief exchange when she'd explained that she had returned to university part-time now that her two boys were in their teens and she had time on her hands, and that psychology was her favorite subject, she came to the real reason for her visit. She was worried about Jason and wondered if I could help. Over the last few months he seemed to have lost his zest for life, and she thought he might be depressed. Her husband, Andrew, even wondered if Jason was experimenting with drugs, although Becky was pretty sure he wouldn't be so silly. Two weeks earlier, the situation had come to a head when Jason became very drunk at a party after the Saturday rugby game and had been delivered home at 3 a.m., semicomatose, by two of his friends. And last week the school headmaster had asked Becky and Andrew to come in for a chat, where he told them that Jason's work standards had plummeted over the past few weeks and he had been missing some of his rugby practices. Becky and Andrew had tried talking to Jason, but with no success; he was sullen and rude and told them to get off his back before locking himself in his room for hours. Then Jason had been called in to see the school counselor, and that had caused more upset. Jason refused to go to school the following day, saying he was sick. By this point in her story, Becky was almost in tears, and I could see this would need more than a brief discussion with me.

"Do you think Jason's behavior might just be a case of 'teenage angst'?" I asked her.

"I wish it were, but he's so different than he's ever been before that we think there must be something else going on. I think he's depressed, and he has always been such an optimistic and balanced person. And he's always been avidly against drugs because of his sport and keeping fit."

"It does sound as if it would be a good thing for him to see someone. Are you wondering whether he could come to the psychology clinic?"

"Yes, I think he might accept that. Having to go to the counselor at school was too embarrassing. And Andrew told him he had no option: He had to either tell us what was wrong with him or go to see someone who could help him."

"And what was his reaction to that?"

"At first, he said he didn't need to see anyone and went and shut himself in his room again. But in the middle of the night Andrew got up because he couldn't sleep for worrying about him—neither of us could—and then he heard Jason crying in his room. He never cries, so it was very distressing. But thank goodness Andrew heard him. Anyway, he went in and after a while Jason did talk a bit, and said he was worried about himself. He thought he was going crazy. He said he'd never touched drugs and didn't get drunk as much as most of his friends and didn't know what was the matter with him. In the end he said he would go to see a psychologist as long as no one at the school had to know."

The psychology clinic is a training clinic for our clinical psychology interns, but on the day of Jason's first appointment, the intern who was scheduled to see him under my supervision went home sick just an hour before Jason was due to arrive. Jason was already on his way, so rather than postponing his initial session—at the risk of his deciding never to return—I decided to see him myself. Becky brought him in and introduced us and then, on my suggestion, went off to the library, saying she would be back to pick him up at the end of the session.

Jason was a tall, good-looking young man, mature for his age; he could easily have passed for 18 or 19. He looked miserable, and answered my questions politely but with minimal effort. He told me in a monotone that he was in the top class at school but could no longer be bothered with it, and that he was in the First Fifteen, played cricket and tennis in the summer, and was a fairly good snowboarder. I asked him how he thought his best friend would describe him. He looked at me in surprise.

"How would I know? I suppose he thinks I'm all right. We get on OK most of the time."

"How do you think he might describe your personality?"

"I don't know."

"Do you think you're seen as an outgoing sort of person, or studious, or shy, or pushy?"

"I used to be outgoing, but not anymore. I can't be bothered."

"What does that feel like, not being able to be bothered?"

"Like shit."

"And that's different from how you used to feel most of the time?"

"Yeah."

"Have you any theories about why you've started to feel like shit?"

"No." Jason's head was down and I could see he was struggling not to cry. Neither of us spoke. Then Jason's fists clenched and he burst out: "There's something wrong with my head. I think I'm going nuts."

That was the breakthrough, and for the rest of that first session, another session three days later, and then a family meeting with Jason and his parents—Jason refused to have his younger brother involved—together we were able to build up a picture of Jason's life over the past few years and the time sequence of the distressing changes he had been experiencing. Of course, as a neuropsychologist, I always had in mind the possibility of mild traumatic brain injury as a possible factor in any client who played rugby. However, as a clinical psychologist I was also alert to the many other possible causes for Jason's problems, not least family stresses, drug and alcohol issues, depression or another psychological or even more serious psychiatric problem, a physical illness, or simply being a teenager.

Jason's relevant "history" was unusually straightforward. His family life was happy; his parents were caring and had an excellent relationship with their sons; Jason was popular, extroverted, good with people of all ages—including his grandparents and his small cousins—a keen sportsman, and academically high-achieving. He only occasionally got drunk, did not take drugs, had never smoked, and had been as "healthy as a horse" all his life. In short, Jason was—or had been until recently—a dream son. Over the past few months he had been feeling terribly tired, found it difficult to concentrate in class, struggled with his homework—especially where he had to learn facts—couldn't stand being around his brother and his rowdy friends, and was irritable with his own friends, parents, and grandparents. Worst of all, his rugby game had deteriorated to the point where his coach had told him that if he didn't improve his attitude on the field and off, he could say goodbye to the First Fifteen. This was a revelation to his parents, as Jason had not told them. So I was not surprised by Jason's answer to my question, "Have you ever been knocked out, or even just dazed, during a rugby match or at any other time?" I might just as well have asked "How many times have you been knocked out," but of course that would have been a leading question.

"I've been dazed a few times, I suppose, but I've only actually had concussions two or three times when I've had to sit out the rest of the game and wasn't allowed to play for three weeks."

It took some careful detective work to discover that Jason had in fact been helped off the field three times over the past two years, twice in the current rugby season, which was by now nearly over. On each occasion he was unconscious for no more than a minute or two, was checked by his GP, and was not allowed to play on the next two Saturdays. Becky said that she had been worried after the last two knocks, as he had seemed confused and muddled for a few hours after each concussion. After a night's sleep, Jason had no longer felt confused, but had a hellish headache. He said he had headaches quite often now, especially when he was trying to concentrate in class, and that was one of the reasons he couldn't be bothered with school anymore.

By early evening he felt so tired he fell asleep over his homework. He used to be a sound sleeper, but he often woke two or three times in the night now, and struggled to get back to sleep. When I asked him if that's when he got to worrying about everything, he admitted it was, and that he knew he was depressed. He couldn't be bothered with parties, because the noise got to him and obviously he couldn't hold his drink. He hated being drunk; he liked to be in control. His girlfriend had practically given up on him anyway, as he was such a morose bastard these days. On the positive side, his appetite hadn't changed—he still ate like a horse—and he was adamant that he didn't have any suicidal thoughts. I felt confident that he was not in danger of self-harm and probably didn't require medication for his depressed mood—at least not until we had tried therapy. I suspected that just learning that there was a physical explanation for his changed feelings and behaviors would go a long way toward relieving Jason's worries.

All Jason's symptoms pointed toward a *postconcussional syndrome* (PCS). So as the next step, I scheduled a neuropsychological assessment to see if he displayed the pattern of results typical of PCS. In the meantime I explained what a PCS was, and we discussed some simple strategies he could use to help him manage his symptoms. First on the list was the importance of taking a long break from rugby and all other activities that might lead to another knock on the head. He also agreed to avoid alcohol completely after I explained that because of the PCS, he would become drunk much more rapidly. He should try to avoid situations where there was a lot of noise and sleep as much as possible. Jason left the clinic armed with some information booklets on concussion and the PCS, as well as a book written for the layperson covering all aspects of mild traumatic brain injury (TBI) and its rehabilitation.

*****

No universal standard exists for defining mild closed TBI—an injury to the brain caused by a blow to the head that doesn't pierce the skull—but it is commonly defined as a loss of consciousness for less than 20 minutes with a *posttraumatic amnesia* (PTA) of less than 24 hours. PTA refers to the period of interrupted ability to form new memories following a concussion; for example, the concussed person may not remember that his parents visited him the previous day, even though he had a perfectly reasonable conversation with them at the time. Many people who sustain a mild TBI may lose consciousness for a few minutes only, or sometimes just feel dazed and confused, and have a PTA of only a few seconds. But even these people can occasionally develop a PCS.

Immediately following a mild TBI, the victim may suffer headaches and feel nauseated, extremely tired, and possibly confused and disoriented for hours to days after the accident. The best treatment at this stage is to sleep and rest. Most people feel fully recovered two weeks later, and many are able to return to work without difficulty, especially if the work is not too taxing mentally or physically. Twenty-five percent or more, however, suffer some symptoms that constitute the PCS for varying lengths of time and in varying degrees of severity. The most common of the cognitive symptoms are a decreased ability to focus on the task at hand, especially in a noisy or distracting environment; an impairment in processing complex information; and problems with recent memory. These deficits are usually assessed by performance on standard neuropsychological tests of attention, information processing, and new learning and recall. In day-to-day life, sufferers notice that they have to put much greater effort into learning and recalling names of new friends and facts in school; that they become irritable in noisy environments; and if they need to do tasks requiring concentration, memorizing information, or processing new information, that they tire very quickly, develop headaches, and soon find themselves falling behind in their work or schooling.

The physical and psychosocial symptoms of mild TBI have a neuropathological basis (lowered cortical arousal from frontal lobe dysfunction) but can be exacerbated if the TBI victim and others misunderstand the cognitive and behavioral changes typical of the PCS. Common symptoms include fatigue, nausea, changes in sleep and eating patterns, periods of dizziness, hypersensitivity to noise, lessened tolerance for alcohol, irritability, anxiety, and depression. If the PCS continues for many weeks or months, sufferers may gradually lose confidence in their ability to work and maintain relationships, resulting in frustration, irritability, and a lowering of self-esteem.

Family disruption often occurs as family members struggle to cope with the problems of the head-injured person. Some sufferers may even come to believe they are going crazy or become so depressed that they feel suicidal, especially if they have not obtained information about PCS and do not relate their problems to the mild TBI they sustained weeks ago.

Because the symptoms of the PCS are common to many disorders, including depression with a psychological cause, the very existence of a PCS is controversial in some medical circles. Some doctors believe that the symptoms that make up the PCS are purely psychological and have no organic—physical—basis. Indeed, for many years the evidence from low-resolution computerized tomography (CT) brain scans corroborating the claims of a neuropathological cause for the symptoms of the PCS was rather slight, but this has changed with high-resolution magnetic resonance imaging (MRI) brain scans. Research studies using MRI have found that shortly after a concussion lasting less than 10 minutes a high proportion of people have small contusions and subcortical hemorrhages, usually located in the temporal lobes and the inferior anterior frontal cortex—the brain matter just above the eyes. Diffuse axonal injuries caused by stretching and tearing of nerve axons (the elongated projection attached to each neuron) are also a possible consequence of mild TBI, although these injuries are minimal compared with severe head injury. This type of damage can nevertheless result in a transient disruption of the *reticular formation*—a diffuse nerve network that connects the brain stem to the prefrontal lobes—causing lowered cortical arousal and the consequent common problems of fatigue, hypersensitivity to noise, and mood swings. Other research has shown that the effects of mild TBI can be cumulative, with patients who have sustained two or more mild concussions taking longer to recover than those sustaining a single mild concussion.

Another aspect of the PCS that fuels controversy over its very existence is that it is idiosyncratic in its choice of victims. Some people seem able to have multiple concussions without developing any of the symptoms of the PCS and others may have the smallest knock on the head and yet suffer a PCS. Why this might be is still unknown, but it is likely that interactions of many organic and psychological factors are responsible for the variable susceptibility of individuals to what appear to be relatively mild blows to the head. Multiple head injuries, a history of serious emotional or psychiatric problems, alcohol or solvent abuse, a demanding occupation, and the individual's age—children, teenagers, and the elderly are more vulnerable—all increase the potential for a significant PCS. In some cases, malingering can be a factor in apparent PCS, especially where there is monetary compensation for problems related to the head injury. In many such cases, a PCS can be viewed as a psychological construct without an organic basis. In true cases of PCS, where there is an underlying organic cause, there is very often some psychological overlay, and it is as important to prevent these psychological symptoms from developing as it is to manage the rehabilitation of the organically mediated symptoms. Whereas some cases of extended PCS may be primarily the result of neurological damage—as supported by MRI findings of diffuse lesions following mild TBI—it is possible that many cases of PCS that continue for months or years have become almost purely psychological. These people should not, however, be viewed as malingerers but as suffering from a poorly managed PCS.

*****

When Jason returned the following week for his neuropsychological assessment—scheduled on a school day at 9 a.m. to ensure that he was not tired before he even began—he seemed a little less down, and told me that after reading the information I had given him on the PCS, he figured that this might be what was wrong with him. On the whole it was a relief, he said, because at least it was something that he could do something about. But when I asked him how the past few days had gone, he looked at me glumly.

"Dad phoned my rugby coach and explained that I probably had these problems because of my concussions, so he banned me from games or even practices for the rest of the season."

"That's tough, but it is the only option if you want to get better. And the season is almost over, isn't it?"

"Yeah, I suppose. But are you sure I'll be cured in time for next season?"

"Until we get the results of your neuropsychology tests we won't know for sure if you have a PCS. But if you do, then we'll need to work out a rehabilitation plan. All going well, I would think you'd be back to normal within a few months, but recovery from PCS is very variable and it could take longer. I'm afraid that it's going to take a lot of patience." I didn't add that returning to rugby at all might prove to be a very bad idea; at this point Jason needed to hang onto hope rather than be battered with what would probably seem to him to be the worst possible scenario.

"Right. Let's get on with these tests then," Jason said, sounding a little less glum.

Jason was easy to assess; he picked up the instructions for each test quickly and refused to stop for breaks. In fact, at the halfway point I insisted we stop for a 15-minute rest and sent him outside with a cup of coffee to sit in the sun. I could see he was tired but determined to stick at it, and I wanted to see how well he did on the tests when he wasn't exhausted. We completed the assessment in two-and-a-half hours, and at the end Jason admitted he was "stuffed" and was happy to agree to my suggestion that he take the rest of the day off from school and go home to sleep. He returned with his parents two days later to discuss the results—he had asked if I could score the tests quickly, as he didn't want to wait for ages before he "knew the worst."

I was able to tell them that Jason's pattern of results strongly supported my preliminary diagnosis: Jason was suffering from a PCS as a consequence of his multiple mild head injuries and concussions. His performance on the general knowledge, vocabulary, verbal comprehension, and verbal abstraction tests placed him in the "superior" range for verbal abilities, which was congruent with his schooling history. But on a test where he was given mathematical problems and asked to work them out in his head, he scored in the average range. This was clearly an impairment for him, as math had been one of his best subjects. His difficulty was being unable to hold long problems in memory while he worked them out, and his performance improved when I gave him the written problem and an unlimited time in which to solve it using pen and paper. He also lost points for slowness when asked to perform speeded tests of visuospatial ability, such as copying a pattern by putting blocks together. But he was able to perform the tasks to a high level if given sufficient time.

On a test of "information processing capacity" specifically designed for TBI victims, Jason's performance was below average. This test, which involves listening to a long string of numbers and adding each number to the previous one while not forgetting the number you just heard, places demands on sustained attention and concentration, working memory, and performing multiple mental tasks under time pressure. The trials of the test are given at increasingly faster speeds. Performance correlates highly with the symptoms of PCS, and repeated assessments with the test over time can provide a good indication of rate of recovery from the concussion. When performance nears normal levels, the individual is usually ready to return in a graduated way to work or school. Jason found this test very frustrating, and almost gave up on it. At the fastest two speeds he was unable to do it at all.

His scores on tests of new learning and memory fell in the average range; he found these tests very tiring as well. Although he drew an excellent copy of a complex figure, his recall of it from memory 45 minutes later was just average. All these average scores marked a considerable drop for Jason, given his position near the top of the academic ranking in his school. On the positive side, on tests of verbal abstraction and other frontal lobe abilities such as organization, planning ahead, and insight into his performance, Jason performed very well.

After a discussion of his results, Jason and his parents agreed that I should talk with Jason's school headmaster and explain the situation. Jason had his end-of-year exams coming up in just over two months, and he was concerned that he would fail them, given his difficulty in concentrating in class and staying awake in the evenings long enough to do his homework. I thought the strategy most likely to assist his rehabilitation was for him to reduce his school hours to mornings only and perhaps drop some of the more taxing subjects completely. Jason looked relieved when I suggested this and said he could drop math and physics, because they were the subjects he now struggled with the most. His father expressed concern that it would put him back a year if he didn't take all his exams, but Becky was quick to disagree, pointing out that even if he had to repeat the year—and this would surely be the worst scenario—that was vastly preferable to having him fail and on top of that not get better.

The school headmaster was receptive to my concerns and said he would discuss with Jason's teachers the best way they could help him reduce his schoolwork without entirely sacrificing the year's work so far. The following week Becky and Jason returned to the psychology clinic and showed me his new schedule. Jason would continue to attend English, biology, and chemistry classes, but he would only be expected to do the homework he felt he could manage. At most he was to do no more than one hour's homework each day. When his classes were in the afternoon or he had a free period between classes, he could go and rest in the "sick bay." Jason's teachers had assured him that if he passed the three subjects he was continuing with, the following year he would be able to advance with his peer group to the next class for everything but math and physics. He could either repeat those subjects this year, or if he was completely back to normal, he could take some extra, catch-up classes to get him up to speed. When the time came to take his exams, he could take them in a separate quiet room and would be given additional time to complete each exam.

This was an excellent start to his rehabilitation program, and Jason seemed reasonably happy with it except for one aspect: He was concerned that he would lose all his fitness, as it had been decided that he should give up all competitive sports for the time being. So together we looked for ways to work some pleasure into his life. This is what we came up with. To keep up some fitness, Jason was permitted to swim in the school pool for 30 minutes each day if he felt like it. He would also begin walking rather than cycling to and from school—a 30-minute walk—with the proviso that if he felt tired after school he would phone his mother to come and pick him up in the car. Cycling and driving within the busy city were off limits for a while because of his slowed reaction times, and to avoid any possibility of another knock on the head!

He should try to get to bed as early as possible each night, and to encourage good sleeping patterns—he had been having trouble getting to sleep even though he felt exhausted—he would complete his homework before the evening meal, and after dinner would do something relaxing, like listening to music or reading a novel, followed by a bath and a hot drink. Once in bed he would put the light out rather than reading or doing anything else. The idea here was to establish his bedroom and bed as a place he associated with sleep rather than, for example, messing around on his computer. In fact his computer was to be moved to the family room, which would allow Becky to keep an eye on Jason's tendency to sit in front of it for hours on end. If he felt like it he could go out with his friends in the weekend to watch sports or go to a movie, with the proviso that he would not drink any alcohol and the suggestion that he avoid noisy situations or parties where he would be bombarded by too much information—situations very stressful for PCS victims, who have an impaired ability to filter out background noise. Jason was amenable to these suggestions, as he had no interest in being anywhere noisy; he couldn't even cope with the TV anymore.

*****

Within a week of first seeing Jason, I received a referral to assess another 16-year-old schoolboy with suspected PCS. The referral came from the New Zealand Government Accident Compensation Corporation—the ACC—which provided national insurance for accident victims, including funding medical treatments, counseling, assessments, rehabilitation, retraining, and financial compensation. Howie was brought into my office by his ACC caseworker, who explained that he had been referred to the ACC by his GP after his school rugby coach had expressed concerns about his slow recovery from a concussion during a match.

Howie was a fine-looking and very solid young man who at 16 towered above me. He had a lovely smile and quickly put me at ease. After his caseworker left, we spent the next half-hour talking about Howie's background and the problems he'd been having before beginning the neuropsychological assessment. Like Jason, he had sustained multiple mild head injuries over the preceding two years: three during rugby games and one as a result of falling off his motorcycle 12 months before I met him. Although he was in the same school year as Jason, Howie's school, in an area of low socioeconomic status, had less ambitious educational aims. Howie usually managed to achieve grades in the average range in English and math, although this was often a struggle, but he did better in his favorite subjects of art, Maori language, and practical mechanics. After his most recent concussion eight weeks ago, when he was unconscious for almost five minutes and spent a night in the local hospital before being discharged home, he had suffered from most of the typical symptoms of the PCS. Now, he said, his worst problems were tiredness, difficulty in concentrating, losing his temper with his brothers and sisters, and awful headaches.

His home environment was much less conducive to rehabilitation than Jason's. Howie shared a small bedroom with three of his brothers, and the noise levels in the small state house where he lived with his parents, his grandmother, and his seven siblings, ranging from three to 18 years, were extreme and continuous. Howie's mother worked two jobs, the first cleaning hotel rooms from 9 a.m. to 1 p.m., and the second cleaning offices from 7 p.m. to midnight. When I asked what his father did, Howie grimaced and replied that he had been unemployed for years and spent his time either at home watching sports on the TV or in the local bar getting drunk. His grandmother got the kids off to school and looked after the two preschoolers, and the older kids—Howie was the third oldest—were kept pretty busy doing odd jobs to earn a bit of extra cash and making *kai* (food) for the family in the evening.

Howie said getting any homework done was pretty impossible in their house, and since his last concussion even the simplest school work was a mission. He'd planned to leave school and get a job as a mechanic at the end of that year, but was thinking he might as well leave right now. I suggested we complete his assessment and see if we could come up with a more feasible rehabilitation plan first and then look at his options, and he said he'd go along with that, as he didn't think he could handle a mechanic's job anyway in his current state.

I was aware that Howie might be disadvantaged by being given the standard battery of tests, developed for white people, and that because of his close connections with his mother's extended Maori *whanau* (family), Howie strongly identified himself as Maori rather than as *pakeha* (white New Zealander) like his father. However, because he had been in the Western, "white" school system all his life and his first language was English, on balance I decided to give him the same tests I had given Jason, although I did use the Maori-friendly test instructions and more culturally appropriate "Maori" examples where I had these available. Howie's overall results showed quite a similar pattern to those of Jason, although, on the basis of his school performance over the past four years, the scores that I considered "unimpaired" for Howie fell in the low average to average range, and his "impaired" scores fell in the range lower than this. He was unimpaired on general knowledge, vocabulary, and verbal comprehension. But he had a lot of difficulty with the mental arithmetic test, although he improved marginally when given more time to solve the problems using pen and paper. Like Jason, he lost points for slowness when asked to perform speeded tests of visuospatial ability, such as making patterns with blocks and drawing a complex figure, but given unlimited time he actually scored in the high average range, which was congruent with his performance in art at school.

Howie was completely stumped by the difficult test of information processing capacity, and early in the very first, slowest trial lost track of the string of numbers he had to hold in his head while adding up others. He flatly refused to attempt any of the faster trials. I didn't contradict him when he excused his poor performance by saying he'd always been hopeless at sums, but I suspected that he would have performed a good deal better, at least on the slower trials, if he didn't have a PCS. On the tests of new learning and memory his scores fell in the low average range or lower, and his recall of the complex figure 45 minutes after his good copy of it was also below average. Like Jason, he was unimpaired on tests of executive abilities such as verbal abstraction, organization, planning ahead, and insight into his performance.

It proved difficult to find a time when Howie and his mother, Rosie, could come in to talk about Howie's results and the best way to set up a rehabilitation program, but we finally managed to schedule a meeting. Rosie looked tired and harassed, but said she was grateful that Howie was being looked after, as she had been worried about him. It soon became clear that Howie's father was not interested in participating in his son's rehabilitation, and that Howie's tiredness after school and reduced ability to help out increased the burden on Rosie and his grandmother. In spite of this, we did manage to establish some goals that Rosie and Howie thought might be attainable. I would discuss with the school headmaster how to reduce Howie's school program and see if he could rest at school during the day. Rosie would ask her eldest son if he would give up his trailer in the garden where he slept to Howie for a few months until he was back to normal. Howie shared a bedroom with his other three brothers, and he said it was impossible to sleep or do any schoolwork there, and he was constantly getting into fights with his brothers because he was so bad-tempered these days. The other children would be asked to help Howie by taking on some of the household tasks he usually did. Rosie said that her kids all loved Howie, and she thought they would help out once they understood he was not well.

Over the next six weeks, Howie's ACC caseworker visited Howie regularly, and every week he came in to see me or we had a phone conversation. His brother did vacate his trailer for Howie, and this according to Howie was a "lifesaver"; he was able to get away from the noise and disruption of the house, although he still had trouble sleeping through the night. Like Jason, he was able to reduce his schoolwork considerably, and he reluctantly gave up rugby and his motorcycle for the remainder of the year. But when, six weeks after I first saw him, I assessed him again on a small number of the tests he had been impaired on, he showed little improvement. I was also concerned about his low mood. Howie talked for a while about the problems he was still experiencing—fatigue, headaches, and depression—and how his problems didn't seem very important in their family when compared with his father's drunkenness, his mother's constant exhaustion, and the ongoing problems his mother and grandmother had looking after his younger brother who had attention deficit disorder. He rarely saw his mates anymore now that he couldn't play rugby or ride his motorcycle, and he admitted that the only way he could cope was to smoke a joint of marijuana every night. He told me in a glum tone that if he was never going to be able to play rugby again he couldn't see the point of staying at school, and added that that was the only reason he was there anyway, as he was pretty dumb. Perhaps, he said, he should leave school and try to get some sort of a job to help his mother out.

After this session, through his ACC case manager, I referred him to a male Maori clinical psychologist whose practice was close to Howie's school and who had enjoyed considerable success with young people like Howie. It seemed particularly important to expand Howie's support networks and explore ways he could reconnect with his friends. I managed to convince him to go to a head-injury support group for teenagers who met once a week to share their experiences and to join in recreational activities such as pool and card games. There, quite by chance, he met up with Jason, whose rehabilitation program was now overseen by the ACC. The two boys recognized each other from their past meetings on the rugby field and quickly discovered they had a lot in common despite their very different backgrounds.

One day, out of the blue, Jason and Howie showed up at my office. I had heard from each of them earlier that they had met at the head-injury support group but didn't know they had become close friends, going—as spectators—to sports events and to the gymnasium four nights a week. They had come to tell me that Jason's family was going away to their beach house for the long summer break and Howie was joining them. Both boys were going to have a complete break from schoolwork and spend their time fishing, swimming, snorkeling—the beach house was close to a marine park—and eating lots of seafood. Howie grinned and added that they had made a pact to keep their alcohol consumption to two beers on Saturdays and that he had given up marijuana to please Jason, who was totally against all drugs. When they returned in time for the next school year, Jason was planning to go on to his final year at school while taking catch-up classes in math and physics, and Howie, encouraged by Jason, was also keen to spend another year at his school.

I was delighted. They had come up with the perfect rehabilitation program for a PCS: rest from tasks that tax the damaged systems of the brain, giving those systems time to recover; a quiet environment with no pressure to "perform" and plenty of time to sleep; minimal alcohol intake; enjoyable and varied activities; and regular, manageable exercise that would not put them at risk of further head injuries. But best of all, their "program" was sure to work because they would be doing it together. Mild TBI has been dubbed "the unseen injury," as to outsiders the PCS seems almost unbelievable. Jason and Howie's relationship had begun because of their common understanding and experience of the debilitating effects that can occur after mild TBI, but had grown into a true and enduring friendship that would far outlast their PCS symptoms.

They had promised me they would drop by when they returned to Auckland, and true to their word, they did. They had had a wonderful summer and both boys were now keen amateur marine biologists. They had spent most of the summer snorkeling, and Jason had been told by his doctor that if his neuropsychological assessment demonstrated that he was "cured," he would be able to take up diving with a tank. Howie figured that the same rule should apply to him!

I reassessed both boys, and as I suspected simply from their happy faces and renewed energy levels, both were now back to normal. Even Howie managed to perform at an unimpaired level on the challenging information processing task. They had decided they would not persevere with their rugby dreams but stick to noncontact sports, although Howie said he could not give up his motorcycle.

Jason did go on to university and became a secondary school teacher of biology and physical education, in his spare time coaching schoolchildren in rugby—but not playing it. Howie also remained at school another year and then scored a job as a technician in the marine biology department of the university, where he was able to indulge his love and knowledge of engines—now in boats—as well as diving, regularly accompanying students on their marine biology field trips. In the summer months, Jason and Howie went diving together most weekends, afterward sharing a beer or two over a barbecue with their partners, and later their children. When I last talked with them they said that they had managed to avoid any further knocks on the head, and Howie added that the very thought of having to do that bloody number-crunching test again was enough to make sure they kept it that way!

■ Further Reading

Ogden, J. A. 2005. The unseen injury: Mild traumatic brain injury. In: *Fractured Minds: A Case-Study Approach to Clinical Neuropsychology, 2nd Ed.* (pp. 193–203). New York: Oxford University Press.

11 ■

How to Get There: The Far Side of Severe Brain Injury

I first heard about Kim's accident from my daughter. She knew Kim only as one of the older girls in a class two years ahead of her, but she was still shocked by the news the headmistress had given them at their morning assembly. Kim's small car, a 16th birthday present from her father, had collided with a streetlamp late on a wet Saturday night. Kim had been driving her two girlfriends—also from the school—home from a party. The other two girls had suffered only cuts and bruises, but Kim now lay unconscious in the hospital. Rumors were flying: Kim had been drunk; she had been speeding; the road had been wet and greasy; she didn't have her seat belt on; she shouldn't have been driving at night as she had only just got her driver's license.

Three weeks later Kim's name appeared on the patient board in Neurosurgery. I felt relieved; her transfer here meant that she was no longer in a coma and was out of danger. I checked her file and read that on admission to Critical Care she was deeply unconscious, with a Glasgow Coma Score (GCS) of 5. The GCS is a 15-point standard rating scale to measure the severity of a coma based on the patient's motor responses, verbal responses, and the stimulus necessary to provoke eye opening. A score of 13–15 along with a loss of consciousness of 20 minutes or less is usually considered to represent a mild traumatic brain injury (TBI); a score of 9–12, a moderate TBI; and a score of 8 or less, a severe TBI. The lowest score possible is 3.

Kim's computed tomography (CT) brain scan initially showed some hemorrhage in the posterior parts of the lateral ventricles and in the fourth ventricle (the sacs filled with CSF in the middle of the brain). There was also some bleeding around the brain stem, an upward extension of the spinal cord extending into the *midbrain* in the center of the brain. The brain stem is the life-support part of the brain, and controls respiration, cardiovascular function, and gastrointestinal function. If it is badly damaged the patient is unlikely to survive, but fortunately for Kim, the damage to her brain stem was not severe. There was evidence of *contusion* (bruising) in the frontal region of the brain on both sides, as well as in the right parietal and temporal lobes. On admission to Critical Care, Kim had her vital functions taken over; she was intubated and ventilated. She had no skull fractures, but had fractured some ribs. After being weaned from the ventilator on the 12th day, over the next week she slowly regained consciousness and was transferred to the neurosurgery ward when her *posttraumatic amnesia* (PTA) had resolved. A magnetic resonance imaging (MRI) brain scan taken 13 days after the accident showed slightly enlarged lateral ventricles, small areas of lowered density—signifying some patchy loss of neurons—in both frontal lobes, and more significant *infarcts* (areas of dead brain tissue) in the right parietal and temporal lobes. A neurological examination carried out on her admission to Neurosurgery showed that she had a significant weakness in her left arm and leg (a left hemiplegia), and a slight weakness of her right arm. Her speech was slow but along with her comprehension appeared normal; she was fully oriented—she knew who she was, where she was, and what time of day it was—and apart from a loss of memory for the drive from the party and the accident itself her memory for the past seemed normal.

This account of Kim's progress gave me some grounds for optimism, especially the statement about the rapid resolution of her PTA. PTA refers to the state of disorientation and confusion that often follows a return to consciousness, when the patient seems unable to attend to and acquire new information. Thus the patient will often not be able to remember what she did or whom she saw yesterday or earlier that same day. The duration of PTA is related to the severity of the TBI, and along with the period of coma gives an indication of the level of recovery that might be expected. The coma and the PTA are the observable signs of the diffuse damage that occurs to the brain when the head collides with a hard object—especially if one or both are moving at high speed—causing the soft brain inside the skull to vibrate on the spinal cord, bruising itself on the bony protuberances on the inside of the skull and shearing and tearing the brain tissue and the axons that permit neurons to communicate with one another. Much of this damage is so small and diffuse that it can't be picked up on a CT scan, and some of it can't even be picked up on an MRI scan, but because of the number of damaged areas and axons, it can cause a lot of trouble.

I returned Kim's file to its slot and went to see her. She was still in the intensive care room, where patients can be watched 24 hours of the day, but she was sitting up and talking with her visitor. I introduced myself, and Kim grinned at me: an engaging grin accompanied by two deep dimples. Her visitor introduced himself as Kim's father, Paul. In spite of his tired eyes and worried expression, he looked almost too young to be the father of a 16-year-old. He explained that Kim's mother, Joanna, would be in after work; she was a building manager and was working on a big project at the moment. He added that they were divorced and were both remarried.

So begins my story of Kim and her family, and their struggle to become "normal" once again. But before entering into their world of pain—emotional pain much more than physical pain, now that Kim was out of danger and on the rocky road to recovery—I want you to read this speech, given by a 22-year-old former university student to a head-injury support group.[1]

> This time three years ago, I was an A student at university studying third-year engineering. I was a good sportsman and enjoyed a great social life. One afternoon while riding my motorcycle home from university, I hit the center lane of the motorway for some reason. I broke my neck, badly damaged my right arm, and I suffered severe head injuries. For the nonmedical of you, that means I bashed shit out of my head.
>
> I don't know much about the rest of that year, but I'm told that I spent three months in hospital, which included one month in the hospital's critical care ward, at $4000 a day. I came out of hospital in a wheelchair to live with my parents, and my mother was given leave from her job to look after her 25-year-old baby. I say baby, because that was about the level I was at. I needed help with everything. I needed constant attention. I needed to be retaught everything. Mum was given a break on the

---

[1] This speech is included with the generous permission of the writer, Neil G., and Jude Hay, who first printed the speech in her University of Auckland master's thesis .

weekends when she returned to her job and Dad relieved her of nursing duties. On two mornings a week, I went to the hospital for occupational and physiotherapy. I made good progress, but then even this minimal rehabilitation was stopped once I had got to the stage that I could beat my therapist at chess. They said that there wasn't much more they could do for me. As I said before, I don't know much about the rest of that year; I spent my time popping in and out of reality, but I do know that I hated being so dependent on my parents, and I hated what this must have been doing to them.

Everyone was amazed at the progress I was making. By the end of the year, I could walk without the walking stick, and apart from the arm, there didn't seem anything wrong with me except that I couldn't say a whole sentence before I had forgotten what I was going to say, forgotten what we were talking about, forgotten who I was talking to. I had no short-term memory at all.

Over the following year, I continued to make good progress. I went to Australia with my brother and cousins for the World Cup rugby matches. That trip gave me a great deal more confidence, and by the end of it I was walking quite confidently amongst big crowds of people. However, on my return to my parents' home, I sank further and further into depression. Where was I heading? What will I be doing in 10 years' time? What will I do today?

I was given a computer so that I could finish my degree, a $4000 machine that took me six months to learn to operate even the simplest programs. I tried hard and I remained very determined, but there wasn't one day I didn't think about suicide. A friend took me up to the YMCA, and he got me to join the gym there, which was probably the best thing I could have done. I was embarrassed about my appearance, but I went there every day and I improved each time, until I had got to the stage where I felt quite proud of what I could do. My arm was amputated at the end of that year, and what a relief that was. It had just been an albatross to me and I now felt a lot better.

At the beginning of the following year I tried to get back into university by redoing my last full year. However, it soon became obvious that it was still far too early even for that and I stopped going. The neurosurgeon suggested that I should start going to the Concussion Clinic at the hospital, where I went for three mornings a week. I'd never heard of a head injury before my accident, so going to this place certainly opened my eyes to it. Sure I'd played rugby for nearly 20 years and had been knocked out quite often, but only for seconds at a time. With this accident I was out for more than three months. Being able to talk with people who knew what I was going through helped me a lot.

I still had a lot of time that I wanted help filling. I was finally referred to the Rehabilitation League to learn how to do simple jobs all over again, so that one day someone might want to employ me. Since starting there I have been a lot happier. Everyone has got to have a reason to get out of bed each day, and I feel that I am making progress again. Being able to stand here and give this speech to you is a big achievement for me now. I am sure that you would all appreciate that the old nut is a pretty complicated system, and that every head-injured person is affected differently by it, but like any injury it requires stimulation for it to heal. Before the Rehabilitation League took me in hand, I wasn't going anywhere; just sitting at home each day.

The point I am wanting to make to you with this speech is that if the system is going to spend this huge amount of money just to keep us alive, then they have got to spend that extra bit to give us some proper rehabilitation, or if money is the main concern here, then they should just let us die with some pride.

I could have chosen many case studies to illustrate the all-too-common problems and frustrations experienced by patients who have had a severe head injury. Many, like Neil—the writer of this moving speech—have suffered when the therapists reach a point when they can do no more, leaving the patient in limbo. But many get through the almost inevitable times of depression and, one day at a time, find ways to bring pleasure back into their lives. Of the dozens of TBI patients I have assessed and worked with, Kim found a special place in my heart, perhaps because she was a student from the school my own daughters attended, perhaps because she was a female in a world of males—most TBI victims are young men—or perhaps because of her exuberant personality and cheeky grin, unsuppressed by her head injury. All of these contributed to my unprofessional fondness for Kim, but on reflection, whenever I think of Kim, I think of her family as well, and it is her family—a complex family even without the added stress of Kim's head injury—that makes her case especially moving. Kim's family had many advantages over the families of most of the survivors of TBI I have known. Her parents had university degrees and were financially well-off. True, they were divorced, and that led to complications when it came to looking after Kim, but they each had new partners who wanted to be involved in her rehabilitation. Kim's siblings and half-siblings, along with their various parental combinations, were willing to do anything to help her. Kim was truly loved, and love would be this family's greatest strength in the difficult times ahead.

Kim spent five weeks in Neurosurgery and then, on the insistence of her father, her family took her home. He felt she would do better there than in a live-in rehabilitation unit. He would make sure she got to the outpatient unit at the hospital for daily physical and occupational therapy. When she was discharged from Neurosurgery two months after her accident, Kim could move her wheelchair about, feed herself rather clumsily, understand speech quite well, and speak fluently, although in a rather flat monotone. Her family and friends said that her personality had changed. When I asked them how, her sister Olive, just 18 months older than Kim, gave this description: "It's as if she's regressed to being a little kid again in some ways. She's always giggling, even when there is nothing funny going on. Before, she was a real extrovert and the life of the party and all that, but she had a serious side too. I would have thought she'd be depressed by what's happened, not amused. Stuck in a wheelchair, hardly able to feed herself without dropping food down her front; what's funny about that? And she used to be very bright at school and interested in serious stuff as well as having fun. Now, if you try to get her to discuss anything serious, like whether she thinks she should start doing some schoolwork again so she won't get too far behind, she gets a sort of vacuous look and either just giggles or says something idiotic like "Silly old school, who cares!" Then for no reason at all she'll start crying and crying. I can understand that better than the giggling, but even her crying seems sort of odd. Yesterday I was watching this comedy on TV with her and all of a sudden she is bawling, but when I asked her what was wrong she had no idea."

The day before Kim's discharge from Neurosurgery, I set up a family meeting to discuss "Where to from here?" The aim of this early meeting was to provide information, predict future problems, and come up with strategies that might prevent some of these or at least ameliorate them. This was the first time I had met all of Kim's immediate family, and at last they were all seated in a large semicircle, crowding the small room. To my left were Kim's father, Paul, his wife, Kathy, and Kathy's 15-year-old daughter.

Paul and Kathy's three-year-old twins spent much of the session running around the periphery of the room and playing hide-and-seek under the chairs. To my right were Kim's mother, Joanna, her husband, Craig, Kim's sister, Olive, and Joanna and Craig's very well-behaved six-year-old son. In the middle of her two families sat Kim in her wheelchair. In stark contrast to her family, she looked happy, giggling from time to time, answering direct questions but never volunteering any information.

In spite of the rather chaotic impression the family projected, I was delighted to see them all there. Kim's future already looked more promising with this great team of potential rehabilitation experts demonstrating their willingness to roll up their sleeves and get working, and perhaps even have some fun in the process. At this point I'm sure none of the people in the room knew what was in store for them. They were still in the honeymoon phase, where their relief that Kim was alive, able to communicate, and even cheerful did much to nurture the hope they held in their hearts—hope that soon the girl in the wheelchair would once more be their bright, funny Kim with the world at her feet. Yes, they thought, she might be left with a limp, and perhaps her left arm would never be completely strong again, but they didn't care about that. So this was the optimal time for me to harness the family's hope and enthusiasm and help them work out how they could share in Kim's care and rehabilitation while supporting—practically and emotionally—each other. The first task was to identify the family members who would take on most of the caregiving and "give permission" for them to ask for help long before they burned out. I wanted to encourage every family member to be proactive and plan from the outset specific ways and times they could help. I wanted to encourage the family to make a list of support people and groups, and to call on these when needed. I would try to prevent future guilt from creeping in by discussing the importance of all family members gradually returning to their own full lives.

"Family centered" counseling is my preferred way to work with anyone who has a neurological disorder. The "family" can include friends; in fact it should include as many people as possible who are willing to be involved in the rehabilitation process. The size of the group will fluctuate as the weeks and months pass and some people leave and others are recruited. Community groups might become involved, and loyal friends might recruit other friends to help out.

In this first meeting, I was careful not to get into too many emotions. That would come later, when the family had had time to recover from the initial trauma and had established a schedule that included the many new activities they would need to do to help Kim. Everyone was still very fragile, and on top of that the two families were all together for the first time. I wanted to keep the discussion practical and as positive as possible without being unrealistic. I gave them examples of problems to spot in the early stages and how to cope with these before they became overwhelming. I predicted hopeful outcomes wherever possible. I mentioned some of the common needs other families like theirs have had, including finding ways to express feelings, coping with disagreements in the family about the rehabilitation process, dealing with rehabilitation and medical systems, coping with changed roles in the family, helping the patient to reach full potential—even if in some cases that is different from before the injury—and feel good about himself or herself, and finding ways for all family members to learn and grow through the process. I was pleased that none of the family seemed to have an extreme denial of the seriousness of Kim's problems and what lay ahead, and none of them appeared to have been severely traumatized. Kim and her three-year-old half-siblings stood out as the only ones in the room who did not have a care in the world. Even the six-year-old joined in the family discussion, saying that he would help Kim with her physical therapy (and indeed he did, spending hours after school throwing her balls and keeping her company).

Two weeks later I met again for an extended session with most of the family—including Kim but not the three youngest members. The family had had time to settle into a routine and already had a long list of problems they wanted to solve. Not least of these was whether Kim should live full-time with Paul and Kathy or spend alternate weeks with each parent. Fortunately the two families lived only two streets from each other, so it was easy for all the family to share in Kim's activities wherever she lived. It soon became clear that Joanna was reluctant to have Kim live with her for the next few months, as she was in the midst of a major building project that took her away from home for long hours. In contrast, Paul had already decided to reduce his work hours at his law practice so that he could spend more time at home, and Kathy was a full-time mother. So it was decided that Kim would live with Paul and Kathy and spend weekends at Joanna's whenever possible. Kim's sister, stepsister, and two best friends each volunteered to spend specific afternoons after school each week with Kim, helping with her schoolwork and rehabilitation and generally just hanging out with her. All four parents agreed to share, as much as possible, the considerable driving necessary to transport Kim back and forth to her physical and occupational therapy sessions every day.

That settled, I decided it was time to broach the emotional minefield that lay in wait below the bustling business of the practicalities of taking care of Kim. My sense was that the two halves of Kim's complex family had, up until Kim's accident, lived separate lives. From now on they would have to find a way to work together, united by their love for Kim. Already Paul had shown some frustration when Joanna insisted that she could not take time off work, and she had displayed her annoyance at his lack of understanding. Perhaps this family needed to step back a little and take time to process their feelings about Kim's accident and her survival, and to understand each other's feelings. Over the next 90 minutes I asked each member of the family in turn to talk about how he or she felt on hearing about Kim's accident, as she lay in a coma and as she then gradually began to recover. This tough assignment was a turning point—or the start of a turning point—for the family. There were tears—many tears—but no recriminations. Here was a group of people who had much more in common than any one of them could have imagined. With the exception of Kim, who remained tear-free and smiling throughout, everyone in the room left that day feeling fragile but no longer alone in their nightmare of fear, desperation, and sadness. I knew that there would be many times over the next months and even years when Paul and Joanna would disagree, despair, and refuse to see each other's point of view, and when their respective partners felt like leaving, and when Kim's siblings and friends got tired and bored with her slow progress and wanted to get on with their own lives. When those times came, they all would need to remind themselves of the feelings they shared, take a deep breath, and take the next step forward.

*****

Now that you have some idea about the beginning stages of the long process of rehabilitation after a severe TBI, it is time for a more detailed description of the head injury itself—what happens to your brain when your head smashes into another object. Once you understand this you will have no difficulty understanding why survivors face so many serious problems for a very long time. Whenever I have described the mechanics of head injury to my university classes I have felt their attention; they were only too well aware that as adults in their late teens and early twenties, they, especially the men, were the primary target group for head injuries. This was not some academic exercise. This was personal.

Traumatic brain injuries can be of three types: *penetrating, crushing,* and *closed.* In a penetrating TBI the skull is pierced or broken—for example, from a bullet wound or by a sharp object in a car accident—and the brain beneath damaged. A crushing TBI, in which the head is caught between two objects—for example, under the wheel of a car—is the rarest type of TBI; often the most serious damage is to the base of the skull and the nerves that run through it rather than to the brain itself.

Closed head injuries like the one Kim had are by far the most common. They occur when the head suddenly accelerates (as when a car runs into your car from behind), decelerates (as when your car hits a telegraph pole), or oscillates (as when you receive a punch to the head that is hard enough to knock you out). There is no penetrating wound and the damage is caused by the movement of the soft brain mass inside the bony skull. *Diffuse axonal injury* (diffuse damage to nerve fibers) occurs because of the stretching and shearing of the fibers as the brain vibrates and rotates on its axis. This type of damage is widespread but is often most severe at the level of the brain stem. The *reticular formation* (RF)—the network of nerve fibers that travel from the base of the brain to the prefrontal lobes (the most anterior part of the frontal lobes)—is especially vulnerable at this point. Damage to the RF results in lowered arousal of the prefrontal cortex, which contributes to many of the frontal lobe symptoms of closed head injury. Arteries and veins may also be torn, leaking blood into brain tissue and causing diffuse disruption or sometimes resulting in a significant area of focal damage where there is a substantial hemorrhage. (Strangely, if the damage from a penetrating

TBI is restricted to a small part of the brain, the consequences may be less severe than in a severe closed head injury, as the impairments will be restricted to the abilities mediated by that damaged area of the brain.)

Further areas of focal damage can be caused by the brain surface's rubbing on the sharp ridges and edges inside the skull as the brain continues to move after the skull comes to an abrupt halt. The sites most commonly damaged are the undersides of the frontal lobes just above the eyes and the temporal lobes. Focal injuries also occur as the brain hits the skull on impact. These include *coup* injuries, in which the damage is at the site of the impact, and *contrecoup* injuries, in which the impact causes the brain to accelerate inside the skull, resulting in its hitting the skull opposite the point of impact. Thus when a car is hit from behind, frontal lesions may result from a contrecoup injury as the brain accelerates inside the skull and hits the bony skull around the eye orbits; from a deceleration injury when the head hits the windshield; from the brain's moving inside the skull after impact; and from the RF's shearing and tearing when the brain vibrates and rotates at the level of the brain stem. It is therefore little wonder that frontal lobe deficits are so common after closed head injury. Damage to the temporal lobes, situated just above each ear, results in the memory deficits that underlie many of the most difficult rehabilitation problems following closed head injury.

The damage in the first few seconds of an accident is sometimes called the *first injury*. Unfortunately, in severe closed head injury, the neurological damage often does not stop there. A *second injury* can occur if the victim is trapped in a way that blocks breathing—perhaps because of vomit that blocks the airways or from an injury to the nose or face—reducing the oxygen supply to the brain. Other injuries may result in the loss of a significant amount of blood, lowering blood pressure and reducing the supply of blood and oxygen to the brain. Rapid acute care at the site of the accident thus involves clearing the airways, stopping bleeding, and replacing lost blood by transfusion to protect the brain from second injury while the patient is transported to hospital.

Many people who sustain a severe closed head injury do not die on impact but days or even weeks later. These deaths or a worsening of the patient's condition are often the result of the *third injury*. Such complications include swelling of the brain from the fluids escaping from damaged cells and blood from torn vessels, which raises intracranial pressure as the brain fills more of the skull. If the brain becomes too tight within the skull, blood has difficulty circulating through it, which can result in *ischemia* (loss of oxygen), causing areas of the brain to die. If the intracranial pressure rises too much, the blood circulation can be cut off entirely and the brain dies. Many of the technologies used in critical care units are designed to minimize brain swelling, keep blood pressure at the correct level, ensure an adequate intake of air and oxygen and the removal of waste products like carbon monoxide, and restrict the levels of water and salt in the body to limit the flow of tissue fluid into the brain.

Blood clots can also accumulate in the days immediately following the accident, and if not controlled or evacuated they too can elevate intracranial pressure, with the same devastating results. Blood clots that form rapidly outside the coverings of the brain (*acute extradural hematomas*) need to be evacuated immediately by a neurosurgeon or they will quickly result in the brain's being pushed down through the small hole in the base of the skull where the brain becomes the spinal cord, causing death. In some cases *chronic subdural hematomas* form slowly within the brain coverings over a period of days; these are not usually life-threatening. They are particularly common in elderly people and can follow quite a minor head injury. Posttraumatic *hydrocephalus* can also occur days or even weeks after the accident when the CSF circulation is blocked by blood or scarring, causing the lateral ventricles to overfill. Sometimes hydrocephalus resolves without intervention, or sometimes the neurosurgeon removes the blockage or inserts a shunt into the ventricle to drain the CSF into a body cavity. The vastly improved technologies now used in critical care units to control the complications that constitute the third injury have significantly increased the numbers of severely head-injured people who survive. As Neil pleaded in his speech, the important quest now is to find ways to improve the long-term outcome for these "lucky" survivors.

There are many models of rehabilitation, but there is no definitive research on which is most likely to result in a decrease in the number and severity of cognitive and emotional problems, an increase in the quality of life—including happiness—and a return to employment or school. Rehabilitation can be focused at different levels. The term *impairment* encompasses symptoms such as a memory problem or a weak leg; *disabilities* are the problems the person experiences as a result of the impairments, such as forgetting to take medication because of the memory problem and as a result having more seizures; and *handicaps* are the social or environmental inadequacies that cause problems for the client with disabilities—for example, the person in a wheelchair is handicapped if there is no ramp at the entrance to a building, and the person with a memory problem is handicapped if expected to memorize the instructions for working the photocopy machine rather than having the instructions printed on the machine.

Intensive, long-term rehabilitation programs are probably best for TBI survivors and should include physical therapy, education for both the survivor and family on the psychological and social problems that commonly follow TBI, and training in personal care, everyday living, and social skills. Cognitive rehabilitation, including relearning to read and write, speech therapy, and problem solving exercises, is often necessary, along with training in using practical strategies, such as keeping a diary, to assist with impaired memory and organizational abilities. Programs should also offer individual, family, and group psychotherapy to address poor self-esteem, depression, anxiety, socially inappropriate behaviors, anger management, and other psychological problems the patient experiences, as well as grief counseling—for the loss of many abilities once taken for granted—for the TBI survivor and the family. The establishment of community support networks is important throughout rehabilitation, because severe TBI lasts a lifetime but the funding for therapists often disappears after the first few months. In the happy situation where the TBI survivor recovers to the level where work is possible, vocational retraining on the job is important, ideally with a system in place for infrequent but regular "maintenance checks" of work performance for the remainder of the individual's working life.

Family and friends also need support, assistance, and sometimes even "permission" to live their own lives without guilt once the critical stages of the head injury have passed. Families who are supportive in the early stages after the head injury may become discouraged and burned out as the years go by and the head-injured person's progress slows down, almost seeming to stop. Psychological and social problems are often significant for one or more years after the head injury, and in severe cases, especially where there has been extensive frontal lobe damage, depression, inappropriate social behaviors, displays of uncontrolled violence and aggression, and poor motivation to work or participate in hobbies can last a lifetime. It is hardly surprising that in such cases families commonly break up.

*****

Three months after her accident I gave Kim a full neuropsychological assessment. There had been no point in doing this earlier, while her brain was still recovering from the acute effects of the TBI. She had come a long way in her physical rehabilitation. For example, she could catch and throw a basketball with two hands, a major improvement showing that her left arm and hand were much stronger. With her right hand she could write slowly. With help from the physical therapist she could stand up and balance on both legs while holding on to a walking frame. She had just begun to learn how to push it along in front of her, helping her to walk. Although Kim had been slowly improving on tests of sustained attention, it still took four sessions to get through a basic neuropsychological assessment; if I could get her to concentrate for ten minutes before a break I was doing well. The giggling her sister had described was still very apparent, and this didn't help either. Nevertheless, I managed to get some sort of profile of her cognitive and memory abilities. I had very detailed information on her abilities before the accident from her school records. She had been in the "superior" range for English, art, and French, and in the "high average" range for math and science. So these were my baselines.

One of the major problems following TBI is a slowing of response speed, and some neuropsychological tests, while scored on their solutions, have points removed if patients take longer to complete them than would be expected for their age. Kim's performance was obviously slowed, so I decided to score these timed tests—primarily the visuospatial tests—in two ways: the standard way, so I could compare her scores directly with the normative scores for people of Kim's age and gender, and also without taking points off for slowness. My main aim at this stage was to see if she could do the tasks and how she went about solving them, not if she could complete them as fast as she would have before her accident. This approach to assessment has a qualitative as well as a quantitative aspect; it enhanced the information I could gather about Kim's thinking processes as well as her emotional responses. For example, I noted whether she tried different solutions if her first was incorrect (she didn't); whether she became upset or frustrated when she couldn't do a task (she just giggled); whether she went about solving a problem methodically or simply attacked it randomly, as by forcing the pieces of a jigsaw puzzle into positions even if they didn't fit (she used the second strategy).

Overall, Kim's verbal abilities—vocabulary, comprehension, and reading—had fallen from "superior" but were still in the "high average" range, so she was doing well given the severity of her TBI. Her writing was still quite clumsy but was vastly improved from her early attempts, mainly because her right hand was almost back to its normal strength. I expected that she would continue to improve with time and practice on all these verbal tests. Kim was lucky: although her more recent MRI scans had shown only minimal damage to her left, "language" hemisphere, in TBI cases the appearance of the MRI can be deceptive. Sometimes diffuse, "unseen" damage lurks and shows up later through impaired performance in verbal tests.

But the MRI scans had indicated more right hemisphere damage, so I was not surprised when she did more poorly on visuospatial tasks. Given that art had been one of her best subjects, the fact that she just scraped into the "low average" range on most of the visuospatial tests, even when I didn't remove points for her slow times, indicated a significant impairment. The way she went about trying to solve many of these tests highlighted two general areas of difficulty: her ability to conceptualize visual objects in space was impaired, most likely a result of the contusion to her right parietal lobe, and she lacked a consistent, planned, or strategic approach to problem solving, probably as a consequence of the diffuse frontal lobe damage she had sustained.

On tests of verbal memory—learning new verbal material—she was just "average," and on nonverbal memory tests such as drawing a complex pattern from memory after just copying it or remembering where objects were located in a display of objects she had just seen, she was "low average." Given her school achievements, these scores demonstrated considerable memory impairment. These types of memory—remembering or learning new material—rely on the temporal lobes, and unfortunately these are two of the brain areas most vulnerable to damage in a closed head injury where the brain is shaken around inside the skull. According to her family, Kim did have some memory problems. She could never remember what rehabilitation activities she was scheduled to do each day, and she had been forbidden to use the gas stove when alone, even to make herself a cup of tea, because she often forgot to turn the gas off. Nevertheless, as her sister pronounced, she had improved "out of sight" on these sorts of memory tasks over the weeks since her discharge from the hospital. As I would expect, her memories for her past were intact, as these don't rely heavily on the temporal lobes. But she did have a gap in her memory for the minutes just before the accident. This time period would be lost forever—probably a good thing—as the brain can't store memories when it is in a coma.

What concerned her family most was Kim's "personality change." This is the shorthand label they used to encompass her inappropriate giggling and sometimes crying and her rather juvenile comments and behaviors—all symptoms stemming from her frontal lobe contusions. The effects of this damage showed up on more formal tests of executive or abstraction skills as well. Her estimated level on these skills before her accident would have been in the "superior" range. Now her scores on executive function tests were in the "low average" range. When she was asked to give the meanings of proverbs, she got many of them correct but on others gave very concrete answers. For example, when asked the meaning of "One swallow doesn't make a summer," she replied, "Swallows always fly about in groups in the summer."

Kim also showed little spontaneous initiative and would not do her physical therapy exercises unless someone was there doing them with her. It wasn't that she refused or that she seemed to mind doing them. When she was told to practice bouncing a ball for five minutes she would do it a couple of times and then just let the ball drop. "Why won't you keep practicing?" Olive asked her. "You know it is the only way to improve your coordination." But Kim just smiled her lovely smile, and said with a giggle, "Can't be bothered."

This lack of initiative is very typical of TBI patients and is also a "frontal lobe" impairment. It is easy to see why these frontal lobe problems are called executive impairments. A CEO without initiative or the ability to think abstractly would soon be out of a job—and probably wouldn't care! Another of these executive impairments is a lack of insight into one's own performance and behavior. Thus Kim had poor insight, and this made her rehabilitation much more difficult. Because she was not concerned about her poor performance, she saw no reason to strive to do better. Her other executive impairments, all very common following a severe TBI, included inappropriate and "roller-coaster" emotions and an inability to organize her time and to plan ahead.

Overall, Kim had come out of this TBI remarkably well. She certainly had the profile of someone with a severe TBI, but her impairments were relatively mild. In particular, although her "frontal" behaviors—her giggling and lack of initiative—were frustrating for her therapists and family, these were quite mild examples of these sorts of difficulties.

Unlike some patients with much more severe frontal lobe damage, she didn't undress in front of her visitors, wander away and get lost, have aggressive and violent outbursts, or sit almost mute and expressionless day after day.[2]

*****

As the weeks wore on, it became clear that Paul and Olive, Kim's father and sister, were the primary caregivers and "rehabilitation experts." Kim stayed most weekends at her mother's house, and Joanna spent at least one full day with her then, but she was unable to take time off work during the rest of the week to help with her daughter. She said that instead she would pay for a professional caregiver to spend time with Kim, and not surprisingly this caused Paul and Kathy considerable distress and anger. But after two sessions of counseling Paul gave up his anger and decided that he couldn't change his ex-wife, and agreed that she could employ a young mother who had trained as a physical therapist to stay with Kim three days a week while her own children were at school. This gave Kathy a break and allowed Paul to return to work full-time. After this, Kim's physical abilities improved rapidly and she and the caregiver became good friends. Olive developed into an expert rehabilitation "therapist," and, with an efficiency and compassion that she had perhaps inherited from Joanna and Paul, respectively, ensured that the schedule involving herself, Kim's friends, and her stepsister worked like clockwork. It had been decided that it was too soon for Kim to return to her school, as she was academically far from ready and became tired very easily. In fact she slept every day from 1 to 3 p.m. and was often asleep by 8 at night. So Kim's sisters and friends spent after-school hours

---

[2] Phillipa, the woman with very severe frontal lobe damage described in Chapter 4, has an extreme "frontal lobe syndrome."

and weekends helping her with schoolwork carefully selected and checked by her teachers and involving Kim in activities essential to teenagers—playing music, doing their hair, and gossiping. On weekends they would take Kim out, in the summer to the beach and in the winter to a movie, or just into the city to wander around the shops. Kim could now walk with a walking frame, but on these outings she would go in her wheelchair.

But if her caregiver or friends weren't around, Kim found it hard to get motivated; if not told to get dressed she would stay in her pajamas until midday, her hair unbrushed, sitting in front of the TV until someone turned it off. The first time her friends wanted to take her to a party at one of their schoolmate's houses, Kim refused and became quite tearful. Joanna contacted me, concerned that Kim was becoming isolated and lazy, and I set up a meeting. Joanna and Olive came along with Kim, and I was amazed at how far Kim had progressed since I had last seen her six weeks previously. In particular I was pleased by her much improved insight; indeed, this was the reason she didn't want to go to the party. She was embarrassed by her inability to walk unaided and her still clumsy left arm. But the return of insight into her problems brought distress and the possibility of depression. When Joanna voiced her concerns that Kim was "letting herself go" and getting lazy, Kim giggled and then started to cry. But when she had calmed down, she did a good job of explaining how she felt, feelings very common in people who have suffered a severe TBI.

"I just feel sort of blank, as if I haven't got any energy even when I've had a bloody long sleep," she said. "I love it when Olive or one of my friends comes over after school because I am sooooo bored, but I just can't seem to get started on anything by myself. And I forget things all the time, like what I meant to do. I know I'm meant to keep a diary but I sometimes forget to write stuff in it or look at it.

My friends seem to give me energy and then I want to do things, as long as they're with me. But I can't do it by myself." She was crying again now and Olive went over and gave her a hug.

It was time for some "psychoeducation," and I explained that Kim's lack of motivation and difficulty initiating activities were not a sign of laziness but a result of her frontal lobe damage, which made it tricky for her to mentally structure her life. The best way to help would be to provide external structure by keeping to routines and by providing written schedules of activities and then organizing the activities for her.

The memory problems resulting from temporal lobe damage caused by a closed head injury are less likely to be helped by the provision of external structure. Problems with *prospective memory*, that is, "remembering to remember," cause the most difficulty for people recovering from a closed head injury. For example, Kim forgets that Paul has asked her to telephone him at lunchtime on the occasional day she is left alone in the house. She forgets that she is going to the movies with her friends on Saturday. Prospective memory problems are best helped by training the patient in using a diary in a consistent and logical manner to substitute for the memory they have lost. Of course it is important to keep the diary on hand all the time and look in it regularly, a very challenging task for a TBI survivor. We decided to try out an electronic diary for Kim, and Crystal, Kim's stepsister, agreed to spend five minutes with her every morning before going to school helping her to program it to bleep at the times when she had to remember important activities. When she heard a bleep, she knew to look in her diary to see what activity she was meant to remember. She was also encouraged to look in her diary at every mealtime and before going to bed. In addition, her friends and family frequently called her on her cell phone—this was before the invention of texting—to chat or to remind her of things she should be doing. It is quite likely that Kim will always have trouble with prospective memory and organizing her life, and her diary, whether paper or electronic, will need to become an essential appendage. We talked about the importance of living one day at a time, appreciating what she can do rather than what she can't do, and focusing on the small steps forward rather than the small steps back. I gave Kim a copy of a wonderful Michael Leunig cartoon called "How to Get There" (shown in Figure 11.1) to put somewhere she would see it every day.

The session finished on a good note, with Joanna responding to Kim's complaint that her mother hardly seemed to know she existed. Joanna apologized for not telling her daughter more often how proud she was of her,

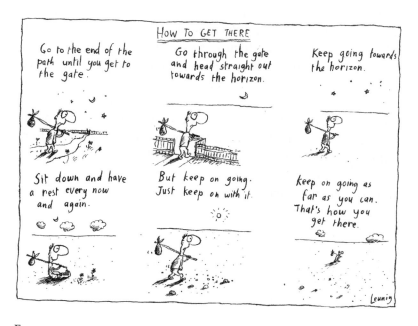

FIGURE 11.1
The cartoon I gave Kim. (Reprinted with the kind permission of Michael Leunig, from his book Leunig, M. 1992. *A Bunch of Poesy*, pp. 9–11. Australia: Collins Angus & Robertson.)

and assured her that she was very aware of how hard she worked at her rehabilitation. When Kim looked unconvinced, Joanna hugged her, and they were both crying when Joanna promised she'd try to be better and tell Kim more often how much she loved her, and not assume Kim could read her mind. Kim seemed relieved when I suggested that she and I could meet alone for a few sessions to talk over some of her worries about her future. I felt she had reached the stage where she could begin to look at who she was now. But before that she would need to grieve for what—and whom—she had lost.

In our individual therapy sessions we began by talking about the "old" Kim, using photographs and even some of Kim's old diaries to help her remember her past self. Kim said she was still thinking she might get back to being pretty similar to the old Kim, even if she had to give up her two ambitions: to be an Olympic skier and to go to medical school to train as a doctor. Over time and with many tears—and some laughter—Kim was able to say "goodbye for now" to her old self. Five sessions into our individual therapy, Kim said she was ready to work out who she was now. She tried drawing her new self, but this usually ended in giggles, so then she began writing something about herself every day; some new personality characteristic she had discovered she had, some new food she liked, how she was or was not like various TV characters. We got a notebook in which to keep a careful record of every new thing she accomplished, from physical activities like walking across the room on her father's arm, to managing not to eat chocolate for two nights in a row, to finishing a novel, to going to a party and dancing with a boy for the first time since her car accident. She asked her family and friends to join in and add things they noticed her achieving. The day that she could write "I returned to school today" was such a highlight that Joanna put on a celebration party that weekend for all the family and Kim's friends.

By this stage, I was no longer needed in Kim's life—the best outcome a therapist could ask for. But just before I bowed out, I assessed Kim again on all the same tests I had given her ten months previously. She had improved on every one, although on none of the tests had she returned to her pre-accident levels. It was very unlikely that she would ever reach the high academic standard required for medical school or have the drive to succeed in that sort of career. Fortunately this no longer concerned Kim, perhaps because of her frontal lobe damage and decreased motivation,. She was happy just to be able to return to school, even though she could only attend in the mornings and still needed to sleep in the afternoons. It did not even appear to upset her too much that she was repeating the year she had been in when she had her accident and was now nearer the bottom than the top of the class.

Recovery from a severe TBI can continue for a lifetime, and I invited Kim and her family to call me if they needed a "maintenance" session, perhaps if a problem, issue, or question came up that they couldn't solve within their now very experienced family rehabilitation team. From time to time I would receive a phone call from Paul or Joanna about some worry they had. A phone discussion was all that was necessary most of the time, until one day about a year after I had last seen the family, Paul called me saying they really needed a family meeting. It was almost a déjà vu experience when they crowded into the therapy room at the university, although this time the three youngest members of the tribe weren't there and Kim walked in with the support of Olive. Her limp was still obvious and she was very unsteady walking alone, but she could manage with two walking sticks and now rarely used a wheelchair. Everyone looked tired and grim, and Kim's smile when I hugged her did not light up her pretty face.

After the initial catching up, Paul told me what was concerning the family. Kim seemed to have stopped wanting to improve. She appeared to have lost interest in every-thing, and they were at their wits' end. Joanna broke in and said, her voice sounding irritated: "She's just plain lazy and spoilt. You spoil her far too much, Paul; you always have." She turned to me. "First he bought her a guitar and she got sick of that in five minutes, and now he wants to take her skiing with the other girls and she's got the sulks and won't go."

Paul took up the story, looking annoyed. "I think you know that before her accident, Kim was a superb skier, by far the best in the family, and we're all pretty good. Every August I always took the three girls for a week's skiing in Queenstown, and I thought that would be a great thing to do again. I've had these special skis made for Kim that she'll be able to use, even with her weak leg and poor bal-ance, and I've found a ski instructor who is experienced in training the disabled to teach her when we get there. I've even asked her best friend to come as well; the girls will have a fantastic time with all their mates. But Kim's decided she's not coming. She'll never get any better if she doesn't put more effort in." Kim was looking sullen, and after a silence, Olive spoke up.

"I can understand why Kim doesn't want to come, Dad. She was such a great skier and she doesn't want to be learning again, that's all. It's not that she's ungrateful for all you're doing for her."

"Is that true, Kim?" asked her father.

"Yes, I suppose," replied Kim, looking at the floor.

"But you'll love it when you get there. Just trust me. You don't even have to ski if you don't want to; just party with the others afterwards."

"Oh Dad, that would be worse, watching them all skiing and me just sitting around. I'm not going. You and Mum just have to get used to the fact that this is as good as I am going to get. Get over it, you've got a cripple for a daughter."

Kim had reached a plateau in her recovery, and she and most members of her family believed that no further change would occur. As we talked more about what had been happening and each family member revealed more of his or her feelings, it became clear that they thought there had been very little real change and progress in the past year. Living with Kim as she made tiny steps meant that those steps went unnoticed or were easily forgotten. When this happens, one therapy technique is to collapse time so that the family can see again just how much progress has been made since the accident. I remembered that I had a video of Kim made by the physical and occupational therapists as a record of her progress. Every week for the first three months and then once a month after that, they had filmed her for five minutes or so doing some of her physical exercises or a neuropsychological test, writing or drawing, or sometimes just talking, beginning with her very first session a few days after she came out of her coma and continuing until her physical therapy stopped, almost nine months later. The family might have seen it in the early stages of Kim's rehabilitation but I decided it was time for us to view it again.

I pulled the curtains and we sat in the dim room and watched as Kim appeared, slumped in her wheelchair like a giggling rag doll. The therapist threw her a large ball, but she made no move to catch it. The date of the next week flashed on the screen, and we watched as the therapist asked Kim some simple questions and some simple sums, getting only blank looks or giggles in reply. The therapist wiped dribble from Kim's chin. Over the 90 minutes of the video, we watched in silence as Kim failed to make a simple pattern out of colored blocks, wrote her name in large, child-like letters but failed to write anything else, failed to add 2 plus 4, began to catch the ball, began to throw the ball, began to make sense out of the colored blocks and laughed with delight, succeeded in adding 2 plus 4 and then managed to subtract and multiply as well, wrote her name easily and began to write simple sentences, held up her diary to the camera, grinning as she pointed to the pages covered by her writing, stood for a few seconds supported by the therapist, walked with the walker, walked with two sticks, and, in the last scene, walked across the room on her father's arm, the pride in Paul's face almost outshining the triumph of Kim's smile. I hadn't seen the video for a long time, and through my own tears I looked around at Kim and her family. Every one of them—including Kim—was crying, her father most of all.

Kim walked out of the therapy room that day holding hands with Paul on one side of her and Joanna on the other. Paul phoned me the next day and asked if he could have a copy of the video. On meeting him by chance years later, he thanked me again for my help, and especially the last session we had together. For me, his words encapsulate many of the essentials of a good rehabilitation process and outcome—the permanent symptoms of the TBI that have become part of the survivor's new personality and identity, the involvement of the family in the rehabilitation process, the emotional lows and highs along the way, the courage, hope, and resilience of everyone involved, and the long months and years of stumbling and making the thousands of small steps that lead to enormous achievements.

"I sometimes get frustrated with Kim's laid-back attitude and lack of initiative, and just want to shake her," Paul told me. "So then I watch the video again. But I always watch it alone and in the dark, because I always cry. And our Kim, she's doing really well. She completed her training as a preschool teacher and she loves it; she's like a kid herself in some ways, so perhaps that's why the little ones love her so much. She lives with her very nice boyfriend, and they seem to be pretty happy. We see her about once a week, and she visits her mother reasonably often. And she still has the "How to Get There" cartoon hanging on the wall in her bathroom, where she sees it first thing every morning and last thing at night. But can you believe it, she still refuses to ski!"

■ Further Reading

Ogden, J. A. 2005. Traumatic brain injury and the importance of ongoing rehabilitation. In: *Fractured Minds: A Case-Study Approach to Clinical Neuropsychology, 2nd Ed.* (pp. 171–192). New York: Oxford University Press.

Osborn, C. L. 1998. *Over My Head: A Doctor's Own Story of Head Injury from the Inside Looking Out.* Kansas City, MO: Andrews McMeel.

Vandergriff, R. 2008. *A Family's Journey Through Traumatic Brain Injury.* Kansas City, MO: Bear's Nest Press.

Wilson, B. A. 1999. *Case Studies in Neuropsychological Rehabilitation.* New York: Oxford University Press.

12

Shaken Up: Taking Control of
Parkinson's Disease

Robert Jacobs, MD, enjoyed the monthly meetings of the
Medical Historical Society, where a group of doctors and
other health professionals met to listen to a lecture on a
medical topic or medical figure of historical interest.
Tonight it was his turn to give the talk, and he had carefully prepared his PowerPoint presentation on James
Parkinson, the doctor who in 1817 first described the "shaking palsy," the illness later called Parkinson's disease (PD).[1]
Robert was a confident speaker, but on this occasion found
himself worrying about the slight tremor that occasionally
plagued his left hand. He was strongly left-handed, and he
was concerned that when he used the laser pointer, any
minor hand tremor would be translated on the big projection

[1]Parkinson, J. 1817. *An Essay on the Shaking Palsy*. London: Sherwood, Nesly
and Jones.

screen to a very obvious shaking of the red dot. He cringed at the thought of his peers thinking he was shaking with nerves. So to be on the safe side he held the pointer awkwardly in his right hand, imprisoning his disobedient left hand in his pocket. On a couple of occasions his left hand escaped, picked up the laser pointer, and to his surprise showed no sign of trembling. But during the wine-and-cheese supper after his talk, the tremor returned. He quickly stuck the offending hand back in his pocket and held his glass in his right hand.

Driving home later that evening he forced himself to consider the awful possibility that he might be one of the sad cases of shaking palsy that he had spoken about this evening. He tried to convince himself that, at only 58 years old, he was surely too young for Parkinson's disease to strike. It was probably just a benign familial tremor. Robert vaguely remembered that his father had a problem with a shaking hand, but he lived to a healthy 85 without any signs of PD; perhaps Robert had inherited the same problem. With that comforting thought, he dismissed any possibility of PD from his mind and went on with his busy life as a general practitioner, husband, and father of two adult sons.

Nevertheless, every now and then the anxiety would creep back as the spasmodic tremor returned. He noted that this usually occurred at the end of a busy day and was most apparent when his left hand was at rest. About four months after his talk to the Medical Historical Society, his son Peter, who had graduated from medical school himself two years previously and was working as a registrar on the neurology ward of the city hospital, joined him one Sunday for a round of golf. Neither man was a serious golfer, and they played more to force themselves to take some exercise and to spend some father–son time together than out of love for the sport. At the ninth hole Peter broached his concern about his father. He told Robert that he'd been aware of his tremor for some months now, and that Lillian, his mother, had also been concerned about Robert, especially since he became irritated when she suggested that he should get a checkup. Because of his "doctor" status, Peter had been given the short straw and had agreed to raise the issue with his father.

Robert made an effort to listen as his son pointed out that in addition to his hand tremor, his movements were a good deal slower than they used to be, and it might be more than just simple aging. As soon as Robert agreed to see his GP for a checkup "when he had time," Peter played his trump card and said that he had mentioned his concerns to Dr. Bracken, the senior neurology consultant on the ward Peter worked on. He had a specialist interest in neurological motor disorders and had made a tentative appointment to see Robert at 7:30 p.m. the following evening in his private clinic; Robert need only phone in if he couldn't make it. Robert was decidedly annoyed by this going behind his back, but reluctantly agreed to keep the appointment, firmly declining Peter's offer to accompany him!

That evening Robert and Lillian had an emotional argument, where he accused her of treating him like a child by talking about him to Peter (and everyone else, he supposed). An upset Lillian told him that he had been snappy and unkind to her lately, and that she had talked to Peter— and no one else—because she was becoming increasingly worried about him. An uneasy truce was finally reached, and Robert promised he would pass on everything the neurologist said when he got back from his appointment.

Next day he duly showed up at Dr. Bracken's rooms, following a reminder call from Peter—which, as he told Peter, he did not require! He had met Dr. Bracken on a couple of occasions in the past but did not really know him. Fortunately, Dr. Bracken had a very easy and relaxing manner, and treated Robert more like a colleague than a patient. He began by asking him about his own observations of his tremor and any other symptoms he was aware of, and what hypotheses Robert had about these. Robert admitted that he had wondered about early PD but thought that he was too young for that, and believed his symptoms were too mild to be used to diagnose PD—even if in time that turned out to be their cause. Dr. Bracken commented that while 58 was quite young for PD, early symptoms could certainly begin to show then. He suggested that even if it were too early to diagnose PD, deciding that it might be a possibility could be helpful to Robert in a number of ways. First, it would allay the anxiety attached to trying to suppress his concerns, it would certainly allay his family's anxieties to know that he was being monitored, and it would allow Robert to be alert for any symptoms, given his own expertise as a doctor. Second, if he did turn out to have PD, they could use every possible treatment when necessary, but not before necessary. Finally, as a doctor, Robert would want to be extra careful that he was on top of his job, as PD often resulted in some cognitive problems. While this possibility would obviously be a concern, being aware of potential problems would allow him to monitor himself and to do what he could to compensate for mild cognitive deficits if they developed.

Robert could hardly disagree with such a reasoned approach and, trying to disguise his increasing anxiety, submitted to Dr. Bracken's examination. He knew that the most common early symptom of PD was tremor, afflicting about seventy percent of sufferers, often seen first in one hand when it was resting rather than active, and progressing to the other side as the disease advanced. Robert's tremor—which he hoped had nothing to do with PD—was limited to his left hand at rest. He knew that in some PD patients, tremor involved other parts of the body as well, including the head. The other main motor symptoms of PD were *muscle rigidity*, which in severe cases resulted in a "frozen" state, *bradykinesia*, a fancy word for slowed movement, and *postural instability*, or easily losing one's balance. Apart perhaps from a slight slowing down, he didn't think he had those symptoms.

Dr. Bracken began his examination with a standard neurological assessment of the 12 cranial nerves and Robert's reflexes, all of which seemed normal. It was a strange feeling being the patient, and Robert found himself almost dissociating from the experience by switching into his "doctor" mode and observing his own examination from that safer perspective. Next Dr. Bracken asked Robert to walk back and forth across the room, and then had him walk heel to toe. He explained that he was interested in Robert's ability to walk with a normal gait and stride, swinging his arms and turning fluently. Apparently Robert did not swing his left arm as much as his right, and when he turned he got a little stuck before he could begin walking again. To assess postural stability, Dr. Bracken asked Robert to stand with his eyes closed and pushed him gently on each shoulder to see if he lost balance. He wobbled but managed to stay upright. Still with his eyes closed, Robert then had to hold his arms and hands out steadily in front of him—but he was aware of his left hand trembling. With his eyes open he then had to use the index finger of each hand in turn to touch his own nose and then to touch Dr. Bracken's finger as fast as possible as he moved it to different positions. Again Robert's left hand let him down; it was too slow to keep up with Dr. Bracken's moving finger, although his right hand had no problem. On a task where he had to place pegs in holes in a board as fast as possible, first with the right and then with the left hand, again he was slow and clumsy with his left hand. Robert valiantly tried to retain his objective stance as Dr. Bracken explained that Robert's slowed left-sided movements and difficulty initiating movements—as he clearly demonstrated after making a turn when walking—were indicative of mild bradykinesia.

Dr. Bracken then moved Robert's arms passively back and forth from the elbow. Robert could see that his left arm stopped and started in a stuttering fashion, a PD symptom called *cogwheel rigidity*. Finally Robert had to write a few sentences across a page and was relieved to find that his writing seemed quite normal. Dr. Bracken agreed; Robert showed no sign of slowed writing—even though he was using his left hand—or *micrographia*, where the PD patient's writing becomes smaller and more cramped as it moves across the page.

By the time the examination was over, Robert was feeling tired and glum, because he could see for himself that all was not normal. Dr. Bracken was straightforward in his summing up and confirmed what Robert had observed for himself: he had Parkinsonian signs restricted to his left side. He had a resting tremor of the left hand, some minor rigidity of his left arm, and a slowed left arm swing when walking, and he was slower at placing pegs in the holes with his left hand than his right, even though he was left-handed. On the positive side, he had no signs of postural instability or micrographia. Thus it would appear that he had one-sided, or unilateral, tremor, bradykinesia, and rigidity—three of the signs of early *idiopathic* (lacking a known cause) Parkinson's disease.

Robert realized he wasn't surprised by Dr. Bracken's diagnosis; deep down he had known he had more than just a benign hand tremor, but he had been in denial. "So what's the latest research on the cause of PD?" he asked, struggling to keep his voice calm.

Dr. Bracken's careful explanation included a lot of information Robert already knew, but he listened intently; this was now about him. Dr. Bracken told him that in PD there is a loss of the neurotransmitter dopamine as a result of a loss of dopaminergic neurons (nerve cells that produce the neurotransmitter dopamine) in the substantia nigra, a part of the basal ganglia lying deep in the brain. Dopamine has been found to contribute to many functions including voluntary movement and some aspects of cognition.

Most cases of PD are idiopathic as no definitive cause can be found. A number of environmental factors are likely to be implicated, but these are, as yet, unknown. At least two genetic forms have been identified that account for a very small number of PD cases, and there may be genetic factors that increase the vulnerability of certain people to developing PD if they are exposed to some environmental influence. The multiple brain traumas of the kind boxers get can result in a form of PD called "pugilistic parkinsonism." When Dr. Bracken told him about the survivors of an encephalitis epidemic in 1918 who developed severe PD, Robert nodded. He had mentioned that in his lecture to the Medical Historical Society.

"And have you read about that tragic drug-related PD outbreak in 1982?" Dr. Bracken continued. "A number of young Californian drug addicts took a heroin-derivative designer drug called MPTP, and it resulted in the rapid onset of severe PD. Their main symptom was severe rigidity, and when they were given L-dopa (another term for levodopa) their PD symptoms were relieved. That was what confirmed that it was a form of PD. In fact a positive response to L-dopa is one of the ways we confirm PD in patients where we can find no obvious cause for the disease as in your case."

Robert knew of course that L-dopa was the drug of choice for idiopathic PD. "Are you sure my type is idiopathic?" he asked, fascinated in spite of his anxiety about his own status.

"Well, I can't rule out some underlying genetic factor entirely, but given that you have no history of PD in your family, idiopathic PD is by far the most likely label for your cluster of symptoms."

"So what's my prognosis?"

"The onset of symptoms is gradual, and the disease progresses in severity over time, but at different rates and with different clusters of parkinsonian symptoms across individuals. Given that you are at the younger age for PD—in most cases the first symptoms appear in the sixties, although there are cases before the age of 40—you are less likely to experience a rapid progression of symptoms than if your symptoms had not become apparent until your late sixties or seventies. In fact, rates of dementia as part of the PD profile increase rapidly when the disease onset is after the age of 70 years."

"And there's no cure?" Robert asked glumly, knowing full well what the answer was.

"Not yet, I'm afraid, although new research on treatments, as well as a cure, are a hot topic in neuroscience. But current treatments result in major improvements of symptoms, and most sufferers will not have a reduced life span as a result of the disease."

"So, what do you suggest for me?"

"I think it would be best to delay starting medication for as long as possible, but you will need to monitor your symptoms carefully so that we can begin medication if the symptoms start to interfere with your medical practice."

"Tell me the worst," Robert said. "What should I expect down the track?"

"Are you sure you wouldn't rather wait a while before worrying about that?" Dr. Bracken asked.

"Well, I already know a lot about PD, but I would appreciate hearing the facts from you. I'm not sure I really understand just how the symptoms will affect my everyday life." Robert sat on his trembling left hand and forced himself to listen, now as a patient rather than as a doctor, as Dr. Bracken described how the PD signs and symptoms tended to develop as the disease progressed.

Robert learned that rigidity was a common early symptom and could result in the patient becoming "stuck" in his chair or when turning around, turning over in bed, or making fine finger movements such as fastening buttons. Body rigidity was one of the most unpleasant symptoms because it resulted in a feeling of helplessness for the patient and could cause considerable discomfort and muscular pain. Posture often became stooped, and the face stiff so that it appeared to lack expression—called a "masked face"—and this frequently caused communication difficulties and misunderstandings. Bradykinesia resulted in a slowness to initiate movements and in carrying out motor tasks. Rapid limb movements became slowed and coordination impaired. Walking was often impaired as well, with the stride length shortening so that the patient wound up taking small, shuffling steps. Sometimes the gait became unbalanced, and to compensate, the shuffling gait got faster and faster and not entirely under the patient's control. Bradykinesia also contributed to the expressionless face, sometimes resulting in social difficulties if others didn't realize that the person's face *couldn't* express their emotions.

A loss of balance, resulting in falls, usually occurred later in the disease. Dystonias, which are persistent muscle spasms of body parts, could look very awkward and were often very painful. Dystonias could be a complication of medication or in some cases a symptom of the PD itself. Some sufferers experienced varying degrees of unusual skin sensations, such as an "electrical" tingling sensation in the limbs. Constipation was common as a result of the reduced ability of the bowel to contract. Fatigue is an ongoing problem for people with PD as it is for many neurological conditions. Anyone constantly on the move or who holds the body in awkward and stiff positions would get tired, and unfortunately the tremor and muscle rigidity of PD exacerbates the patient's fatigue.

"I've read that PD patients are often depressed," Robert said when Dr. Bracken had finished his explanation.

"A significant proportion do suffer from depression, and it seems to be in part organically based; that is, a result of the disease itself. But depression can also be an understandable psychological response to the illness. Do you think it's been a problem for you?" Dr. Bracken asked.

"I don't think so. I've been worried that I might have Parkinson's but I haven't had any of the symptoms of clinical depression, like eating problems, waking up in the early hours and feeling down, or feeling hopeless, thank goodness. What about dementia? Will that be something to look forward to later, even though my symptoms started early?" Robert asked, trying to keep his voice light.

"Hopefully not. Only about ten to fifteen percent of PD patients become demented, and there is no substantial evidence that dementia is closely tied to the progression of motor symptoms. Although a few patients with quite mild PD symptoms show signs of early dementia I have wheelchair-bound PD patients with very advanced motor symptoms who have intellects sharper than mine."

"That's a relief at least," Robert said.

"Yes, but as you probably know, in most PD patients the mind doesn't escape damage entirely. Many develop some mild and specific cognitive deficits that it pays to be aware of, especially if you are in a vocation that requires sharp thinking like you are."

"What sort of problems?" Robert asked, swallowing.

"Symptoms vary, but executive impairments seem to be most common, although these are usually quite subtle. The loss of dopamine in the basal ganglia primarily causes motor symptoms, but the basal ganglia also have rich connections with the prefrontal cortex—the anterior part of the frontal lobes. So a disruption of these pathways probably explains the executive difficulties. In particular, when PD sufferers have to rely upon their own spontaneous internal strategies, they can have difficulties with organizing and planning ahead, and carrying out cognitive and motor plans. For example it is difficult for them to think about how they would prepare a reasonably complex meal, and performing the required tasks in the right sequence. When they're given external visual cues, such as written step-by-step instructions, the executive difficulties don't seem to occur.

One family of deficits that have also been linked to frontal executive dysfunction involves the ordering of events in the correct time sequence, and knowing which event occurred most recently. For example, it's been shown that, compared with healthy people the same age, some PD patients have more difficulty putting past public events such as the assassination of John Kennedy, Watergate, and the explosion of the *Challenger* space shuttle into the correct time sequence, although they can describe each of those events accurately. Some PD patients also find they can no longer easily shift their thoughts from one topic to another."

"What do you mean?" Robert asked.

"Well, perhaps if you were dealing with your e-mails and your wife wanted to discuss what the two of you might do in the weekend, you might find it difficult to stop thinking about your last e-mail and focus on what she was telling you." Dr. Bracken paused, but continued when Robert nodded at him to go on.

"Unfortunately, executive problems can affect many other cognitive abilities. Often patients even in the early stages of PD have a lot of trouble copying complex figures, but it seems that this isn't because of their motor impairment or a visuospatial impairment, but rather because they don't think out a sensible strategy to ensure that they copy systematically, and as a consequence can get in a right mess. Strategic forward planning is an executive ability that is pretty important in all sorts of tasks we do every day."

"What about memory?" Robert asked. "I have a bit of trouble remembering people's names these days."

"Tell me about it!" Dr. Bracken said, grinning at him. "That's a common problem as we age, I'm afraid. However, PD patients do have a few memory problems beyond the fact that they are aging. Like all us older people, they have problems—but greater than normal—with recalling memories spontaneously, without cues, although they can readily recognize and pick out items they have previously learned if they are given a list to choose from. That's called recognition memory. Some researchers think PD patients also have difficulty with working memory: That's the memory system that allows us to work on information in our mind for a brief time. For example we use our working memory when we're working out an arithmetic problem in our heads. But I think that rather than speculating about which of these cognitive problems you might have, you should have a neuropsychological assessment. Then we'll have a baseline of your performance at this early stage to compare with future assessments."

"I suppose so, but I'd like to talk it all over with my wife and sons, and then I'll get back to you, if that's OK," Robert replied. He had just about reached the end of his day's supply of bravery and no longer seemed to have the ability to look at PD objectively.

"That's a good idea. There's no urgency at all. Take all the time you need."

The sympathy in Dr. Bracken's tone was almost too much for Robert and he left the room quickly before he broke down in tears. But the tears came that evening, when he told Lillian about his diagnosis. After a good sleep, helped along by a sleeping pill, he felt calmer, at least until he had to relay it all again to his two sons that evening. But the next week he contacted Dr. Bracken and told him he would go ahead with the neuropsychological assessment. Once that was over and he knew the worst, he would decide whether he should begin medication.

The neuropsychological assessment was incredibly difficult for him even though he thought he performed normally on most of the tests.[2] The clinical neuropsychologist seemed very competent and professional, but Robert was acutely aware of his extreme anxiety and that he was perspiring profusely throughout the two-hour ordeal. His tremor constantly betrayed him, and on one occasion he froze and could not complete a task where he had to copy a simple pattern drawn on a card by putting red and white blocks together. When he was asked to copy a complex figure he lost his way in the maze of lines and became very confused about which ended where. He could see by the end that he had made a right muck of his drawing. He was even more disheartened after his miserable attempt to draw the figure from memory later in the assessment. (Figure 12.1 shows the complex figure and his attempts to draw it.)

He felt happier when given some verbal memory tests that didn't involve motor skills, and afterward was certain he'd performed reasonably well on them. But then the neuropsychologist gave him a test where he had to sort cards according to secret rules that he had to infer from the "right" or "wrong" responses the neuropsychologist gave each time he placed a new card on a pile. Sometimes the rules changed, and Robert had to figure this out from the neuropsychologist's feedback as well. He did well at figuring out the first few rules but then became increasingly frustrated as the neuropsychologist told him repeatedly he was wrong. He began to think that it was a trick test designed to see whether he could cope with frustration rather than a test of any cognitive skill. As he said to the neuropsychologist at the end of the session, many of the tasks were hardly fair tests of his thinking, as his tremor

---

[2] I was Robert's neuropsychologist but have chosen to write Robert's story from his own point of view, reconstructed from many conversations we had.

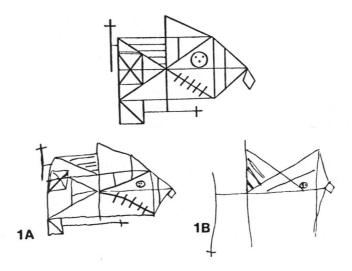

Figure 12.1
When Robert copied the Rey Complex Figure (top), he produced drawing 1A, but 45 minutes later, his drawing of the figure from memory, IB, was very impoverished.

and slowness prevented him from demonstrating his full cognitive abilities. She agreed that this was an issue and assured him that when she scored and interpreted the tests she would take this into consideration, and in some cases the test scores would probably be unhelpful. She promised to send a report to him and Dr. Bracken within a week.

It was a long week for Robert, and he did not feel much better when the report arrived. It was written clearly and emphasized his superior cognitive abilities in many areas, especially on tests of general knowledge, comprehension, arithmetic, and verbal memory. However, even when his tremor was taken into consideration, Robert did have mild impairment on tasks involving motor actions, mainly because he was slower than other people of his age and intellectual ability. On the test where Robert had to copy a complex figure, his performance demonstrated that he had possible visuospatial perceptual deficits as well as executive deficits, including poor organization and forward planning. This was certainly no surprise to Robert, as he knew he'd done badly on that test. Apparently on the card-sorting task, also a test of executive functioning, he was unable as the test wore on to change mental set and learn from his errors that the rules had changed. The neuropsychological report concluded that his mild deficits were consistent with a diagnosis of Parkinson's disease and that his mild to moderate executive difficulties, while probably not a major problem now, should be monitored very carefully over time given his occupation. The report ended with the suggestion that Robert would be wise to consider whether he should continue to work as a sole practitioner, and to think about taking on a partner with whom he could consult over any difficult or unusual cases.

After discussing the neuropsychological report with Dr. Bracken, Robert decided he should begin medication immediately, as his tremor was starting to be a problem. Dr. Bracken cautioned him that the sooner he began medication, the sooner the drug would become ineffective, so delaying medication for as long as possible was worth considering. He reminded Robert that he was only in the earliest stage of the disease, but would go on to have symptoms on both sides of his body, then begin to suffer balance problems while still being independent, and after many years could become severely disabled and possibly require a wheelchair. Taking medication now could make it harder to control those symptoms later. But Robert remained firm and said he wanted to control his hand tremor now so he could continue confidently in his medical practice while he was still cognitively relatively unaffected by the disease.

So Dr. Bracken started him on Sinemet, a medication that combines L-dopa and carbidopa. L-dopa is a precursor of dopamine that, unlike dopamine, can cross the *blood–brain barrier* (a physiological mechanism in the blood vessels that acts as a filter and prevents some substances from entering the brain from the circulating blood). Once in the brain the L-dopa converts to dopamine. Carbidopa is added to the L-dopa to inhibit the peripheral conversion of L-dopa to dopamine and so allow more to cross the blood–brain barrier. It has the added advantage of reducing such side effects of L-dopa as nausea and vomiting. As Dr. Bracken explained, there are many other drugs that treat various PD symptoms, including amantadine, an antiviral agent that strengthens the effect of dopamine, and COMT (catechol-O-methyltransferase), which can prevent dopamine from being broken down. At some point these might be helpful for Robert. But Sinemet would very likely be effective for a number of years in reducing his movement disorders, and there was evidence that it might also alleviate some of the cognitive symptoms.

Starting medication turned out to be the right decision for Robert. His symptoms rapidly improved, and he felt much happier about continuing in his practice. With encouragement from Peter, he advertised for a partner, and within two months a pleasant young woman doctor joined him. As the months went by, Robert became accustomed to the fact that he had PD, and most of the time never gave it a thought. He had checkups with Dr. Bracken every three months, and over the next four years, apart from some changes in his medication, felt he was on top of his disease. He learned exactly when he needed to take his Sinemet to perform at his best. He made a decision not to stress himself by giving any more lectures to the Medical Historical Society, but still enjoyed attending the meetings. He continued to play golf for a few years and actually found that swinging his golf club back and forth helped him overcome his rigidity. He found that family, friends, and colleagues were very understanding and did not make a big issue of his condition. Peter, who now worked as a general practitioner in a large community practice, had developed a special interest in PD, primarily as a result of his father's illness, and Robert found he was able to talk about his symptoms and concerns with his son without embarrassment.

A year after his diagnosis, Robert's symptoms had spread to his right side, and to control his increasing bradykinesia and rigidity his medication had to be increased. Shortly after this he became quite depressed, and his GP started him on the antidepressant Prozac. This did seem to relieve his depression, and he remained on it. He had a follow-up neuropsychological assessment two years after his diagnosis, and to his relief the report concluded that his visuospatial and executive impairments had not worsened significantly and his verbal memory was still within normal limits. However he did give up driving soon after his diagnosis, when he found that he sometimes had difficulty changing traffic lanes when he should, and the neuropsychologist suggested this might be a result of his difficulty in changing mental set.

Sleeping was another problem, mainly because of his inability to move into a comfortable position in bed. He often got stuck in one position and was unable to turn over or even get out of bed if he needed to in the night. As a result he occasionally ended up wetting the bed, much to his embarrassment. He and Lillian decided to sleep in separate rooms so that she at least could get some sleep, and they had an alarm system installed so that if necessary, Robert could push a button attached to the side of his bed and a buzzer would sound in Lillian's room. Lillian coped remarkably well most of the time, although it took a lot of strength to pull or push Robert into a position where he could start moving again—especially first thing in the morning before his first dose of Sinemet—so she was often tired. She also had to suffer considerable frustration when Robert became irrational and illogical during some argument, usually when he was tired. This was a complete personality change for him; he had previously been a very nonjudgmental person, always ready to listen to the other side of an issue. His neuropsychologist thought that this new inflexibility was also a result of executive problems.

Three years after his diagnosis, Robert and his practice partner took on a third, part-time doctor so that Robert could work mornings only, when he felt at his best. Their receptionist/practice nurse became very skilled at finding out what patients were coming in for and ensuring that Robert saw only those who had straightforward illnesses like flu or who needed a basic checkup or a repeat prescription for a chronic illness. By this time his voice had become very quiet—another PD symptom—and when he was writing his words became smaller and smaller until they could hardly be read. Fortunately, writing that was almost impossible to read was fairly standard for doctors, and the local pharmacist was able to interpret most of his prescriptions!

*****

Robert decided against joining the local PD support group, as he felt that would only depress him, but he keenly kept abreast of new research on PD via the Internet and medical library and through Peter, Dr. Bracken, and the neuropsychologist, who had now become an important support person. He became fascinated by the many famous people who had suffered from PD, and devoured books about the subject, especially those written by PD sufferers themselves. As PD is the second most common neurodegenerative disease after Alzheimer's disease, affecting 1 in 500 people in the population, with 1 in every 100 people over 60 years old suffering from it, the number of famous—and infamous—people with it didn't surprise Robert, and made him feel much more normal. It cheered him to know that the late Johnny Cash and the late Pope John Paul II, as well as the former US attorney general, Janet Reno, had risen above the disease to do great things. The boxer Muhammad Ali was probably a victim of PD, although his parkinsonian symptoms might be a case of pugilist's encephalopathy, or widespread brain damage caused by multiple head traumas. Certainly his severe hand tremor was apparent for the world to see when he lit the Olympic flame at the Olympic Games in Atlanta in 1996.

Robert read Oliver Sacks's book *Awakenings*, based on the story of a group of survivors of von Economo's encephalitis, the epidemic of viral encephalitis that began in Europe in 1918.[3] Some survivors developed what was known as "sleeping sickness," a severe form of PD, the main symptom of which was rigidity. Sacks's book dramatized the administration in 1966 of the then experimental drug levodopa to these sufferers, who had been frozen like statues for decades—resulting in their rapid "awakening" into walking, talking individuals. Sadly, as the effects of the medication wore off, the sufferers returned to their frozen state. Robert and Lillian borrowed the DVD of the 1990 film based on the book, starring Robin Williams and Robert De Niro, and Robert was amused to see the patients using some of the same tricks he used to help overcome his slowness in initiating movement, like swinging his arms back and forth a few times to begin walking. He thought he might try the trick shown in *Awakenings* where lines drawn on the floor like railroad ties provided the external visual stimulus the PD patients often needed to start walking. Once movement was initiated, often with great difficulty, it could become fluid and automatic for a brief period as long as there was no interruption to the flow, either by the person's consciously thinking about what he was doing or by someone or something else distracting him. But as the film neared its sad end, Robert and Lillian

[3] The Further Readings section at the end of this chapter gives full references for this book and the other books mentioned in the chapter.

sat in the dark with tears rolling down their faces as the "awakened" PD patients relapsed back into rigidity when the levodopa lost its effectiveness.

Robert was intrigued to discover that there was considerable evidence that Hitler was a PD sufferer: for example, as early as 1934, when he was only 45 years old, he had a left hand tremor. One theory is that he developed parkinsonism as a consequence of suffering from von Economo's encephalitis in 1918. By 1944 his symptoms were more marked and included tremor, bradykinesia, postural instability, a wooden facial expression, an increasingly quiet voice, and episodes of severe depression. It also seems likely that he was becoming severely cognitively impaired and possibly demented by the end of his life. The mental inflexibility associated with PD might well have been a factor in Hitler's slow response to the D-Day landings in Normandy in 1944, as he was convinced that the Allies would launch their attack at Calais. Hitler's Minister of Armaments, Albert Speer, wrote of Hitler in 1944, a year before he committed suicide: "Hitler was shriveling up like an old man. His limbs trembled, he walked stooped with dragging footsteps....His uniform, which in the past he kept scrupulously neat, was stained by the food he had eaten with a shaking hand."[4]

Robert even tracked down novels that included a main character with Parkinson's, often ones where the sufferer remained intellectually alert while struggling with a disobedient body. He was delighted when the book club he and Lillian belonged to decided to discuss Jonathan Franzen's *The Corrections* and Rohinton Mistry's *Family Matters* at their monthly meeting. They all agreed that the Parkinson's disease itself was not the central theme of these novels, but the way the symptoms of the disorder

[4]Stolk, P. J. 1968. Adolf Hitler: His life and his illness. *Psychiatria, Neurologia, Neurochirurgia, 71*, 381–398.

challenged the victim and his family were used as a pivot—or perhaps excuse—for family disarray and dysfunction. *The Corrections* centered on an all-American family, in contrast to *Family Matters*, which revolved around an Indian family living in Britain. However, in spite of the books being very different, both in style and in context, there were many similarities in the ways in which these two families from vastly different cultures tried to cope with and understand their parkinsonian relative. The descriptions of the sufferings of the PD victims, often from the point of view of the sufferers themselves, could be grueling but, as Robert said, gave a very accurate picture of what it was like to live with the disease. Lillian thought the struggles and emotions that the different family members went through when trying to empathize and put up with a progressively incapacitated elderly man seemed an accurate reflection of the situation in real life, although she added quickly that she had not found it too difficult yet dealing with "young" Robert!

For some reason, PD seemed to lend itself to literary endeavors, and Robert particularly enjoyed autobiographical accounts written by people with PD about their struggle with the disease. They invariably illustrated the deep involvement, both emotional and scientific, that many PD sufferers developed with their disease, as well as proving that many remain intellectually able in spite of it. He discovered that often the main theme of these memoirs was that of taking control of the symptoms, and the authors of these narratives accomplished this control in many creative ways. One book, *Injured Brains of Medical Minds: Views from Within*, included accounts of PD written by medical and health professionals and reflected many of his own feelings and thoughts. But his favorite memoir was *Ivan: Living with Parkinson's Disease*. The author, Ivan Vaughan, a college professor, showed his creativity in a way that Robert found moving, humorous, and informative, and he often reread bits of it when he needed a confidence boost or new ideas about how to take control of his own symptoms. For example, Ivan would time his medication to maximize the possibility that his drugs would be at their most effective when he was scheduled to give a lecture or perform some other social role.

And of course he purchased each of actor Michael J. Fox's autobiographical books as soon as it was published. Surely Fox's amazing efforts to raise the profile of PD and the funds to research it must be the ultimate example of taking control of the disease. This star of the TV show *Family Ties* and the *Back to the Future* movies had become the most prominent modern face of PD. In 1998 Fox revealed that he had been diagnosed seven years earlier—when he was just 30 years old—with young-onset PD. After disclosing his condition he committed himself to fighting it, and in the 10 years since the Michael J. Fox Foundation for Parkinson's Research was launched in 2000, over 200 million US dollars had been raised. The mission of the foundation—"to find a cure for PD through an aggressively funded research agenda and to ensure the development of improved therapies for those living with Parkinson's today"—gave Robert and his family hope. With such enthusiasm and the funding to support cutting-edge research, new therapeutic medications and surgical techniques were being developed regularly to treat the disease's symptoms, and in the not too distant future a cure, perhaps via gene transfer or genetic engineering, was a real possibility.

*****

Of course, Robert knew that his "honeymoon" period of being able to keep his parkinsonian symptoms under control to a reasonable degree with medication would not last forever. Sure enough, five years after his diagnosis, he began to experience one of the worst side effects of L-dopa treatment, the "on/off" syndrome. Some thirty minutes after taking his medication his arms and head would begin to writhe, and these *dyskinesias* would go on for about another thirty minutes. If he was lucky he would then enjoy about an hour of relative normality, but after that his parkinsonian symptoms would take over, and if he did not take his next dose in time he often found himself stuck, immobile in his chair. At this point he could no longer work as a GP. By now he had reached the age of 63, and because he and Lillian had made considerable efforts to put in place some additional investments when he was diagnosed with PD, he was in a good financial position to retire. The other two doctors in the practice were sad to see him go, but were able to buy Robert's share of the practice.

Relieved to have the responsibility of the practice off his shoulders, Robert now felt able to concentrate on coping with his ever-increasing disability and trying to ensure that he and Lillian also continued to enjoy some social life as well as enjoy time with their grandchildren. He followed a careful and healthy diet and made an effort to go for a walk every morning before breakfast. Unfortunately, this became increasingly difficult because of his rigidity in the morning, and he found he needed to wait one hour after taking his medication until his dyskinesias abated and then go for his walk before his rigidity took over. His walk was more of a shuffle and often he would end up shuffling faster and faster until he either fell over or collided with a wall. If he was particularly unlucky he would then freeze and have trouble getting up. This resulted in his younger son, Jack, joining him every morning for his walk. By this stage Robert's interest in surgical treatments for parkinsonian symptoms had begun to dominate his thoughts.

Currently these included the use of stereotactic functional neurosurgery to place a tiny lesion using heat (a radiofrequency lesion) unilaterally in either the part of the deep brain called the thalamus—a procedure called *thalamotomy*—or in the globus pallidus interna, a part of the basal ganglia—called a *pallidotomy*. These procedures were first introduced in the 1950s. Thalamotomy was used for the relief of tremor on the side opposite the surgical lesion and pallidotomy could reduce awkward movements—dyskinesias—bradykinesia, rigidity, and to some extent tremor, and was probably the more common operation. Sometimes both operations were carried out during the same procedure on the same side, and some PD sufferers underwent a second operation on the opposite side after an interval of three months or longer. With carefully selected, nondemented PD patients who no longer responded well to drugs, these operations could result in a dramatic and immediate cessation of symptoms that lasted for at least two years. Robert was excited by these treatments, especially pallidotomy, and tried to dismiss from his mind the caution that further longitudinal studies of pallidotomy were needed to assess the very long-term alleviation of parkinsonian symptoms, the effects of later carrying out a second operation on the other side of the brain, and possible unwanted side effects including permanent subtle cognitive deficits, especially in older patients.

He was even more hopeful about an even newer procedure called deep brain stimulation (DBS). This required a multielectrode lead to be implanted into part of the thalamus and connected to a pulse generator surgically implanted under the skin of the upper chest. To turn it on and off, the PD sufferer passed a handheld magnet over the chest. When the device was on, the thalamus was electrically stimulated, blocking the tremor; most sufferers turned the stimulator off overnight or when their tremor was not a problem. The very expensive battery needed replacing about every five years, requiring another small operation. Unfortunately, DBS could lead to some unpleasant side effects including tingling in the head and hands, depression, a slight paralysis, slurred speech, a loss of balance, and a loss of muscle tone. Current research was also experimenting on implanting a deep brain stimulator in other areas of the brain circuits implicated in PD, including the globus pallidus interna and the subthalamic nuclei. So far there had been some promising results, including reduction of bradykinesia, tremor, and dystonia.

Dr. Bracken agreed to enrol him in the assessment program for a pallidotomy, and to Robert's relief, he was pronounced a suitable candidate. After being on the waiting list for six months his day in the operating theater finally came, and he had a right-sided pallidotomy. The results were excellent. Robert's left-sided bradykinesia and rigidity were immediately much reduced, and he was able to decrease his medication so that his on/off syndrome was much less disabling. Though his voice remained quiet, to Lillian's delight the operation improved Robert's ability to show facial expressions; he had shown the world a very wooden face for the last three years. He now had a slightly lopsided expression, but she thought it very attractive when compared with his previous bland one. To celebrate Robert's newfound mobility, Lillian and Robert embarked on a two-month trip to England and Ireland to visit relatives and on the whole had a good time.

One year after the pallidotomy, Dr. Bracken asked Robert if he would like to try DBS on the left side of his brain to see if this would reduce his right-sided symptoms. Dr. Bracken was involved in a research trial of DBS of the subthalamic nuclei, and this meant that the operation, including the pulse generator and battery, would be funded through the research project. Robert gladly underwent the numerous research tests to see if he was a suitable candidate, including another of the dreaded neuropsychological assessments. Although this demonstrated some worsening of his previous cognitive problems as well as a new problem, a mild difficulty with new verbal learning, these were not considered bad enough to make him ineligible for the research trial, and he soon had his second day in the operating theater. He was well aware that he might suffer some side effects from the DBS and that it might take him a while to get the hang of it. Indeed, he did find that his speech became a little slurred when he turned on the pulse generator, but this was a minor price to pay for the ability he now had to "turn off" his tremor and reduce his bradykinesia and rigidity on his right side simply by waving a magnet—or magic wand as Robert called it—across his chest where the pulse generator was implanted.

Robert was well aware that the positive effects of his two surgical interventions might not last forever, and that in time his illness would probably result in his becoming wheelchair-bound. But on the bright side, there were many exciting therapeutic advances in the experimentation stage. In the surgical field, research was being carried out on ways to produce brain lesions in PD patients without opening the skull or using a scalpel. These nuclear techniques used tiny pulses of radiation to precisely target and destroy the same neurons destroyed in pallidotomy and thalamotomy operations, aided by 3-D computerized images of the brain. These methods could not yet produce clearly defined brain lesions, but in time would be able to improve on the more invasive neurosurgical procedures Robert underwent when he had his pallidotomy.

The news contained frequent mentions of other techniques like implantation of dopamine-producing cells from the human fetal brain into the brains of PD patients and the use of transplanted stem cells. Of course there were difficult ethical issues involved in using human fetal material, and to circumvent these, researchers were exploring the use of other sources of transplant tissue, including the transplantation of tissues from other animals into humans. This brought with it another set of problems: The rejection of the transplanted tissue by the recipient had to be overcome, and the possibility that viruses might be transferred from the donor animals to humans had to be considered. But clinical trials were already in progress where PD sufferers in the advanced stages of the disease received fetal neural cells from pathogen-free pigs.

In the more distant future—probably too late for Robert—genetic engineering was likely to play a major role in the treatment and even the cure of PD. Perhaps designer cells producing dopamine and other neurotransmitters relevant to PD would be developed over the next few years. Genetically engineered neural growth factors able to prevent the degeneration of dopaminergic neurons might be injected into the PD sufferer or drip-fed via implantable pumps directly into the cerebrospinal fluid in the ventricles of the brain.

But for now, Robert felt blessed by the fact that at 65, seven years after his diagnosis, his cognitive impairments, while certainly more marked than previously, were still largely restricted to visuospatial and mental flexibility problems, with his verbal memory being, in his opinion, not much worse than the memory of many of his friends of advancing age! As far as Robert was concerned, he had not lost the abilities most important for his quality of life: he was still able to enjoy reading, listening to music, and playing with his grandchildren, and with careful planning of his medication, could even occasionally make love to his wife. And on that positive note, we will leave Robert and Lillian enjoying their retirement, one day at a time.

■ Further Reading

Fox, M. J. 2002. *Lucky Man: A Memoir.* New York: Hyperion.
Fox, M. J. 2009. *Always Looking Up: The Adventures of an Incurable Optimist.* New York: Hyperion.

Franzen, J. 2001. *The Corrections*. London: 4th Estate.

Kapur, N., ed. 1997. *Injured Brains of Medical Minds: Views From Within*. Oxford: Oxford University Press.

Mistry, R. 2002. *Family Matters*. London: Faber & Faber.

Ogden, J. A. 2005. Mind over matter. Coping with Parkinson's disease. In: *Fractured Minds: A Case-Study Approach to Clinical Neuropsychology, 2nd Ed.* (pp. 254–275). New York: Oxford University Press.

Sacks, O. 1991. *Awakenings (Revised Edition)*. London: Picador.

Vaughan, I. 1986. *Ivan: Living with Parkinson's Disease*. London: Macmillan.

13 ■
Hard, Ain't It Hard: A Family's Fight with Huntington's Disease

Christine's childhood was about as good as it gets. She was the eldest of four children, and the family lived in a beautiful home with large gardens overlooking a river in a leafy suburb of Melbourne. Her father, Paul, was a successful architect, and Helen, her mother, was a homemaker in every sense of the word, having willingly given up her teaching position when Christine was born in 1945. With the births of Mark, Sara, and David over the next nine years, Helen had her hands full, although Paul—a man well ahead of his time—cooked meals on the weekends, washed dishes, and took his wife away from her mothering and domestic roles for a week of golfing or skiing at least once a year. The family traveled to England and Europe on two extended trips when the children were still school age, and every summer they would set off on a three-week camping and hiking trip in the Australian bush, giving Paul the opportunity to pass his enormous love and knowledge of the wilderness onto his offspring. Christine remembers him as the rock of the family, very warm and loving, free-spirited, and full of energy and joy.

Paul's life hadn't always been so privileged. Born in 1915, he was the eldest of four brothers. The family was poor, and after Paul's father died in his early forties, his mother struggled to bring up the four boys alone. According to the death certificate, Paul's father died of malaria contracted as a young man working in New Guinea, although in retrospect there were indications of possible neurological problems in the months before his death. Paul trained as a teacher, and he and Helen married when Paul was 25. When World War II was declared, he went to war, and he was discharged in 1943 with a badly damaged leg. He decided to retrain as an architect, which he did by attending university part-time while still working as a teacher. Christine was born when he was at university. By the time she was eight and had two siblings, Paul had earned a reputation as one of the most sought-after architects in Melbourne, and they had moved into their beautiful home by the river.

When Christine was 17 and her father in his late forties, Paul's personality began to change. He became increasingly solitary and withdrew from his friends and even from his family. Most obvious and upsetting were his sudden explosive rages precipitated by trivial incidents that previously would not have concerned him at all. For example, Christine recalled an occasion when her father smashed a milk bottle on the table in front of the children just because her brother had used the last of the milk, leaving none for Paul's cup of tea. After these explosions Paul would quickly return to his normal, stable self, leaving the family shaken and upset. Nine-year-old David still occasionally wet his bed at night, and if this occurred when Paul was tired or stressed he would sometimes take a belt to his son; previously physical punishment was unheard of in this family. Helen often took the brunt of Paul's rages and their marriage was now under serious strain.

All four children were very bright and did exceptionally well at school. Christine entered medical school when she was 18, but when she was 20 the family's financial situation changed dramatically. Paul had complete control of the family finances and gave Helen a weekly allowance for domestic spending. Thus it came as a shock when their bank contacted her with the news that they were deeply in debt. After some investigation it became apparent that for the past three years Paul had earned no income, and his costs to run his architect's office as well as the family's costs had been coming out of their savings. Every day Paul had been dressing in his suit and driving to his office, where he sat all day, doing nothing. He had dismissed his secretary and no one had realized his predicament. So his office was closed down, and, still only 52, Paul found himself officially "retired." Fortunately, the house was in Helen's name and mortgage-free, and the family was able to remain there. But when Helen revealed she was looking for a teaching position, Paul exploded, and fearful for her and the children's safety, she gave up her efforts. To add to the family's stress, Paul was at this time diagnosed with a lymphoma, which was treated successfully with radiotherapy through his neck. This didn't help his behavior, which grew steadily worse. Sometimes he was his normal, affectionate old self, but then, without obvious cause, he would become apathetic and withdrawn, or he would erupt in a violent rage, sometimes physically attacking Helen. No cajoling or tears from his family would move him from his stubborn refusal to see a doctor or get any help.

Frightened by her father's increasingly violent rages and personality change, in desperation Christine telephoned a professor of psychiatry at her university to ask his advice. She did not know the professor personally, but had attended a lecture he gave where he showed a therapy video of himself with a psychiatric patient. His compassionate attitude on the video had impressed Christine, and thus she was distraught when he responded to her initial explanation about her situation with an abrupt statement that he hadn't time to discuss students' personal problems and rudely terminated the conversation. As Christine said to me many years later, he could at the very least have given her the name of a health professional she could contact. Christine never forgot that feeling of being pushed aside and left alone, and made a silent pact with herself that when she qualified as a doctor she would always listen very carefully to her patients' concerns and take special care with young people, never turning them away when they needed time and support.

Mark, four years younger than Christine, was the most academically gifted of the four children. At 18, in his first year at university, he received exceptionally high marks in all his courses. But in his second year, Helen received a letter from one of Mark's tutors telling her that his essays were "gobbledygook" and she should try and find out what was going on. She took Mark to a psychiatrist, who diagnosed him with paranoid schizophrenia, admitted him to a psychiatric hospital, and told Helen that she could not see him or contact him for six months, as his schizophrenia was rooted in a dysfunctional relationship with her. Not long after this, following a dreadful scene when Paul tried to strangle Helen, Christine called the psychiatric crisis team, a free service set up to respond to difficult situations involving people with psychiatric conditions. When the crisis team arrived at the door Paul sent them away, telling them they were trespassing. It was time for Helen to leave for her own safety, and she rented an apartment for herself and the two younger children, Sara, now aged 17, and David, 14. Helen never saw Paul again, and although she was able to build a new life for herself and return to her teaching career, she was dogged with feelings of guilt, especially because her children had to take on the full burden of caring for and coping with their father.

Christine tried to get on with her own life, and after graduating from medical school she married Stephen. Eighteen months later their son, Ian, was born. In spite of her busy schedule Christine kept in close contact with her family, now scattered and in deep trouble. She, along with Sara and David, visited Mark at the psychiatric hospital regularly, reporting back to Helen, who was desperate to see him but remained banned in accordance with the backward thinking of that time. Mark improved somewhat on medication and after six months was transferred to a halfway house. Although he coped reasonably well some of the time, he became a regular user of marijuana and alcohol. Most of his good friends faded out of his life, but one staunch mate found him a small apartment close to a biscuit factory, where Mark was able to obtain a simple job. The routine of walking to the factory every day and working kept him on a reasonably even keel for two years, but then his alcoholism resulted in his dismissal.

Left to himself, Paul did nothing in the house or garden and his home became a hovel. Christine took leave from her medical practice and with her three-month-old son moved in for three months to try to tidy it up. Paul barred anyone else from entering the property and continued to refuse to see a doctor or go into the hospital. Christine thought that he must have sustained some brain damage when he received the radiation treatment for his lymphoma, but was unable to get this checked out owing to her father's intransigence. Around this time, when her father was 55, she noticed that he had a tremor, but again thought this must be a consequence either of his radiation therapy or perhaps secondary tumors seeded from his lymphoma.

After Christine returned from staying with her father, Stephen's job took the family overseas for a year—a year when they were able to put aside the responsibilities of looking out for Paul and Mark, freeing them to enjoy their small son, now joined by a baby sister, Jill. On their rather reluctant return to Australia, within minutes of stepping inside her childhood home it became apparent to Christine that her father's condition had deteriorated. Although he was able to hold an intelligent conversation and was still quite mobile, Paul now walked with a wide-based gait and had quite significant *dysarthria*—slurred speech as a result of poor muscle control—which made it difficult for people who were not used to him to understand him. Although she was reluctant to voice her fears, Christine was beginning to suspect her father had Huntington's disease, and that this might explain Mark's psychiatric symptoms as well.

With Sara and David still in Melbourne and able to keep an eye on their father and Mark, Christine and Stephen moved to a town about a hundred miles from Melbourne, where Christine joined a general practice. It wasn't until Paul was 60 that Christine was finally able to confirm his diagnosis. She managed to get her stubborn father, now suffering from spontaneous writhing movements—*chorea*—as well as tremor, to stay with them for a holiday. While he was there, she had him surreptitiously "diagnosed" by a neurologist friend who came to their home for dinner. He had no doubt that Paul was suffering from Huntington's disease, and Christine was now convinced that this would also explain Mark's illness. Paul continued to refuse any formal examination or tests, and denied that he had a problem.

*****

As a doctor, Christine knew that Huntington's disease (HD) was a chronic, progressive hereditary disease typified by a number of motor abnormalities, most obviously the excessive, irregular movements called chorea, and that a progressive decline to a severe dementia was almost inevitable if the patient lived long enough. As a GP Christine had never treated a HD patient, but now she wanted to know everything about the condition.

She found that HD was the focus of one of the most remarkable stories of discovery in medical history. In 1872 George Huntington, a North American general practitioner, published the first unambiguous description of the unrelenting neurodegenerative disorder in *The Medical and Surgical Reporter*.[1] The title of his article was simply "On Chorea," and his description of this type of chorea as a specific hereditary disorder became quickly and widely accepted. Careful pedigrees of generations of HD families around the world have since confirmed his theory by documenting that half of the children of a parent with HD will also develop HD if they live long enough. That is, HD is an *autosomal dominant hereditary disorder*.

Simply put, HD is caused when one gene (or allele) of a usually healthy gene pair we all carry is abnormally elongated. This HD gene mutation is dominant, so that anyone who carries it will develop HD. Each child has a 50% chance of inheriting the mutated allele from a parent who has it, even if the parent has not yet developed any HD symptoms. On the bright side, the child also has a 50% chance of inheriting the HD parent's healthy allele, in which case the child will never develop HD and will never pass it on. Until it is known for certain whether or not a descendant of a person with HD has inherited the HD mutation that individual is said to be "at risk." When Christine's father was diagnosed with HD, her risk for developing HD became 50%, and each of her children immediately became at risk as well, but their risk was 25%.

[1] Huntington, G. 1872. On Chorea. *Medical and Surgical Reporter, 26*, 320–321.

If Christine were to develop HD symptoms and be diagnosed with the disease, her children's risk would increase to 50%. If Christine had predictive genetic testing before showing any symptoms and discovered that she did carry her father's mutated HD allele, her risk of developing HD would increase to 100% and her children's risk to 50%. The hoped-for outcome of course would be that predictive testing would show that Christine had inherited her father's healthy allele and not his mutated one, in which case her risk would reduce to zero and all her descendants would also be at zero risk.

Prior to the availability of a specific molecular genetic predictive test for HD, neuropathology at autopsy was the accepted gold standard for its firm diagnosis. The primary anatomic finding is a generalized shrinkage of the brain with cell loss in the corpus striatum, part of the basal ganglia lying deep within the brain. This cell death results in altered neurotransmitter levels, including reduced levels of the inhibitory neurotransmitter GABA (gamma-aminobutyric acid). Because of the basal ganglia involvement, the most obvious symptoms of HD are severe abnormal motor movements, some of which are similar to those seen in Parkinson's disease (PD), although PD is caused by cell loss in a different part of the basal ganglia, the substantia nigra.[2] As HD progresses, other parts of the brain are affected, including the cortex, and especially the frontal cortex. In addition, the connections between the basal ganglia and the prefrontal cortex are damaged, resulting in patients experiencing ever-worsening "executive" impairments, such as difficulties in abstract thinking and planning ahead, and problems shifting their thoughts from one topic to another.

Chorea is the most common and prominent motor symptom and is usually among the earliest symptoms to

[2] Read more about Parkinson's disease in Chapter 12.

develop. These random and abrupt movements usually progress over the course of the disease from restlessness with only a mild, intermittent exaggeration of expression and gesture, to fidgeting movements of the hands, to an unstable, writhing, dance-like gait, or a continuous flow of disabling, violent, "crazy-looking" movements. Sustained muscle contractions resulting in twisting, repetitive movements, and abnormal postures—called *dystonias*—are also common. Tremor can occur in HD, although this is more often associated with PD. Other motor abnormalities that HD and PD have in common are rigidity and *bradykinesia*—a slowness of movement—that can result in freezing, a terrible symptom where the HD patient is unable to move. Gait abnormalities are obvious in patients who have had HD for some years, with a wide-based staggering gait being a common feature.

Eye movement abnormalities occur early in the disease in most patients and gradually worsen. Patients have difficulty in initiating eye movements (*saccades*) within the field of vision and show a decrease in saccade velocity. They are often unable to suppress blinks and head movements during saccades, and the accuracy of saccades is also impaired, resulting in undershooting of the target. Dysarthrias like Paul's slurred speech are common, and early in the disease speech rate and rhythm is often abnormal, worsening over time until speech becomes unintelligible. Some patients become mute even before their motor disability is very severe. *Dysphagia*—abnormal ingestion—is another distressing and common symptom, and can involve inappropriate selection of food, inappropriate rate of eating, retention of food in the mouth after swallowing, regurgitation, choking, and asphyxia.

In the latter stages of HD serious loss of weight and muscle bulk occur in spite of an adequate diet and feeding. This is not simply the result of constant excessive movement but appears to be an integral aspect of HD.

Fortunately, choreic movements largely cease during sleep, although in the latter stages of HD the patient may be sleepy during the day and wakeful at night. In the final stage, patients are severely physically disabled and demented, and thus totally dependent on others. About twenty percent of HD patients become incontinent near the end. Death usually results from a combination of weight loss, immobility, a tendency to aspirate food, and an increased vulnerability to pneumonia, cardiovascular disease, and other diseases.

Nearly all patients with HD experience psychiatric symptoms. Depression is common, especially in the early stage of HD when the patient is fully aware of their condition and their grim and unalterable prognosis. Suicide rates are almost four times higher than in the healthy population. Many other psychiatric and behavioral problems are also common; the vast majority of HD sufferers regularly show signs of one or more of *dysphoria* (low mood), agitation, irritability, apathy, anxiety, *disinhibition* (an inability to inhibit inappropriate behaviors), and euphoria. Delusions and hallucinations are problems for a small number of HD patients. Other symptoms that cause concern for families, and which probably often arise from the psychiatric symptoms already mentioned, include moodiness, aggression, violent behaviors, hypersexuality, paranoid suspicions, lying, stealing, a loss of interest in personal appearance, marked self-neglect, and mutism. There is no clear evidence that any of these neuropsychiatric symptoms correlate significantly with the severity of dementia or chorea or with disease duration, and it may be that other factors, including *premorbid* personality characteristics (personality traits the individual had before showing outward signs of HD), contribute to the presence and severity of affective symptoms. As the patient becomes more demented and loses insight, apathy may increase and depression decrease.

There is considerable overlap between the cognitive symptoms typical of HD, PD, and Alzheimer's disease. PD and HD are similar with respect to some of the executive difficulties their sufferers experience, but HD patients also demonstrate a deficit in skill learning not found in PD, as well as severe memory deficits more similar to those seen in Alzheimer's disease than to those of PD. In HD the cognitive impairments worsen and gradually spread to more areas of cognition as the atrophy of both subcortical and cortical structures becomes more widespread. Neuropsychological testing becomes increasingly difficult and probably pointless as the motor symptoms and psychiatric and behavioral problems, especially apathy, increase. Thus quite soon in the disease neuropsychological testing may be limited to gathering a gross measure of deterioration with the use of dementia scales, and patients may remain severely demented for years until death, on average about fifteen years after the first HD symptoms become apparent.

In the grand scheme of things, HD is a rare disease, occurring in about one to five people in every 100,000, with an equal likelihood of affecting males and females, although its prevalence varies across countries and ethnicities. But for a disease like HD, caused entirely by genetic inheritance, statistics like these aren't very useful given that they don't highlight the fact that the disease is restricted to family groups. Christine was already discovering that HD is more than a gene mutation; it is a family matter that challenges families in every way. The physical, psychological, social, and economic stresses on every member of an HD family are enormous and unrelenting. Not only do all family members have to live for many years with the knowledge that they or their relatives might develop the disease; they must also watch and care for their grandparents, parents, and sometimes their children as they struggle through the stages of HD.

Christine was both saddened and heartened to read about the experiences of these stresses on Marjorie Guthrie, the wife of the iconic American folksinger, Woody Guthrie, who developed HD symptoms around 1952 and died in 1967, when he was only 55. Following Woody's death, his widow founded the Committee to Combat Huntington's Disease, which led to the formation of the Huntington's Disease Society of America. The aim of this society is to promote education, research, and services for families of HD sufferers. The current research on HD is exciting and advancing rapidly, and there is hope that in the future this disease might be treatable, and with predictive testing of the fetus now available, that it will be more frequently prevented from passing down through the generations. But in the meantime, HD families could well take Woody Guthrie's classic blues "Hard, Ain't It Hard" as their anthem.

*****

For Christine, Mark was proving to be an even greater problem than Paul as Mark's HD symptoms worsened, fueled by alcohol and marijuana. The disgusting state of his apartment finally became too much for the landlord and neighbors to ignore, and Mark was thrown out. He decided to go back home to live with his father, which, given Paul's poor health and the state of the house, was an even greater nightmare for Christine. The two men were incapable of caring for themselves or each other, and as Helen was banned from the house she couldn't help. On one occasion two men broke into the house and sexually abused Mark while Paul sat in his deck chair outside in the garden, gazing at the river. Even later, when he was told about the rape by Christine, Paul appeared unaffected by his son's distress.

Christine often wondered whether her father's refusal to venture outside his lonely house and garden was his way of protecting himself from the hurtful prejudice that HD victims frequently have to suffer. Perhaps he had been embarrassed and shamed too many times. Even before his motor symptoms were severe and when his mind was still quite sharp, he had been accused of being drunk and disorderly. On one occasion when Christine, Stephen, and their two small children were staying with him, Paul suggested he take the children for a walk in their double baby stroller. The house was in a very quiet street, it was a beautiful day, and the baby stroller helped Paul's stability, so Christine thought it would be a nice bonding experience for her father and his grandchildren. When Paul had not returned in an hour, Christine and Stephen went to look for him, but to no avail; he had disappeared. After they'd searched for Christine's lost father and babies for a number of hours and telephoned hospitals and police, a police sergeant who knew Paul recognized him as the man being held in their suburban police station. It transpired that a policeman had seen him with the baby stroller in the small park at the end of the street and had thought that he was drunk. He and the children had been held in the police station while the police attempted to find out who they were. Because of Paul's slurred speech, they could not understand him when he tried to explain who he was. Apparently communication between suburban police stations in Melbourne was not very efficient; while police were out searching in one area, Paul was locked up as a drunken vagrant in another.

After that, Christine knew to check out individual police stations as well as hospitals when her father or brother disappeared. Mark was frequently picked up by the police, and at times the family spent 24 hours or more searching for him before they discovered him in a police cell. The worst incident occurred when he was arrested for armed robbery after his car was found abandoned in a seedy part of town. It was some days and a court appearance later before fingerprints at the scene of the crime were found to belong to a known violent offender and Mark was released. As Christine discovered when she befriended other HD families, it is common for the police to pick up HD sufferers, assuming they are drunk.

Christine was never happy seeing her father isolated in his big house, and one weekend, not long before he died, she and Stephen bundled Paul into the car with the children and set off for a weekend break at the coast. They had booked a motel right on the beach and thought the sea air and sun would do them all good. But shortly after their arrival at the motel, Paul fell through the plateglass window, cutting himself, but fortunately not too badly. Christine cleaned and stitched up his wounds but Paul was very upset and insisted that they couldn't stay there. They put their bags back in the car and went to the motel office to explain about the broken window and give the proprietor a check that would more than cover the replacement cost. In front of Paul and the children the proprietor let fly with abusive language, shouting at them that he knew he should never have let them stay in the first place with their crazy father. The family drove off with Christine in tears, Stephen angry, and the children upset.

In an attempt to pacify the children, after about an hour's drive they stopped at a café (where they had never been before) in a small town so that the children could have a milkshake and ice cream. Carrie, the sole woman running the café, greeted them warmly and asked them if they would like some lunch. Christine explained that her father had a motor disorder that prevented him from eating any food that was not pureed. On hearing this Carrie sat down with Paul and asked him what his favorite foods were. He replied—with some surprise no doubt—that he loved liver pâté, whereupon Carrie bustled out to the kitchen and made him a delicious pureed liver pâté, as well as pureed fruit salad to follow. She then sat down with them and chatted away to the children while Christine concentrated on feeding Paul, then talked to Paul while the family ate their lunch. By this stage Paul's speech was very slurred, but Carrie concentrated on what he was saying and managed to carry on a perfectly normal conversation with him. The family left, warmed by this other side of human nature and knowing that their memories of this abbreviated weekend break would no longer hold quite so much pain. The memory of Carrie's compassionate and normal interactions at a time when they were desperately needed still brings a lump to Christine's throat more than thirty years later.

Paul never admitted that he had Huntington's disease and continued to refuse all medical help. Finally, when he was almost bedridden, his children were forced to have him committed, and this scared and stubborn man had to be forcibly removed from his house into an ambulance by the police. He spent three weeks in a ward for chronic psychiatric patients, where he continued to refuse all help. He then suffered a stroke and was transferred to a nursing home. He wouldn't eat and died six weeks later at the age of 63. A postmortem showed the brain pathology typical of HD.

*****

When Paul died, Helen was able to sell the house and buy a small apartment for Mark close to an outpatient psychiatric facility. He went there daily for therapy sessions as well as to Alcoholics Anonymous, although he was never able to remain sober for long. He was helped by the social worker at the psychiatric unit, as well as by a music therapist with whom he established a good relationship. But finally this too failed as his behavior became increasingly erratic and motor problems began to show. Helen, now in her late sixties, took him into her apartment to care for him. Mark was 6 foot 2 inches, and although extremely thin and by now very weak, was very difficult for Helen to handle. But her apartment was close to a beach, which he loved, and he would spend long hours swimming and sunbathing in the sand dunes. Mark still retained much of his sense of fun, and when he was feeling relaxed and not plagued by the dreadful fatigue that is so debilitating for HD patients he almost seemed like the witty Mark who had achieved so much in his first year at university.

At this point Christine was desperately trying to find a nursing home that would take him, but with no success. HD patients have very specific nursing needs and none of the nursing homes had the appropriately trained staff or facilities to cope with relatively young mobile patients with psychiatric problems, whose severe motor problems put them in constant danger. The Huntington's Disease Association worked with her to find a suitable nursing home, and finally, after years of struggle, they were able to set up a special ward in a single-story building on the grounds of a general hospital. Mark spent four days a week in the final three years of his life in there, going to stay with Christine or his other sister for three days each week. Christine felt these visits were essential for his well-being, but they were very difficult for the family, as Mark was up all night, was incontinent, and had to be fed pureed food.

In the last year of his life, Mark was mute, blind, and wheelchair-bound. At this point a very difficult decision had to be made about whether to insert a feeding tube directly into his stomach. The purpose of this was to enable the nurses to feed him easily and quickly with a high-calorie substance, as feeding him by mouth at this point with sufficient pureed food to keep him alive took about three hours a day, clearly not possible for busy nurses. The negative side of the feeding tube is that it delays death long past the time when the patient has any quality of life, and indeed has been reduced to a vegetative state. Patients in the final stage of HD usually die from choking—which is why they must be fed with pureed food or gel—from respiratory illnesses such as pneumonia that develop as they become increasingly emaciated, weaker and immobile, or from malnutrition or heart failure. The family made a joint decision that their HD family members would not have feeding tubes inserted, so that they would not suffer the pain and indignity of having their lives prolonged artificially. So for the last years of Mark's life Helen visited twice every day to spend ninety minutes carefully feeding pureed foods to her son—the same son she had once been banned from seeing, accused of dysfunctional mothering and causing her boy's psychiatric problems. When Mark died of pneumonia at the age of 39, the family's grief was tempered with relief that he was finally at rest.

But Helen had one more difficult decision thrust upon her. Within an hour of Mark's death she was shaken by a telephone call from someone she had never spoken to before, asking her without any prior discussion or warning if she would release Mark's body parts for research purposes. Hopefully researchers and clinicians today are no longer this irresponsible and take care to explain research projects at an appropriate time and in a sensitive manner, well before the patient's death, giving ample time for the HD patient and family to consider whether they wish to be involved. Many HD families become participants in research on HD at some point, and this can be rewarding. Most clinical researchers are compassionate and very sensitive, but a small minority of researchers forget that for the family there is a loved person behind what to the researcher may simply be an exciting investigative opportunity.

*****

In common with a number of other medical conditions, the stimulus for setting up research and support institutions for HD came initially from individuals who had themselves been personally affected by the disease. The Hereditary Disease Foundation, which promotes research into HD, was started by Dr. Milton Wexler after his wife died from HD and is continued by his daughter, Dr. Nancy Wexler. The foundation has played a central role in the remarkable study that began in 1979 of a large HD population living by the shores of Lake Maracaibo in Venezuela. This group is the best example of how quickly a dominantly inherited genetic disorder can take over a small, isolated community. Painstaking research has revealed that one ancestor with HD who lived in the early 1800s has so far left more than 18 thousand descendants, 14 thousand of whom are still alive today and many of whom have HD or are at risk for it. This detailed and unique pedigree was a crucial factor in locating, in 1983, the approximate location of the gene involved in HD.[3] In 1993 after further painstaking work by many research groups in the US and UK, a group lead by Harvard Medical School researcher, James Gusella's isolated the precise causal gene and identified the mutation of this gene that causes the disease.[4] At this point an expanded group, called the Huntington's Disease Collaborative Research Group, published its findings.[5] This group was a collaboration of six US and British research teams, and although Gusella's team isolated the gene, the credit was rightly given to the entire collaboration, as the research that preceded the gene's precise identification was an essential aspect of the discovery. This truly collaborative effort is a superb example of how medical and

[3]Wexler, N. S., Young A. B., and Tanzi R. E. 1987. Homozygotes for Huntington's disease. *Nature, 326,* 194—197.

[4]A book written in 1995 by Alice Wexler provides the background to this project and describes the activities of the Hereditary Disease Foundation from the perspective of the Wexler family. The complete reference is in the Further Reading section at the end of this chapter.

[5]Huntington's Disease Collaborative Research Group. 1993. A novel gene containing a trinucleotide repeat that is expanded and unstable on Huntington's Disease chromosomes. *Cell, 72,* 971–983.

other scientific research should be—a cooperative endeavor motivated by the determination to find the truth and make a difference, not by competition and the desire for personal aggrandizement.

*****

One year after Mark's death, Christine became aware that her youngest brother, 35-year-old David, was showing HD symptoms. David was an adventurer and a journalist, a job that enabled him to work overtime for nine months of the year and then take three months off to travel the world. He had been very close to Mark and spent long hours with him throughout his illness. His relationships with women tended to be brief, in many cases ending soon after he introduced his girlfriend to Mark and explained about the Huntington's gene. But he did form one serious relationship, and Lucy, his partner, on discovering she was pregnant, decided to go ahead and have the baby, fully aware that the child could carry the HD gene. Lucy and David's relationship was over before their son, Patrick, was born, but David saw him on a regular basis, and he and Patrick developed a strong father–son relationship over the first 12 years of Patrick's life.

It was when Christine was looking at a video taken at Christmas of David mowing the lawn and playing with her children that she first noticed a subtle movement disorder. That night, she suggested the two of them go for a stroll in the balmy evening air, and, trying to hold back her tears, she gently told him of her suspicions. Deep down, David had been aware that he was having trouble with tremor and choreic movements, especially when he was tired. But with Christine's observations confirming it, denial was no longer an option for this intelligent and gutsy man. For a while he did give in to depression, but he soon forced himself to face up to the disease and do whatever he could to stay healthy and happy, if only for his young son. He managed to hang on to his job for another three years even as his symptoms escalated. He stubbornly refused to stop driving in spite of numerous minor accidents, because he relied on his car for his independence. Perhaps this uncharacteristically selfish behavior was an early sign of the executive problems—poor insight, not learning from his mistakes, concrete thinking—that soon became more obvious as David's ability to organize himself and to plan ahead became severely impaired. At one particularly low time, he obtained a copy of a book that gave instructions for committing suicide, but his executive functions were so poor by then that he was unable to work out how to put these instructions into practice.

Yet like Mark and his father when they were severely disabled, if he was interested in a topic—in David's case, current affairs, politics, and journalism—and he liked the person talking with him, David could converse at a high level. He retained his sense of fun and his wit but he also retained his stubbornness, a trait no doubt inherited from his father. He did not want to live with his mother and so remained alone in a fourth-floor apartment. He refused any help, including "meals on wheels," assistance with housekeeping, or visits by social workers. If his sisters brought him prepared meals he would refuse to open the door, and when they had gone he would retrieve the meal and throw it in the trash. On the positive side, unlike many HD victims, including his brother, he did not try to alleviate his suffering with alcohol or drugs, although he smoked heavily, an ongoing danger in his filthy apartment stacked high with old newspapers.

Christine tried to convince him that he must live with either her or her sister for his own safety and their peace of mind. His response was to lock himself in his apartment for three weeks, after which time Christine was convinced he must have died, as no amount of knocking and calling to him brought forth any sound. The family were forced to take out a guardianship bond that would allow the health authorities to remove him—if he were still alive—to a psychiatric ward for four days once a month so that he and his apartment could be cleaned up. This involved a very public procedure of using a cherry picker to get a fireman and a male psychiatric nurse in through his window. He was brought out alive but kicking and screaming and accusing Christine of letting him down, while she was in tears on the street below.

Once a month this scene was repeated. On his second stay in the psychiatric ward David escaped and hitchhiked five miles back to his apartment, which was being sprayed with pesticide. The sprayer told him he couldn't stay there, as the fumes would do him in. His reply—that he would just sit in the apartment while the spraying continued—resulted in the sprayer's leaving and yet another "HD crisis call" to Christine. Once again she had to catch a flight to Melbourne to sort out the situation, and rely on her partner in her medical practice to see her patients, and on her husband to take care of their children. The HD ward where Mark had ended his days had been shut down by the local government, which needed the land for further development. This had caused a great deal of anguish for the local branch of the Huntington's Disease Association as its members, including Christine and her sister Sara, had put a great deal of time, money, and care into the facility and into the gardens surrounding it, as well as training the staff in the specialist skills required to care for HD patients. It was a relief for Christine and Sara when they finally found another good nursing home for David, who was becoming demented and less mobile.

For the ten years prior to his death, David was unable to care for himself. He spent his last two years immobile on his back, mute, choking on food, and able to use only his eyes to follow his caregivers' movements. This "locked in" state was agony for his family, as it was impossible to know how much he could understand, whether he was in pain, or how they might be able to help him. As she did for her eldest son, in his final years Helen visited David twice a day to sit with him and feed him with gel. He died from pneumonia when he was 49, and at his funeral Helen wondered if this was how so many women in the world wars felt as first their husbands and then their sons died in battle.

*****

For advocates of voluntary euthanasia, HD must provide a clear case for careful consideration. Some people at risk of developing HD or in the early clinical stages of the disease might welcome the legal right to request euthanasia when they reach the final stage of the disease. The problem is, of course, that they could not be considered mentally fit to make this decision at that stage, and thus the decision would have to be made well in advance. The right to have their lives ended with some dignity might relieve some of the psychological stress and anxiety suffered by at-risk and confirmed HD victims, and so could reduce the inflated incidence of suicide and "accidental" deaths in HD families.

Although few asymptomatic family members would be willing to admit to themselves or others that they too would be relieved if euthanasia for their affected family members were legal, nevertheless it seems likely that many family caregivers would prefer this alternative to the current situation of watching their loved ones struggling on through the final stages of HD. These complex ethical issues are of course bound up in moral, religious, spiritual, and cultural beliefs, which serves only to highlight the point that decisions about euthanasia must be made freely and autonomously by the HD sufferer early in the disease course or before symptoms emerge.

The difficult ethical and moral dilemmas that face Huntington's families are seemingly endless. Euthanasia is, for most families, not a real possibility, although this will surely change over time as more countries make it legal. But in most Western cultures, individuals are legally—if not religiously—permitted control over whether or not they should have children, and for a couple who knows that one of them may—or perhaps even does—harbor the Huntington's gene, whether to have children is an immense decision. Christine's first two children were born before she knew her father had HD. When she realized she was pregnant again, five years after her daughter was born, her first thought was that she must have an abortion. By now she knew her father and Mark had HD, that her chance of getting it was 50%, and that her children had a 25% chance of having the mutated HD gene. When Christine shared her concerns with Stephen, he simply asked her if she would have this baby if she knew for certain she didn't have the HD gene. When she nodded mutely, with tears in her eyes, he put his hand on her stomach and said, "The chance of this baby NOT having HD is 75%, and even if he—or she—does draw the short straw, he might not show any symptoms until he is old, and by then researchers might well have discovered how to treat or even cure it."

Back then there was no predictive test for HD, and years later, when a test that did not require samples from family members who had HD and were still alive did become available, Christine's children were growing up. After thinking all the issues through and discussing them with her mother, husband, and sister, Christine and her sister Sara both decided not to have the test at that time. The possibility of either one's being found to have the HD gene was too painful, and the family thought that coping with this in their future would be unbearable on top of caring for Mark and David. When the children reached their teens, Christine offered to have the predictive test so that they would have more certainty on which to base their own decisions about having children of their own. They told her that coping would become impossible for them if they found out that their mother was going to develop HD, and they would rather not know.

All three children grew up with HD relatives and had always been very accepting and natural with their grandfather and their uncles, visiting Mark and David in their nursing homes right up until their deaths. As Christine said with a wry smile, their youngest son was 27 before the family celebrated a Christmas without a family member who had HD. To balance the stress of living with the possibility that Christine might develop HD, Christine and Stephen tried to live as normal a life as possible, and as a result their children did not concern themselves unduly with worrying about what might be. Every member of the family lived life to the full, perhaps a result of harboring the "free-spirited" gene that seemed dominant not only in Christine's gene pool but also in Stephen's.

*****

David's son, Patrick, was the first member of the family to make the difficult decision to have the predictive blood test. Sadly, his test came back positive, increasing his risk from 50% to 100%. After finding out his results, Patrick required counseling for many months while he struggled with depression as well as with high-risk behaviors, including one major car accident when he crashed into a wall on a straight road. Whether this was a suicide attempt was not clear. But with the help of good counseling and finding a partner who wanted to be with him in spite of his HD status, he decided it was time to move on and live life to the full while he was still fit and able. The *genogram* (genealogical family tree) of Christine's family in Figure 13.1, showing each member's relative risk of HD

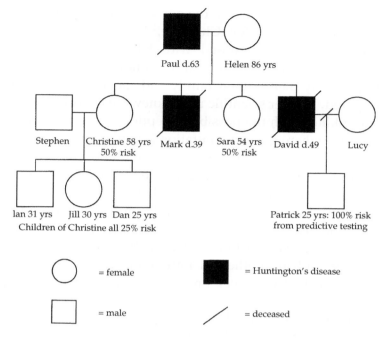

FIGURE 13.1
Genogram of Christine's immediate family, showing members who have died of HD and the risk levels for their descendants. (Reprinted from Ogden, J. A. 2005. *Fractured Minds: A Case-Study Approach to Clinical Neuropsychology, 2nd Ed.*, p. 290, with kind permission from Oxford University Press, New York.)

after Patrick received his results, reflects, with its stark black and white boxes, the terrible emotional burden the HD mutant gene places on families.

As Christine and Sara passed their 60th birthdays, still symptom-free, their risk of getting HD decreased. Christine still had the same clear olive skin she had when I first met her when she was 30, her face remained unlined, and her brown eyes and warm smile conveyed a sense of serenity and well-being. She kept physically fit, swimming and walking most days, and intellectually was as sharp as ever. But the fact that three of her immediate family members showed HD symptoms by the age of 47 at the very latest held little comfort for Christine, because her father's brother was not diagnosed with HD until he was 72. Sometimes she allowed herself to wonder if the HD gene affected only men in their family and she and Sara would be spared. But her scientific mind knew this was just wishful thinking: With the possible exception of juvenile HD, a rare form where the gene mutation is usually passed on by the father, the HD gene is not sex-linked and it is the luck of the draw which children draw the short straw—or in this case the long allele. The 50% rule had already struck in their family, as two of the four children had inherited the gene. But Christine knew this was no protection: 50% was just an average; in one family all four children might inherit the gene and in another all four might escape it. So the shadow of HD was ever present, and instead of feeling uncomplicated joy whenever one of their intelligent, amusing children did something free-spirited, Christine felt a little niggle of concern. Was this an early sign of a changing personality and all that implied? To me, blessed with healthy children of the same age, Christine and Stephen's children seemed as stable, normal, healthy, energetic, and successful as any parent could wish for, but of course living with the challenge of HD can only be understood from personal, painful experience.

One day Christine received a phone call from their son, Ian, now living in Canada, eager to share his news that he and Maureen, his Canadian partner, were planning to marry the following year. By this time, in the opening years of the 21st century, this shouldn't have been a concern for Christine, even though she still didn't know if she carried the HD gene mutation and therefore might have passed it on to Ian. If Maureen became pregnant she could have a prenatal predictive test on the unborn fetus at 9 to 12 weeks, assuming both parents agreed and were prepared to abort the fetus if it carried the HD mutant gene. If the fetus tested positive for the HD gene mutation and was not aborted, this could cause an ethical dilemma, as the child would grow up without the right *not to know* his or her HD status. It was also possible to avoid abortion but still ensure that the HD gene was not carried into the next generation by using in vitro fertilization. In this technique, a number of the father's sperm are injected into a number of the mother's eggs in a laboratory, and each resulting embryo is tested immediately. Those carrying the HD gene mutation are discarded and an embryo without the HD mutation is planted in the mother's womb. This technology is controversial given criticisms that it could lead to "designer babies," although as the advocates of this means of preventing HD point out, neither the sex of the embryo nor any other genetically mediated characteristics are tested for.

A difficult situation can arise when an individual with a 25% risk requests predictive testing. For example, if Ian had decided to have the predictive test himself and discovered he was HD-positive, then Christine would know she also had the mutant gene, and in turn the risk of her other children—Ian's siblings—would increase to 50%. Such situations need to be treated on a case-by-case basis. Careful genetic counseling of both generations, including full explanations of the implications, will often gradually resolve the issue one way or another. However, Maureen was from a strong Roman Catholic background and firmly against abortion and in vitro fertilization. She would not agree to Ian undergoing predictive testing, because if he turned out to carry the mutant HD gene, they would either have to avoid pregnancy altogether or be willing to have any fetus tested, which raised the unacceptable possibility of aborting the fetus if it carried the HD mutation.

So with Stephen's support Christine at last decided to undergo the extensive counseling and testing process that must precede a predictive blood test for HD. Counselors have clear guidelines as to their role. They must ensure that the person requesting predictive testing has not been coerced into this by well-meaning relatives. For example, parents or grandparents may believe that young adults at risk should establish their HD status before marriage or having children, but many young adults do not want to chance knowing their status and possibly constraining their future prospects for marriage, children, employment, health insurance, and psychological well-being. Christine was able to establish that all of her children—as well as Maureen—were now supportive of her finding out her own HD status and therefore finding out how their own risk levels changed. They understood that if she did have the mutant gene, they would all be in jeopardy of losing their houses and health insurance unless they also had a predictive test that proved to be negative.

Test results are always given at a face-to-face meeting, preferably with a support person also present and at a prearranged meeting time to lessen the anxiety of waiting for the telephone call or letter announcing that the result is in. One or more follow-up meetings some weeks or even months after the predictive test results have been released are essential, as this will be a difficult time not only for those who have the HD gene mutation but sometimes also for those who find they do not carry the mutation. In both cases, a major adjustment is necessary—from living with terrible uncertainty to living with the knowledge either that you will develop HD or that you will not, while other family members remain at risk. This latter situation can lead to survivor guilt and a heavy involvement with the affected relatives, sometimes to the serious detriment of the "lucky" one's own lifestyle. Some people who find they do not carry the HD gene mutation suffer a loss of identity with their extended family, where many members either have HD or are at risk of developing it.

All too soon the day set aside for Christine to learn her test results rolled around. She and Stephen traveled to

Melbourne for their appointment with Emma, their social worker. Emma had stood beside Christine and Stephen through hell and back; she had decided to specialize in caring for HD families as a result of working with Mark when he was first admitted to a psychiatric hospital over 35 years ago, and had remained his and then David's social worker throughout their lives. Sitting in Emma's office, holding Stephen's hand, Christine wondered if Emma was thinking that this was the worst task she had ever had to perform for their family. She and Stephen had confessed to each other that they each felt sure that Christine's test results would prove she had the HD mutation. So they were prepared for the very worst, and as Christine explained later, they were both crying as they watched Emma's moving lips, her words making no sense at first.

"Christine, Christine, do you understand what I'm telling you?" Emma was saying. "You have a negative result; you haven't got the mutation. You are clear. You'll never get Huntington's disease. Your children are safe."

Finally her words sank in, and Christine and Stephen looked at each other and across at Emma, who seemed to be crying as hard as they were.

"Phone Ian. He'll want to know immediately," Emma urged.

"But it'll be the middle of the night in Canada!" Christine protested, beginning to smile at last.

"Do it now," Emma said, holding out the phone.

So she did, and her son didn't mind being woken up one bit.

■ Further Reading

Ogden, J. A. 2005. Huntington's disease: A family challenged. In: *Fractured Minds: A Case-Study Approach to Clinical*

Neuropsychology, 2nd Ed. (pp. 276–303). New York: Oxford University Press.

Sulaiman, S. 2007. *Learning to Live with Huntington's Disease: One Family's Story.* London: Jessica Kingsley.

Wexler, A. 1996. *Mapping Fate: A Memoir of Family, Risk, And Genetic Research.* Berkeley: University of California Press.

Wexler, A. 2008. *The Woman Who Walked into the Sea.* New Haven: Yale University Press.

Wexler, N. S. 1979. Genetic Russian roulette: The experience of being at risk for Huntington's disease. In S. Kessler, ed. *Genetic Counselling: Psychological Dimensions* (pp. 201–217). London: Academic Press.

14

The Long Goodbye: Coming to Terms with Alzheimer's Disease

From five years old Sophie had her nose in a book. By 10 she had decided she wanted to be a librarian, but by 15 she had become the leader of her school debating team and was thinking more along the lines of a career as a current affairs journalist and presenter. This idea stuck, and when she left high school she completed first a university degree majoring in English and then a journalism course, graduating with distinction. After a stint as a reporter on the local newspaper, she talked her way into a job as a fact finder in the news and current affairs department of the local radio station. By her 28th birthday she had risen to newsreader, spending the hours when she was not on air researching news stories. Her marriage to Peter, already making his own mark in a small law firm, followed by the births of their three children within five years, put her career on hold for a time. On returning to the workforce when she was 36, her children now aged from one to five, she was offered a position as a radio talk show host. At first she was uncertain that this was where her heart lay, but as she became increasingly popular with her listeners she was given more freedom to develop new programs, including book and music reviews and panel discussions on current affairs.

The next few years were hectic as Sophie juggled her work around her family commitments, and Peter, now a partner in the law firm, slaved long hours. But it was a happy sort of hectic. With the help of Sophie's widowed mother, Prue, who looked after the children three days a week, Sophie's boundless energy and optimism enabled her to work part-time at the radio station and freelance as a journalist yet stay involved in her children's lives. But when Matthew, the youngest, was six, it became increasingly clear that Prue was not coping, frequently forgetting to come over to the house in time for the children's return from school. Prue's ability to look after her own home and herself deteriorated until finally Sophie could no longer ignore her concerns that this was more than old age. Sophie suggested Prue see her GP; this resulted in a referral to a geriatrician and an assessment by a neuropsychologist. Accompanying her mother, still only 65, to a follow-up meeting with the geriatrician, Sophie felt a smidgeon of hope when he explained that Prue's poor memory *might* be a sign of a progressive illness, but that until they had reassessed her in six months' time to see if her difficulties had worsened, he couldn't make a diagnosis. But as the six months wore on and Prue became even more forgetful— Sophie and Peter were no longer comfortable leaving her in charge of the children, even for a brief period—she was not surprised when after the second assessment Prue was diagnosed with probable Alzheimer's disease (AD).

For some months it was a tussle to get Prue to move in with them, as she insisted there was nothing wrong with her. Sophie and Peter took turns checking on Prue at least twice a day, and after Sophie saved the house and probably her mother's life when she arrived one day to the scream of the smoke alarm, a kitchen full of smoke from a pan of fat on fire on the stove, and her mother crouched in the corner of the room, Prue agreed to sell her house and live with her daughter. Sophie decreased her hours at the radio station so she could take care of Prue. They employed a home caregiver for the times when Sophie was at work, and 10-year-old Diane spent hours with her grandmother after school while her younger brothers attended an after-school program. The next five years were stressful for the family as the once happy, intelligent, and smartly groomed Prue become verbally abusive and paranoid, her behavior at times so bizarre that inviting friends around became impossible. When Prue was 68, Sophie reluctantly placed her in a nursing home. Within a year she was mute and incontinent and no longer consistently recognized her daughter or her grandchildren. Struggling with guilt over abandoning Prue, Sophie and Diane, who had been very close to her grandmother, had a few sessions with a psychologist, who listened while they talked and cried. On the psychologist's suggestion Sophie decided to research and write a series of articles for the local newspaper on AD and the issues it raises for family members. This more than anything else helped her to put her guilt into perspective and come to terms with her grief. By the time Prue died at 70, Sophie knew more than she wanted to about dementia.

From then on she was always finding symptoms in herself. Forgetting names became an embarrassment and she began to write the names of people she met in a notebook with short descriptions beside them. Her diary became an essential part of her, and she knew that without it she would not be able to continue as a radio talk show host. Once she was on air, she would be fine, and no one else seemed to notice her memory lapses. With the name of the person she was interviewing printed in large letters at the top of her page of interview questions, she felt safe. But if someone asked her the next day whom she had been interviewing, she struggled to remember the name and sometimes even the face or anything about the interview. She obsessively went over the research notes she had made when her mother was alive and searched the Internet for new information about the causes of and treatments for AD.

Peter was three years older than her, and Sophie was only too aware that he did not have these lapses. She took no comfort when he told her forgetfulness was normal for someone of her age and recounted instances—very few as far as Sophie could see—when he forgot important dates and the names of their acquaintances. Perhaps, Sophie thought, if she were in her sixties she would be less concerned, but she was only 49. Her best friend tried to calm her down by telling her she was probably going into menopause. At first Sophie grasped this possibility with relief, and managed to find Internet articles describing memory lapses as menopausal symptoms.

But when she found herself forgetting the beginnings of novels before she reached the ends, even if she had only started them a day or so previously, she knew she needed help. She had been an avid reader since she was five, and of all her like-minded friends she was the one who remembered for years not only book titles and authors but every detail of the plots, every facet of the characters' personalities, and how the books ended. Sophie made an appointment to see the same psychologist who had helped her and Diane when Prue had been in the final stages of AD. The therapist was the first person who took Sophie's concerns seriously, and although she had only a basic training in neuropsychology, she gave Sophie a neuropsychological assessment. Sophie had no idea how she had done; she had certainly made a fair number of errors. But when she returned to see the psychologist the following week, she got a pleasant surprise. The psychologist was pleased with her results: Sophie had scored in the average range across all the tests of the standard intelligence scale, as well as on memory tests where she had to learn a list of unrelated words over a number of trials and recall some short stories after they were read to her. In fact Sophie's only poor score was on her drawing from memory of a complex geometrical figure she had copied 45 minutes previously. Her score on this fell well below the average score for a woman Sophie's age. The psychologist attributed this to fatigue and anxiety and explained to Sophie that she was probably imagining her memory difficulties since her results on most of the memory tests were quite normal.

Here lies a salient lesson for psychologists who are not fully trained in neuropsychology. Sophie's psychologist made the mistake of thinking that an *average* score is a normal score, whereas she should have compared the scores with an estimate of Sophie's *premorbid* abilities, that is, the level she would have been at well before she ever began to experience memory problems. There are tests that can provide an estimate of premorbid ability level after the client has deteriorated. But even without such tests an experienced neuropsychologist would have assumed that given Sophie's university degrees and her journalistic talents, her premorbid abilities, especially her verbal abilities, would have been well above average and probably in the "superior" range. That is, if she had no problems she would have been expected to score well above the "average" woman of her age. The memory tests the psychologist gave her were very simple, and a different picture would probably have emerged had Sophie been given more difficult verbal memory tests. In retrospect, it was clear that Sophie's average— and so, low for her—scores on some of the verbal tests were due to word-finding difficulties, which were already apparent in Sophie's normal conversation.

Sophie was nevertheless comforted for a time by these "good" results. But over the next 18 months it became apparent even to her family that something was dreadfully wrong. Her current affairs radio show became an embarrassment as her word-finding problem grew worse, and she began to repeat questions she had asked only minutes before. Sophie was a current affairs journalist who had lost her quick wit, a radio talk show host who had lost her words. When one day she forgot not only the name but the political party of the politician she was interviewing, she felt only relief when her boss suggested she take early retirement. Her GP referred her to a geriatrician who specialized in dementia, and the assessment process began in earnest.

*****

The doctor's first task was to assess whether there were sufficient symptoms of dementia to cause concern. She took note of the memory and word-finding problems observed by Peter, and the possibly relevant fact that Sophie's mother had died of AD. She then gave Sophie the Mini-Mental State Examination, a common screening test for dementia, and because her score fell in the moderately impaired range, the doctor proceeded with exhaustive medical investigations to rule out any causes that could be reversible or that would require a particular treatment regimen. She also referred Sophie to me for a full neuropsychological assessment.

Sophie had no history of hypertension, strokes, heart problems, metabolic imbalances, or endocrine disease that could account for her memory impairment and word-finding difficulties. Her work had never involved substances likely to cause neurotoxic or other physical deficits, and she was not currently in an environment (such as living in a house that was being painted) that can cause transient problems such as headache, loss of concentration, and apparent memory problems for some people. A thorough investigation of medications is always essential and would have been even more so had Sophie been elderly, as it is common for patients in this group to be taking several medications for various ailments. But Sophie took no prescription medications and did not smoke or take recreational drugs, thus ruling out drug side effects, interactions, overdoses, or a gradual toxic buildup of medication. Sophie had also never suffered from psychiatric problems, although she was currently feeling depressed and not sleeping or eating well. Sophie herself attributed these problems to her anxiety about the possibility of being diagnosed with AD.

Sophie's physical examination yielded normal results. It had included an examination of her hearing and vision, as uncorrected poor vision and hearing, again more common in an elderly population, can result in confusion, disorientation, apparent memory impairment, and paranoia and thus be misdiagnosed as dementia. Laboratory screening tests on Sophie's blood, urine, and cerebrospinal fluid ruled out any metabolic disorders that might account for the symptoms. Sophie asked hopefully if her problems could be related to the onset of menopause, but the geriatrician did not think so; her cognitive difficulties were too marked and Sophie did not as yet have any of the physical signs of menopause. A computed tomography (CT) scan of Sophie's brain showed no areas of stroke or any mass such as a tumor. The lateral ventricles—the "lakes" of cerebrospinal fluid in the center of the brain—appeared slightly larger than normal for her age. As the ventricles can expand into the space resulting from neuronal death, this suggested the possibility of some minor cortical atrophy, but this can occur with normal aging. Thus the doctor's preliminary findings were that no clear cause could be found for Sophie's reported cognitive difficulties, and in particular, she ruled out reversible causes of dementia. The paradox is that finding no clear cause for this suite of cognitive impairments is the basis for a diagnosis of a primary progressive dementia, most commonly AD.

Unlike Sophie's case, in many cases of AD the patient is clearly demented by the time of the first assessment. Often the sufferer and family have adapted to the gradual cognitive changes, excused them on grounds of old age, and covered them up by reducing the individual's participation in difficult tasks. Such a "cover-up" is particularly common for people who have retired or who work in the home, where a cognitive decline may be less noticeable than at a job requiring a good memory and the ability to make decisions in novel situations. While a delay in diagnosis can be positive, given that it also delays the anguish the patient and family will surely suffer, there are also reasons favoring an early diagnosis. If the cognitive decline is due to a reversible or treatable cause, over time the disorder may advance too far for optimal treatment. In recent years drugs have been developed that can reduce some of the symptoms of AD, and these are more effective in the early stages. Unfortunately these drugs weren't available in the early 1990s, when Sophie was diagnosed.

*****

Peter and the three children came with Sophie to her first session with me. She was a tiny woman with dark hair and eyes and delicate facial features who looked ten years younger than her 51 years. Her voice was strong and clear, and it quickly became apparent that she had a vibrant personality, even given her understandable anxiety. It was obvious from the outset that her husband and children loved her dearly, and at first they were fiercely protective of her to the extent of minimizing many of her problems.

After spending some time explaining the neuropsycho-logical assessment process, I first talked generally with the family, concentrating on the many positive aspects of their family life and Sophie's numerous achievements. When the family felt more at ease, I commenced a more structured approach by taking a careful history from each member of the family, including Sophie, regarding the onset of her cognitive symptoms. Important dates such as each of Sophie's birthdays over the past five years were tagged, and Sophie's behaviors and accomplishments at those times were explored. This information enabled me to build a picture of a gradual decline of memory and word-finding abilities and a recent problem with finding her way around. This picture was consistent with a dementing process such as AD, but not with vascular dementia, which is caused by a series of small, barely noticeable strokes. Vascular demen-tia tends to have a more distinct onset than AD and pro-gresses in small steps, as new cognitive difficulties become apparent with each stroke. Similarly, if depression were the primary cause of Sophie's problems, the onset of memory and other cognitive difficulties would probably have been more abrupt. In addition, word-finding problems and dif-ficulties finding one's way around are unlikely to be notice-able problems in cases of mild to moderate depression. At this stage of my assessment I did not offer any opinion, saying only that I needed to assess Sophie's memory and other cognitive abilities before coming to any conclusions.

Sophie came alone to the following three sessions, and I assessed her using a broad range of neuropsychological tests. The results of the cognitive and memory tests carried out 18 months previously by the psychologist made it pos-sible to assess whether any deterioration had occurred since then. Despite her having been told she had no prob-lems in the previous assessment, I believed that given her average scores, Sophie had already been showing symp-toms of verbal and memory impairments as well as word-finding difficulties. Using various methods available to the neuropsychologist—including her past achievements—I estimated her premorbid ability as "superior." This was in stark contrast to her current scores on the standard cognitive tests I gave her; these had now dropped below average. Her responses were also slowed, and her word-finding problem was very apparent, especially in a test where she had to define words. For example, when asked to define "breakfast," she answered, "It is when you eat something like toast or bacon and eggs, not at night but before work." Clearly she knew what breakfast was—the first meal of the day—but she was unable to find simple words to explain it. This strategy of describing the word in a very roundabout way is called *circumlocution*.

I repeated the test Sophie had been given before where she had to first copy and then 45 minutes later draw from memory a complex geometrical figure. Figure 14.1 shows the copies she made of this figure (called the Rey Figure) on the two occasions 18 months apart. The deterioration on this difficult visuospatial task was dramatic, especially given Peter's comment that Sophie used to enjoy sketching and had been very good at it. Sophie took considerable care and time with her copy and refused to stop even when it became apparent she was becoming upset by her performance. When she finally completed it after a five-minute struggle, she was crying as she said: "How can I find that so impossible? Look at it; it is dreadful, dreadful. A small child could do better than that." Her drawing from memory of the Rey Figure after a 45-minute delay consisted of a rectangle and nothing else.

On verbal memory tests, Sophie's scores had also worsened significantly, whether the task was to learn lists of unrelated words or recall simple short stories. Even on much easier recognition tests she did poorly. For example, she was shown 50 unknown faces, one at a time, and then shown pairs of faces, one of which had been in the previous

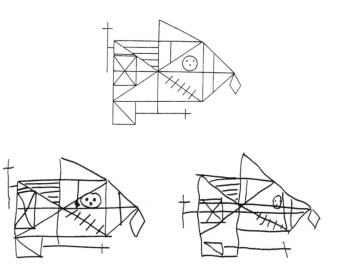

FIGURE 14.1

When Sophie copied the Rey Complex Figure (top) in the early stages of Alzheimer's dementia, she produced the drawing at bottom left. On the same task 18 months later, she drew the picture on the bottom right, demonstrating significant cognitive decline. (Reprinted from Ogden, J. A. 2005. *Fractured Minds: A Case-Study Approach to Clinical Neuropsychology, 2nd Ed.* p. 321, with kind permission from Oxford University Press, New York.)

series, and was asked to point to the face she had previously seen. This sounds difficult, but humans are amazingly good at recognizing faces they have just seen, and most people find this test very easy. Similarly, Sophie was shown 50 simple words one after the other and then had to select the words she had seen from pairs of words. Recognizing that you have seen a word or face is much easier then spontaneously recalling it without having it in front of you. Everyone forgets a name from time to time but as soon as someone gives you three or four to choose from you immediately recognize the one you want. As it is not permitted on these recognition tests to give "right" or "wrong" feedback, Sophie thought she had done quite well, and her mood lifted a little.

I assessed Sophie's memory for past events informally by inviting Peter into the session and asking him to name events they had both attended; I then compared Sophie's recollections with her husband's. She was able to spontaneously recall some details of major events held in the past year, such as her own 51st birthday party and her daughter's 21st birthday party, both large social events, but she was unable to recall any details of a television series she and her husband had watched over a recent six-week period. When Peter described it, she said she experienced a vague feeling of familiarity but could not add any details herself. She remembered that there had been a celebration on her last day at the radio studio but could recall no details. In fact, it was a formal dinner with a presentation to Sophie of a painting, and was attended by about sixty people. When Peter described the painting, she said she could now recall it and could see it in her mind's eye hanging over the fireplace, but her recall of the presentation itself remained vague. When asked to recall the names of her nieces and nephews (whom she knew quite well), she could not. She could, however, remember her own children's names—but she was unable to recall the birth dates of her two sons, and thought each was a year younger than he was.

I then gave Sophie some brief subtests from an aphasia battery to assess her language abilities. Her comprehension was good and she could write letters, numbers, and sentences to dictation. When asked to tell me what was happening in a picture, she gave an impoverished description, listing objects with no indication of the depicted actions. This problem was clearly more than one of word-finding and indicated a marked decline from the previous fluent and rich content of her articles and interviews.

Another important area that is compromised in the middle to later stages of AD, usually after memory problems are well established, is the ability to think abstractly, to modify one's performance in response to feedback, and to strategize and plan ahead. All of these abilities are associated with the frontal lobes, although other areas of the brain are also involved in these "executive" functions. Sophie performed poorly on tests that tapped any of these abilities. In contrast, she showed good insight into her difficulties by becoming upset by her poor performance. Poor insight is also an indicator of frontal lobe dysfunction, so this was a positive sign that Sophie's dementia was not yet advanced. In fact her feelings of depression resulted from her still being able to understand what was happening to her, which requires good insight. This had implications for her care and treatment. First, it could be helpful to treat Sophie's depression with antidepressants or with counseling, and second, Sophie still had the ability to think for herself and make decisions about her treatment and her future, and she should be given every assistance to do this. This type of intervention would also allow Sophie to take some control over her current illness and future treatment, and that in itself should help to diminish feelings of depression, helplessness, and hopelessness.

In summary, the pattern of results from this assessment demonstrated a generalized cognitive decline compared with Sophie's previous assessment and a highly significant decline in relation to her estimated premorbid "superior" cognitive abilities. Sophie was clearly trying her best throughout the assessment and was distressed at times when she realized how poorly she was performing. Sometimes clinical depression is mistaken for the early symptoms of AD, but as Sophie had no history of depression, her current depressed mood appeared to be a direct result of her insight into her deteriorating cognitive abilities. The assessment was spread over three sessions, and great care was taken to ensure that she was not tired; when she became upset, testing was terminated as soon as Sophie would allow. In an attempt to diminish her anxiety, whenever possible difficult tests were followed by tests she was more likely to be able to accomplish. Despite these measures, her distress and anxiety probably had some negative influence on her performance, but these factors were by no means sufficient to explain her low scores.

The results from the medical investigations, the exclusion of other causes for the dementia, and the neuropsychological assessment enabled the geriatrician to make a diagnosis of probable AD. Of particular importance was the fact that the cognitive deficits were progressive and included definite retrograde memory impairments (difficulties remembering past events) and anterograde memory impairments (difficulties retaining newly learned knowledge) as well as deficits in language, abstract thinking, and visuospatial abilities that together made it impossible for Sophie to continue in her work or to interact socially as she used to.

*****

The term "dementia" refers in its most general sense to an irreversible and serious decline of cognitive abilities, including memory, to the extent that the sufferer is unable to take care of themselves. There are many types of dementia, but AD is by far the most common, constituting approximately seventy percent of all dementia cases, and affecting more than 25 million people worldwide. In the US alone it has been estimated that there will be about 13 million people with AD by the year 2050.

The time from diagnosis to death in AD ranges from 3 to 20 years, with an average survival of 7 years. Death is not a result of the AD per se but of other illnesses and infections to which demented people are more susceptible. Although men and women are equally susceptible to AD, because men die, on average, at a younger age than women, the ratio of women to men increases during old age and therefore women are more likely to be affected. AD creeps up on the sufferer gradually and is often quite advanced before the individual is first seen by a doctor or other professional.

In the recent past a certain diagnosis of AD could be made only following a brain biopsy while the sufferer was living—a rare occurrence—or more commonly following a brain autopsy after death. Today, specialist teams working in dementia or memory units are able to make a reasonably firm diagnosis of AD if the patient fits the inclusion criteria for the disease and other possible causes for dementia are excluded. Increasingly sophisticated laboratory tests are being used for the latter purpose, and MRI brain scans taken every year or so can measure whether the progression of cerebral atrophy is greater than would be expected for normal aging. Neuropsychological assessments remain an essential aspect of the diagnosis of AD, as only these can demonstrate the progressive and gradual decline in memory and other cognitive abilities.

The neuropathology of AD, which can only be confirmed by biopsy or autopsy, includes the presence of *neurofibrillary tangles* and *amyloid,* or *senile, plaques* in the brain. Neurofibrillary tangles are twisted masses of protein fibers that displace the normal neurons; although these tangles are present in normal elderly people, they occur in much larger numbers throughout the brains of AD patients and especially affect the functioning of the hippocampus in the medial temporal lobes. The density of these tangles correlates with the degree of psychological disturbance before death. The hippocampus is important for memory, so it seems likely that the high number of neurofibrillary tangles either in the hippocampus or in structures connecting the hippocampus to other important brain structures relates directly to the severe memory deficits that are one of the hallmarks of AD. Amyloid plaques are composed of degenerated nerve cell material with a core filled with the fibrous protein amyloid. They occur in small numbers in the normal elderly but in large numbers throughout the cortex and deeper structures of the brains of AD victims as well as in other dementias, including Kuru and Creutzfeldt-Jakob disease (both "slow virus" dementias related to "mad cow" disease). The brains of AD victims also have large numbers of *granulovacuolar organelles* (small clusters of dead brain cell material that collect in the neurons). These are particularly dense in the hippocampus. At the biochemical level, AD is characterized by a reduction in levels of an enzyme used in the production of the neurotransmitter *choline acetyltransferase*; this finding provides some basis for developing treatments that increase the activity of the cholinergic system, a neurotransmitter system involved in the regulation of memory and learning. Other neurotransmitter abnormalities, including reduced concentrations of *dopamine, serotonin,* and *noradrenaline,* have been found in the brains of some AD victims, but the findings are inconsistent.

Research that measures cerebral atrophy in groups of AD and age-matched control subjects has demonstrated that atrophy is present in many but not all cases of dementia. Because some atrophy occurs with normal aging, it is often difficult to detect pathological atrophy in the individual demented patient from a gross inspection of brain scans.

Sophie was one of a small proportion of cases of AD where the onset of symptoms is between age 40 and 65 years. This form is sometimes labeled presenile AD or early-onset AD. In some cases this is an inherited form of AD called familial Alzheimer's disease (FAD), which is related to mutations of the Alzheimer precursor protein (APP) gene on chromosome 21. Other genes have also been identified as causative factors for early-onset AD. It is possible that such a gene was responsible for Sophie's AD, given that her mother's first AD symptoms were apparent before she was 65. However, the great majority of cases of AD are diagnosed at 65 years or older (senile, or late-onset, AD). Most researchers believe there is insufficient pathological or behavioral evidence to distinguish between early- and late-onset AD.

Theories about nongenetic causes for AD come and go, as do theories about protective factors or ways we can protect ourselves from developing AD. Various lines of research suggest that people who are highly educated or physically and mentally active into old age are less likely to develop AD. A fascinating long-term study reported by David Snowden and his colleagues in 1996, carried out on 93 white American nuns from the School Sisters of Notre Dame religious congregation, demonstrated that the density of ideas expressed in brief handwritten autobiographies by the nuns when they were in their early twenties predicted the likelihood that they would develop the cognitive impairments typical of AD in old age. Those with the lowest density of ideas were much more likely to show severe cognitive impairment 58 years (on average) later. As the findings were the same for a subset of 85 college-educated nuns whose occupation was teaching, it seems unlikely that either education or occupation were relevant factors. In a subset of 25 nuns who died (14 nuns from the main study and a further 11 nuns from another, similar convent who had also written autobiographies as young nuns), a low idea density in their autobiographies at age 22 (on average) predicted the number of neurofibrillary tangles found in the hippocampus and neocortex at autopsy, which confirmed AD neuropathologically. Low idea density in early adulthood was present in 9 of the 10 nuns who had neuropathological evidence of AD, and only 2 of the 15 nuns without AD.

As all of the nuns had lived in very similar environments from young adulthood, Snowdon and his colleagues suggested that the relationship between poor linguistic ability in early adulthood and impaired cognitive performance in later life was likely to be associated with cognitive ability in early life and not with environmental, health, or educational factors in adulthood. He postulated that the nuns with a high density of ideas as young adults had a higher "neurocognitive reserve capacity" and would therefore be less vulnerable to the later neuropathological changes of AD. To support such a hypothesis, it would be expected that some nuns with a high idea density in their twenties and who did not demonstrate severe cognitive impairments in old age would nevertheless show the pathological changes of AD on autopsy. But only one of the 25 nuns who died and was autopsied showed this pattern, and thus Snowdon concluded that the neurocognitive reserve hypothesis was unlikely. An alternative hypothesis is that low linguistic ability in early life is an early expression of later AD. This idea finds some support in the autopsies of individuals aged 20 to 100 years that show that the neurofibrillary tangles characteristic of AD develop over five decades.

*****

Research efforts into the causes, treatment, and prevention of AD are massive, and patients and families can always hope that new and more effective treatments for the symptoms—if only to slow down their progression—are just around the corner. Hope is especially valuable in the early and middle stages of AD, and there are many ways to ease the way for patients and their families. Some of the most useful treatments are those that alleviate coexisting medical conditions or treat the psychiatric symptoms of dementia. Antidepressants can be helpful in the early stages if the patient is severely depressed; antipsychotic medications may reduce psychotic symptoms and decrease aggressive and agitated behaviors; and sleep disturbances can be treated with short-acting hypnotics. Drug therapies must be carefully monitored and introduced slowly to avoid over-medicating and kept to a minimum to avoid unpleasant or even dangerous side effects.

If Sophie were diagnosed in 2010, she might well have been offered drugs that could sharpen her impaired memory and other cognitive abilities in the early stages of the disease. Many of these drugs have the aim of increasing the level of the neurotransmitter acetylcholine in the brain which is reduced in AD and necessary for a healthy cholinergic system. Given as a drug to AD patients it acts a bit like a strong dose of caffeine and doesn't produce unacceptable side effects. Sadly, despite the exponential increase in AD research, no drug or treatment has yet been discovered that has the ability to alter or slow the progression of the disease, and it seems increasingly unlikely that a magic bullet will be found that will cure AD. Hopefully ways to prevent some cases may be found, but the most effective way to treat this disease as it reaches almost epidemic proportions as a result of our aging population will be via a multidisciplinary approach targeting every facet of the illness.

For family members, caring for a person with AD is probably more stressful than actually having AD, especially in the later stages, when patients becomes increasingly unaware of their surroundings and lose the ability to understand what is happening to them. In the early and middle stages of AD, the patient usually continues to be cared for at home, which is desirable because confusion and disorientation are minimized if the patient remains in a familiar environment. Most families need enormous support throughout this period, including good information, respite care, home and nursing help, support from other families of AD sufferers, and psychological support and counseling. Providing good nutrition, encouraging meaningful activities, and providing a familiar and calming environment will help patients in the early and middle stages of AD to cope better. Knowledge about practical strategies caregivers can use to reduce the distress and antisocial behaviors of their AD relative can be both useful for the caregiver and empowering for the patient. For example, caregivers can practice ways to respond to their relative when she becomes agitated and abusive that avoid arguing or correcting her or using logic to counteract her irrational complaints. Often patiently repeating back or "reflecting" the patient's comments and, when possible, attempting to paraphrase in simple language the feelings that underlie the irrational or paranoid statements (perhaps of helplessness, fear, anger, or confusion) will calm the patient, who may quickly forget what upset her. Confusion, forgetfulness, and paranoia can be reduced by keeping the patient's environment and routine as familiar as possible and explaining in advance any changes in routine that are necessary.

In addition to modern and increasingly effective drugs that ameliorate some of the cognitive and behavioral symptoms of AD, a number of studies have demonstrated that in a significant proportion of cases of early and middle stages of dementia there are techniques that can assist patients in regaining some of the skills of daily living they have lost. Such programs include combinations of providing information, assisting with spatial orientation (such as learning to find their own way to the toilet), and teaching communication skills (such as learning to express their feelings of pleasure and displeasure), basic skills including feeding, and even more advanced skills like doing the laundry. Other, equally important programs improve caregivers' self-confidence by teaching them ways of dealing with the patient and the symptoms of the disease as it progresses.

Throughout the earlier stages of AD, it is important to keep a close eye on the patient's emotional state. Suicide risk must be assessed, especially when the patient is depressed, and psychological or drug therapy provided as needed. Patients who are mildly or moderately depressed and still have reasonable cognitive abilities can sometimes find a path out of their depression by "putting their house in order." This could include discussing their future care with their families, making a will, planning the details of their funeral, and writing letters for their children and grandchildren to read after the writer's death. The patient can share family photographs and treasures with family members and be encouraged to talk about the past—perhaps while being recorded—so that these memories can be passed on to younger and as-yet-unborn family members. "Putting one's house in order" may also involve patients making peace with others and with themselves, and it often paves the way to emotional acceptance that life is nearing completion. All these actions can be empowering for the patient and can form a positive part of the grieving process, both for the AD sufferer and the family.

As the dementia worsens, patients lose insight, become increasingly apathetic or behave increasingly inappropriately, are likely to wander without any idea of where they are going or how to find their way back, and require considerable assistance with everyday activities such as washing, dressing, eating, and using the toilet. At this stage, strategies that previously helped to calm the patient are no longer effective. This is the point where families often must make the difficult decision to place their relative in a home, without knowing how many years remain before their death. Understandably this is an intensely stressful time for families. They are physically and emotionally exhausted from years of caring for their loved one while she deteriorates into a person quite alien to the one they have known all their lives; in addition, they feel guilty because they feel they are abandoning the patient in her time of greatest need. If the patient is a parent or partner who once took care of the caregiver, such abandonment cuts very deeply indeed.

Some families—particularly extended families and those from cultures with great respect for their elderly—are able and willing to care for their relative in the home until death, but for many, continuing to care for someone in the last stages of dementia places an intolerable stress on the family or on particular family members. Psychological counseling may be helpful in assisting these families to understand that their relative can no longer appreciate them and sadly is unable to care whether she remains at home or is nursed in a hospital or hospice. The best that can be done for patients at this stage is to make them as comfortable as possible and to ensure that they are not in pain, which often requires professional nursing and medical care.

*****

Telling patients they have a terminal illness is one of the hardest things a clinician has to do. It is probably hardest when the patient is a child or a young to middle-aged adult. People with AD are usually in their seventies and older and have perhaps enjoyed a healthy and rich life. But somehow, when it comes down to it, it is always hard to give someone, however old, a death sentence. And with AD it is more than a death sentence; it is a prediction that the next few years will be increasingly difficult not only for the patient but also for the family.

Sophie and Peter were given the news by the specialist geriatrician—I was present as well—in a meeting arranged a week after the neuropsychological assessment was complete. Sophie, of course, was expecting bad news, but nevertheless had continued to hold a small hope that her symptoms might have some other, less tragic cause. When this final ray of hope was dashed, her immediate reaction was to grimace and comment, "Well, at least I'll have a good excuse for my crazy behavior now." She then fell silent, and after we had arranged a family session in two days' time, her husband took her home. I made it clear to them that they would have ongoing counseling and therapy available to them as well as other more practical help as they required it.

Sophie was the only member of the family who did not come to the next session, which was taken up with listening to the grief and anger of each family member and answering their questions honestly. Sophie had remained almost mute for a day following her return home but had begun to cry when her 17-year-old son, Matthew, hugged her and told her he was going to make sure she was around for his 21st birthday. Since then Sophie had continued to cry and sometimes fall asleep from exhaustion, and the family had decided to leave her in the care of a good friend from the Alzheimer's support group while they attended the counseling session.

They decided to continue the same routine as long as possible but with a roster to ensure that at least one family member or one of Sophie's friends was in the house at all times to be available if Sophie should need them or want to talk, go out, or simply watch television with them. Peter had already decided to take partial leave from his law practice, which fortunately he was financially able to do, so that he could spend as much time with Sophie as possible before her dementia worsened to the point where she could not appreciate her family.

The possibility of suicide was discussed, and all her children said they would make their love and need of their mother so clear that she would not want to take her life. The importance of finding a nursing home or hospice where their mother could be cared for in her final months was brought up by Diane, who had been the family member most involved in her grandmother's illness and care. It was agreed to put this on hold until Sophie felt ready to talk about it.

Within a week, Sophie felt able to see me for her first therapy session. Initially Sophie attended with her husband but then she decided to continue weekly sessions alone. During these sessions with my assistance she wrote letters to her husband and to each of her children to be read after her death. She made a short audiotape recording for the entire family, made difficult by her word-finding problems, especially given her emotional state. With many stops and starts, however, she completed a very moving tape, which later became an important catalyst in the grieving and healing process for her family.

Once these tasks were completed, Sophie decided to have a session with her family, during which she discussed her wish to be placed in a hospice when she needed full-time nursing care. She also spoke about her wishes for her funeral and explained that she had written letters to be given to each of them after her death. This was a very positive session, after which the family members were able to talk at home with one another about what Sophie had shared with them. Sophie did not ask for further therapy sessions, but on her request I visited her at home from time to time.

In the period when Sophie was having her individual sessions with me, the other family members also attended sessions to talk about practical issues and concerns as well as to begin to work through their own grief. Diane found Sophie's decline particularly difficult, because it brought back memories of her grandmother's dementia. All the children had concerns, at first unvoiced, that they too would end their days demented. I discussed this fear with them in terms of statistics, emphasizing the many family members of AD patients who do not develop the disease; the massive research efforts going into finding the cause, a cure, and treatments for AD; the changing societal views and laws about euthanasia; and the many productive years the children had ahead of them before they need worry about the fairly unlikely possibility that they would also develop AD.

Sophie remained at home for four years. As she had requested in the early stages of her illness, she was placed in a hospice when she needed full-time nursing care. While at home she remained relatively easy to look after, and family members quickly learned ways to defuse potentially difficult situations. Sophie's depressed mood improved as her insight decreased, and within a year of diagnosis she no longer experienced periods of depression. She often made inappropriate or insensitive comments, frequently forgot or confused her children's names, and could not be left alone in the house for fear she would hurt herself or set fire to the house by leaving the stove on. The family continued to help her cook simple meals as long as she was able, since this gave her pleasure for a short time.

She sometimes became agitated for no apparent reason, and occasionally threw food or crockery if she did not like the food she was given. Her family didn't argue or correct her but simply removed the offending food, led her to her rocking chair, placed headphones over her ears, and played her her favorite music. Matthew in particular spent many hours reading to her, playing simple card games of "snap" with her (letting her win most of the time), and accompanying her on walks. Sophie retained his face and name in her memory longer than any others. After much soul-searching, Peter returned to his full-time law practice after a year, but he continued to keep most evenings free for Sophie. As he said, this work routine kept him "sane" and gave him the psychological strength to cope with Sophie.

Sophie deteriorated rapidly once in the hospice, and within six weeks she was mute and could recognize no one. Matthew had a small family gathering to celebrate his 21st birthday three months after Sophie entered the hospice, and Sophie came home for the occasion. To an onlooker she might have appeared unaware of what was going on, but Matthew insists that when he said to her, "See, Mum, I knew you would stick around for my 21st," she squeezed his hand and smiled at him. She died a month later, and a postmortem confirmed that she had suffered from AD.

The family came to four therapy sessions following her death and were greatly helped and comforted by the audiotape and letters Sophie had left for them. Their grieving was already well advanced by the time Sophie died, and at the end her death came as a relief. Their support for one another was very strong, and they felt that as a family they had gained much of value from the quality time they had been able to spend not only with Sophie but with each other. Matthew is now a hospice nurse.

*****

Dementia, whatever its cause, is a tragedy for the victim and for family and friends. It is also one of the most difficult areas for professionals, as they too must watch, helpless, as a person with a personality, intellect, and soul deteriorates into a "vegetable." It is perhaps this feeling of being unable to halt the inevitable decline that makes it so stressful to work or live with people with dementia. Therefore, any interventions, however small, that give sufferers some control over their lives—even if it is simply controlling when they go to bed—or that give the caregivers and family some means of improving the quality of the sufferer's daily existence will partially alleviate feelings of helplessness and depression.

Families know the dementia sufferer best, and when given some encouragement, even small children can often come up with new and creative ways to ease the lives of the caregivers and bring some happiness into the patient's day. After the shock of the diagnosis has subsided and a routine of care has been established, it is important that all members of the family continue to live their own lives as well as sharing in the care of the patient if that is their wish. It is all too common for the bulk of the care to fall on the shoulders of one person, usually a woman relative; this situation should be avoided from the outset by the therapist's encouraging the setting up of a roster system and the use of community services as well as family members for caregiving.

Sophie was particularly fortunate in having a supportive family that was financially well-off. Many elderly people who become demented have no family and are placed in a geriatric hospital early in their dementia, which often seems to precipitate their deterioration and death, perhaps because they lack stimulation or because they are still able to feel at some level that no one cares whether they live or die, and they simply give up.

Caregivers also need to have their coping abilities and stress levels monitored so that they can receive assistance with and respite from their roles before they collapse either physically or emotionally. Dementia is ultimately a tragedy for family and friends; their stress and grief continue for the duration of the disease and often long after the sufferer's death. For dementia sufferers, the loss of insight that accompanies the middle and late stages of dementia spares them much emotional pain and embarrassment.

It is perhaps only when we watch a person who was once active, independent, intelligent, humorous, and loving gradually "lose her mind" that we begin to comprehend the magnificence and complexity of the human brain and want to discover more about what it can do, how it works, how it can overcome great adversity—including damage to itself—and how we may someday be able to fix it when it goes wrong. Part of the challenge for neuroscience researchers is to find answers to these questions. For the clinical neuropsychologist and other professionals working with people like Sophie and her family, the human tragedy they see daily becomes one of the most salient reasons for persisting with this difficult but rewarding work.

■ Further Reading

Franzen, J. 2002. My Father's Brain. In: *How to Be Alone* (pp. 7–38). London: Fourth Estate.

Genova, L. 2007. *Still Alice.* New York: Pocket Books.

Ogden, J. A. 2005. Dementia: A Family Tragedy. In: *Fractured Minds: A Case-Study Approach to Clinical Neuropsychology, 2nd Ed.* (pp. 304–327). New York: Oxford University Press.

Snowdon, D. A., S. J. Kemper, J. A. Mortimer, L. H. Greiner, D. R. Wekstein, and W. R. Markesbery. 1996. Linguistic ability in early life and cognitive function and Alzheimer's disease in late life. Findings from the Nun Study. *Journal of the American Medical Association, 275,* 528–532.

Index

language disorders and, as
spectrum, 65
left temporal lobe damage and,
57
MI therapy for, 44–46
multidimensional therapy
programs for, 47
music as therapy for, 48
neologisms with, 59
neuropsychological assessment
for, after therapy, 49
nonverbal memory with, 41
number comprehension with, 41
oral apraxia with, 41, 43
paralysis with, 40
physical therapy for, 47
return to normal life after, 50–52
right hemisphere of brain and, 39
single-subject study designs for,
46–47
speech deficits with, 59
swear words with, 38–39
symbol comprehension with, 41
syntax issues with, 59
therapy strategy assessments for,
46
verbal memory with, 59–60
Wernicke's area damage and, 59
APP. *See* Alzheimer precursor
protein
apraxia
autotopagnosia and, 124–125
constructional, 123
dressing, 25, 117
ideational, 124–125
ideomotor, 124
oral, 41, 43, 124
arachnoid mater, 28, 233
subarachnoid space and, 28
arteries
carotid, 29
vertebral, 29
Asperger's syndrome, 18
assessment, clinical
after aphasia therapy treatment,
49

of brain damage, ethnic
differences as influence on, 53
cultural influences on, 49–50,
52–55
of head injuries, 139
for temporal lobectomy,
psychological profile for,
211–214
from testing, 9–10
astrocytomas, 72
atrophy, of brain, 15
attention, 11–12
absence seizures and, 233
with frontal lobe syndrome, 107
highly focused, 12
for neuropsychological testing,
152–153
prefrontal cortex and, 33
prefrontal lobes and, 98–99, 107
auditory neglect, 80
autism, 18
autosomal dominant hereditary
disorders, 341–342. *See also*
Huntington's disease
autotopagnosia, 119–120
apraxia and, 124–125
body part identification deficits
with, 132–133
constructional apraxia and, 123
detail testing for, 128–130
executive functions and, 122
handedness and, 122
ideational apraxia and, 124–125
ideomotor apraxia and, 124
left parietal lobe damage and,
119
memory deficits with, 124
oral apraxia and, 124
oral language tests and, 122
qualitative data for, 130–132
steroid therapy for, 121
symptoms of, 119
visuospatial testing for,
123–124
Awakenings (Sacks), 325–326
balance. *See* posture, with PD

68
emotional balance with, 41
functional limitations with, 39
from hemorrhagic stroke, 67
language comprehension with, 41
language disorders and, 75
nonverbal memory with, 41
number comprehension with, 41
oral apraxia with, 41, 43
paralysis of right hand with, 40
symptoms of, 40–41
Broca's area, 19
aphasia and, 39
double dissociation and, 20
expressive aphasia and, 39–40
third frontal gyrus, 39–40
burr-hole biopsy, 83–84

Capgras syndrome, 141
carbidopa, 322
caregivers, for dementia patients, 391
carotid arteries, 29
central sulcus fissure, between brain hemispheres, 27
cerebellum, 25
cerebrospinal fluid (CSF), 28
hydrocephalus and, 28
ventricles of, 28, 149–150
cerebrovascular accident (CVA), 37
cerebrovascular system, for brain, 29
aneurysms, 29
carotid arteries, 29
circle of Willis in, 29
deep veins, 29
strokes and, 29
subarachnoid hemorrhage, 29
superficial veins, 29
vertebral arteries, 29
Charcot, Jean-Martin, 142
Freud as student of, 142
hypnotism therapy for, 142
Chen, Pauline, 4
choline acetyltransferase, 380

chorea, with HD, 340, 340–341, 342–343
chronic subdural hematomas, after TBI, 289
circle of Willis, 29
aneurysms and, 29
circumlocution, as speech strategy, 101, 374
clients, as descriptive term, 2
clinical neuropsychology. *See* neuropsychological, clinical
clinical psychology. *See* psychology
closed head injuries, 16–17
blood clots after, 289
causes of, 287
chronic subdural hematomas after, 289
diffuse axonal injury in, 287
first injury in, 288
frontal lobe damage from, 112
hydrocephalus after, 289–290
ischemia from, 289
prospective memory deficits with, 298
RF damage with, 27, 287
second injury in, 288
TBI, 16
third injury, 289
clots. *See* blood clots, after TBI
cognition
executive lobe impairments and, 100, 102, 112
higher, in mind hierarchy, 11–12
cognitive disorders
higher, 81
lower, 81
cognitive neuropsychology, 4–5
cognitive rehabilitation, after TBI, 290–291
cogwheel rigidity, 312
color memory, deficits in
achromatopsia, 162
with visual object agnosia, 162–163
coma, brain damage and, 277

after left hemisphere damage, 63
    PD and, 315–316
developmental brain damage,
    18–20
    developmental brain disorders
        and, 18–20
    Down syndrome and, 18
    fetal alcohol syndrome, 18
developmental brain disorders,
    18–20
    Asperger's syndrome, 18
    autism, 18
diffuse axonal injury, 287
diffuse brain damage, 15–18
    from AD, 15–16
    from brain atrophy, 15
    from edema, 18
    from HD, 17
    from meningitis, 17
    from PD, 17
    TBI, 16
diplopia, 139
disabilities, 290
    handicaps from, 290
disinhibition, 109. See also
        inappropriate emotions
    with HD, 344
dopamines, 312–313
double vision. See diplopia
Down syndrome, 18
drawing tests
    for hemineglect, 76
    for visual object agnosia,
        157–158, 159–160
dressing apraxia, 25
    Gerstmann's syndrome and, 117
drug use, PD from, 313
dura mater, 28
dysarthrias, 340, 343
dysarthric speech, 92
dysexecutive disorder, 108–110
    disinhibition with, 109
    lack of insight of condition, by
        patients, 109–110
    planning deficits with, 110
dyslexic disorders, 65

dysphagias, with HD, 343
dysphoria, with HD, 344
dystonias
    with HD, 343
    with PD, 315

early-onset AD, 380
The Echo Maker (Powers), 141
edema, diffuse brain damage from,
    18
electroencephalogram (EEG)
    for brain activity, 7
    for epileptic seizures, 216
    for Molaison, H., 175
emotions. See also inappropriate
        emotions
    with AD, 384–385
    with aphasia, 41
    with frontal lobe syndrome, 108
    prefrontal lobes and, 98
emotional skills, training for
    for physicians, 3
    for psychologists, 3
emotional withdrawal, with
        aphasia, 62–63
epilepsy, 100, 208
    absence seizures with, 175, 209
    corpus callosum surgery
        for, 208
    drug treatment for, future
        assessment of, 224
    EEG monitoring for, 216
    generalized seizures with, 175,
        208
    hemispherectomy for, 208–209,
        233
    hippocampal removal and, 201
    idiopathic causes of, 210
    pregnancy and, 210
    temporal lobectomy for, 210
    temporal lobe seizures with,
        209–210
    Wada test for, 217–218, 219–221
episodic memory, 186
    for Molaison, H., 186
euthanasia, HD and, 356

258
alcohol use and, 258
cognitive symptoms of, 259
as controversial diagnosis, 260
CT for, 260
family disruption from, 260
malingering as factor in, 261
mild traumatic brain injury and,
16–17, 258–259
MRI for, 260
physical symptoms of, 259
prevalence of, as random, 261
as psychological construct, 261
psychosocial symptoms of, 259
rehabilitation program for,
271–272
reticular formation disruption
and, 260
from sports activities, 258
support groups for, 270–271
posterior lobes, 30–31
posttraumatic amnesia (PTA)
brain damage and, 277
with mild traumatic brain injury,
258
with severe traumatic brain
injury, 276, 277
postural instability, with PD, 315
posture, with PD, 315
instability in, 311, 315
Powers, Richard, 141
predictive testing, for HD, 357–358
prenatal, 360–361
prefrontal cortex, 32–33
attention and, 33
executive functions in, 32
hemineglect and, 80
lobes in, 98–99
RF and, 33
prefrontal lobes. See also frontal
lobe syndrome
anatomy of, 98–99
attention and, 98–99, 107
damage to, 97
emotion and, 98
executive thinking in, 99–100

impairments to, 100, 102, 112
leucotomy for, 101
lobectomies of, 97
lobotomies of, 100–101
pregnancy
epilepsy and, 210
HD and, 357, 360–361
premorbid abilities, in neuropsychological testing, 369
Presley, Elvis, 194–196
prestriate visual cortex, lesions in,
162
procedural memory, 185–186
prosody, 245–246
prosopagnosia, 141
definition of, 87
visual object agnosia and,
143–144, 161–162
prospective memory
with frontal lobe syndrome,
106–107
with TBI, 298
psychologists, emotional skills
training for, 3
psychology
clinical, 5–6
clinical neuropsychology and, 4
psychology clinics, 254
psychomotor seizures. See temporal
lobe seizures
psychomotor skills, after temporal
lobectomy, 222–223
psychosurgery, 100–101
frontal lobotomies in, 100–101
PTA. See posttraumatic amnesia
Pueblo tribe, topographical
orientation among, 52
pugilistic parkinsonism, 313

receptive aphasia, 57, 59
confused oral language with,
60–61
damage location as influence on,
68
receptive aphasia (Cont.)
emotional withdrawal with,

shortsightedness, treatment
evolution for, 224
Sinemet, 321–322
single-subject study designs, for
aphasia, 46–47
multiple therapies within, 46
size discrimination, of shapes, 155
"sleeping sickness," PD as, 325
Snowden, David, 381
soul, memory as, 199–200
spatial agraphia, 85
specialized evolution, 52–53
speech deficits
agrammatical, 40
with aphasia, 40, 59
circumlocution strategy with,
101, 374
dysarthric speech, after
hemineglect, 92
in frontal lobe syndrome, 101
neologism formation, 59
phonemic paraphrasias, 59
semantic paraphrasias, 59
for syntax, with aphasias, 59
Speer, Albert, 326
sports, head injuries from, 256
PCS, 258
static focal damage, 13
steroid therapy
for autotopagnosia, 121
for hemineglect, 92, 93
strokes
cerebrovascular system and, 29
focal damage from, 13–14
hemineglect and, 74
hemorrhagic, 67
ischemic, 67
subarachnoid hemorrhage, 29
subarachnoid space, 28
superficial veins, 29
support groups
for head injuries, 278–281
for PCS patients, 270–271
for TBI survivors, 291
swear words, with aphasia, 38–39
right hemisphere of brain

and, 39
swelling. *See* edema
symbols, comprehension of, with
aphasia, 41
syndromes, definition of, 24

tactile agnosia, 24–25
tactile neglect, 80
frontal lobe syndrome and,
104–105
TBI. *See* traumatic brain injury
temporal lobectomy, for seizures,
210
musical memory after, 217–218
neuropsychological assessment
for, 214–216
psychological assessment for,
211–214
psychomotor skills after,
222–223
unilateral, 215
temporal lobes, 27, 31
bilateral medial temporal
lobectomy, 175–176
under MRI, 149
MTL, damage to, 179
receptive aphasia and, 57
TBI and, 288
temporal neocortex in, 177
temporal lobe seizures, 209–210
in hippocampus, 209–210
indications for, 209
MRI for, 211
temporal neocortex, 177
terminal diagnoses, patient
responses to, 2–3
testing. *See* neuropsychological
testing; predictive testing, for
HD
thalamotomy, 329–330
thalamus, RF and, 27
third frontal gyrus, 39–40. *See also*
Broca's area
third injury, in TBI, 289
traumatic brain injury (TBI), 16. *See
also* closed head injuries; mild

MRI for, 148–150
music as memory cue, 168
object function recognition with, 159
occipital lobe damage and, 144, 150–151
prosopagnosia and, 143–144, 161–162
with retrograde autobiographical memory loss, 163, 163–164
shape recognition with, 159
size discrimination with, 155
verbal intelligence testing with, 153
verbal memory testing, 154–155
visual perception and, 155–157
white brain matter with, 150
visual perception, visual object agnosia and, 155–157
visual sense. *See* sensory visual cortex
visual stimuli, hemineglect and, 80
visual testing, for hemineglect, 86
visuospatial testing
for AD, 374
for autotopagnosia, 123–124
after hemispherectomy, 243–244
for PD, 320–321
for personal orientation, 243
voice, decrease in volume, with PD, 324
von Economo's encephalitis, 325

Wada test, 217–218, 219–221
for musical memory, 219–221
purpose of, 219
weight loss, with HD, 343
Wernicke, Carl, 19, 59
Wernicke's aphasia, 57, 59
confused oral language with,

60–61
damage location as influence on, 68
emotional withdrawal with, 62–63
functional difficulties with, 59
from ischemic stroke, 67
language disorders and, 75
left temporal lobes and, 57
neologisms with, 59
phonemic paraphrasias with, 59
semantic paraphrasias with, 59
syntax with, 59
verbal memory with, 59–60
visual field defects from, 58
Wernicke's area, 19
aphasia and, 59
double dissociation and, 20
in Molaison, H., 177
Weschler Intelligence Scales, 8
Western culture,
neuropsychological assessments influenced by, 53–54
consultants for, 55
morality of offering choice in, 54–55
Native Americans and, 54
Wexler, Alice, 352
Wexler, Milton, 352
Wexler, Nancy, 352
white matter, in brain, 27
with visual object agnosia, 150
Williams, Robin, 325
working memory
with frontal lobe syndrome, 106
PD and, 318

Printed in the USA/Agawam, MA
September 2, 2022

797862.027